Evolving Medical Imaging Techniques

Editors

THOMAS C. KWEE
HABIB ZAIDI

PET CLINICS

www.pet.theclinics.com

Consulting Editor
ABASS ALAVI

July 2013 • Volume 8 • Number 3

ELSEVIER

1600 John F. Kennedy Boulevard • Suite 1800 • Philadelphia, Pennsylvania, 19103-2899

http://www.theclinics.com

PET CLINICS Volume 8, Number 3
July 2013 ISSN 1556-8598, ISBN-13: 978-1-4557-7604-7

Publisher: Adrianne Brigido

PET Clinics (ISSN 1556-8598) is published quarterly by Elsevier Inc., 360 Park Avenue South, New York, NY 10010-1710. Months of issue are January, April, July, and October. Periodicals postage paid at New York, NY, and additional mailing offices. Subscription prices per year are $215.00 (US individuals), $309.00 (US institutions), $110.00 (US students), $244.00 (Canadian individuals), $345.00 (Canadian institutions), $134.00 (Canadian students), $260.00 (foreign individuals), $345.00 (foreign institutions), and $134.00 (foreign students). To receive student and resident rate, orders must be accompanied by name of affiliated institution, date of term, and the signature of program/residency coordinator on institution letterhead. Orders will be billed at individual rate until proof of status is received. Foreign air speed delivery is included in all Clinics subscription prices. All prices are subject to change without notice. POSTMASTER: Send address changes to PET Clinics, Elsevier Health Sciences Division, Subscription Customer Service, 3251 Riverport Lane, Maryland Heights, MO 63043. **Customer Service: 1-800-654-2452 (U.S. and Canada); 314-447-8871 (outside U.S. and Canada). Fax: 314-447-8029. E-mail: journalscustomerservice-usa@elsevier.com (for print support); journalsonlinesupport-usa@elsevier.com (for online support).**

Reprints. For copies of 100 or more of articles in this publication, please contact the Commercial Reprints Department, Elsevier Inc., 360 Park Avenue South, New York, NY 10010-1710. Tel.: 212-633-3812; Fax: 212-462-1935; E-mail: reprints@elsevier.com.

Printed and bound by CPI Group (UK) Ltd, Croydon, CR0 4YY

Transferred to digital print 2012

Contributors

CONSULTING EDITOR

ABASS ALAVI, MD, PhD (Hon), DSc (Hon)
Professor of Radiology, Division of Nuclear Medicine, University of Pennsylvania School of Medicine; Department of Radiology, Hospital of the University of Pennsylvania, Philadelphia, Pennsylvania

EDITORS

THOMAS C. KWEE, MD, PhD
Department of Radiology and Nuclear Medicine, University Medical Center Utrecht, Utrecht, The Netherlands

HABIB ZAIDI, PhD, PD
Division of Nuclear Medicine and Molecular Imaging, Geneva University Hospital, Geneva, Switzerland; Geneva Neuroscience Center, Geneva University, Geneva, Switzerland; Department of Nuclear Medicine and Molecular Imaging, University Medical Center Groningen, University of Groningen, Groningen, The Netherlands

AUTHORS

ABASS ALAVI, MD, PhD (Hon), DSc (Hon)
Division of Nuclear Medicine, Hospital of the University of Pennsylvania, Philadelphia, Pennsylvania

ALEX BHOGAL, MSc
Department of Radiology, University Medical Center Utrecht, Utrecht, The Netherlands

MATTHEW BLACKLEDGE, BSc, MSc, PhD
CRUK EPSRC Imaging Centre, Institute of Cancer Research, Sutton, United Kingdom

DAVID R. BUSCH, PhD
Division of Neurology, Department of Pediatrics, Children's Hospital of Philadelphia; Department of Physics and Astronomy, University of Pennsylvania, Philadelphia, Pennsylvania

REGINE CHOE, PhD
Assistant Professor, Department of Biomedical Engineering, University of Rochester, Rochester, New York

DAVID J. COLLINS, BA, CPhys, MInstP
CRUK EPSRC Imaging Centre, Institute of Cancer Research, Sutton, United Kingdom

BART DE KEIZER, MD, PhD
Department of Radiology; Department of Nuclear Medicine, University Medical Center Utrecht, Utrecht, The Netherlands

JILL B. DE VIS, MD
Department of Radiology, University Medical Center Utrecht, Utrecht, The Netherlands

TURGUT DURDURAN, PhD
Assistant Professor, Medical Optics Department, ICFO - Institut de Ciències Fotòniques, Castelldefels, Barcelona, Spain

JEROEN HENDRIKSE, MD, PhD
Department of Radiology, University Medical Center Utrecht, Utrecht, The Netherlands

JOHANNES MARINUS HOOGDUIN, PhD
Brain Division and Imaging Division, Department of Radiology, University Medical Center Utrecht, Utrecht, The Netherlands

J. MARTIJN JANSMA, PhD
Department of Neurology and Neurosurgery, Rudolf Magnus Institute of Neuroscience, University Medical Center Utrecht, Utrecht, The Netherlands

DENNIS W.J. KLOMP, PhD
Assistant Professor, Department of Radiology, Image Sciences Institute, University Medical Center Utrecht, Utrecht, The Netherlands

DOW-MU KOH, MD, MRCP, FRCR
Department of Radiology, Royal Marsden Hospital, Sutton, Surrey, United Kingdom

THOMAS C. KWEE, MD, PhD
Department of Radiology and Nuclear Medicine, University Medical Center Utrecht, Utrecht, The Netherlands

ALEXANDER LEEMANS, PhD
Image Sciences Institute, University Medical Center Utrecht, Utrecht, The Netherlands

ANNEMIEKE S. LITTOOIJ, MD
Department of Radiology, University Medical Center Utrecht, Utrecht, The Netherlands

PETER R. LUIJTEN, PhD
Department of Radiology, University Medical Center Utrecht, Utrecht, The Netherlands

RUTGER A.J. NIEVELSTEIN, MD, PhD
Department of Radiology, University Medical Center Utrecht, Utrecht, The Netherlands

ESBEN T. PETERSEN, PhD
Department of Radiology, University Medical Center Utrecht, Utrecht, The Netherlands

DANIEL LOUIS POLDERS, PhD
Imaging Division, Department of Radiology, University Medical Center Utrecht, Utrecht, The Netherlands

JEROEN C.W. SIERO, PhD
Department of Radiology, University Medical Center Utrecht, Utrecht, The Netherlands

CHANTAL M.W. TAX, MSc
Image Sciences Institute, University Medical Center Utrecht, Utrecht, The Netherlands

DREW A. TORIGIAN, MD, MA
Department of Radiology, Hospital of the University of Pennsylvania, Philadelphia, Pennsylvania

NINA TUNARIU, MRCP, FRCR
Department of Radiology, Royal Marsden Hospital, Sutton, Surrey, United Kingdom

ANJA G. VAN DER KOLK, MD
Department of Radiology, University Medical Center Utrecht, Utrecht, The Netherlands

SJOERD B. VOS, MSc
Image Sciences Institute, University Medical Center Utrecht, Utrecht, The Netherlands

JANNIE P. WIJNEN, PhD
Post-doc, Department of Radiology, Image Sciences Institute, University Medical Center Utrecht, Utrecht, The Netherlands

ARJUN G. YODH, PhD
Professor, Department of Physics and Astronomy, University of Pennsylvania, Philadelphia, Pennsylvania

JACO J.M. ZWANENBURG, PhD
Department of Radiology, University Medical Center Utrecht, Utrecht, The Netherlands

Contents

Preface: Evolving Medical Imaging Techniques xi

Thomas C. Kwee and Habib Zaidi

Advances in Magnetic Resonance Spectroscopy 237

Jannie P. Wijnen and Dennis W.J. Klomp

Magnetic resonance spectroscopy (MRS) is a noninvasive technique that provides in vivo information about tissue metabolism. This article briefly describes the physical mechanisms of this powerful technique that enables imaging of endogenous markers for disease. Some examples are given of its current application in clinical use, thereby pointing out some pearls and pitfalls. In addition, new techniques for MRS and their potential for and impact on clinical use are discussed.

Chemical Exchange Saturation Transfer MR Imaging: Potential Clinical Applications 245

Daniel Louis Polders and Johannes Marinus Hoogduin

Chemical exchange saturation transfer (CEST) measurements hold great promise as the next step in magnetization transfer imaging and possibly allow for in vivo quantification of many clinically relevant parameters, including pH, temperature, and amide concentration. Therefore, it is a valuable method to add to the MR imaging toolbox. The aim of this article was to review the methods for the acquisition of CEST data and necessary postprocessing. CEST research is very much a field still in development, and initial explorations in clinical applications are shown to illustrate the potential of CEST as a new contrast mechanism.

Competing Technology for PET/Computed Tomography: Diffusion-weighted Magnetic Resonance Imaging 259

Dow-Mu Koh, Nina Tunariu, Matthew Blackledge, and David J. Collins

Whole-body diffusion-weighted (DW) imaging is a recent development. The image contrast is based on differences in mobility of water between tissues and reflects tissue cellularity and integrity of cell membranes. The tissue water diffusivity is quantified by the apparent diffusion coefficient. By performing imaging at multiple imaging stations, whole-body DW imaging has been applied to improve tumor staging, disease characterization, as well as for the assessment of treatment response. Information from DW imaging studies could be combined with those using PET imaging tracers to further refine and improve the assessment of patients with cancer.

Diffusion Magnetic Resonance Imaging and Fiber Tractography: The State of the Art and its Potential Impact on Patient Management 279

Sjoerd B. Vos, Chantal M.W. Tax, and Alexander Leemans

Diffusion magnetic resonance (MR) imaging is sensitive to microstructural changes in tissue. Diffusion tensor MR imaging, the most commonly used method, can estimate the magnitude and anisotropy of diffusion. These tensor-based diffusion parameters have been shown to change in many neuropathologic conditions. Recent advances in diffusion MR imaging techniques may provide quantitative measures that are more specific to the underlying tissue change. Diffusion MR imaging

Potential Clinical Applications of PET/Magnetic Resonance Imaging **367**

Annemieke S. Littooij, Drew A. Torigian, Thomas C. Kwee, Bart de Keizer, Abass Alavi, and Rutger A.J. Nievelstein

Hybrid PET/magnetic resonance (MR) imaging, which combines the excellent anatomic information and functional MR imaging parameters with the metabolic and molecular information obtained with PET, may be superior to PET/computed tomography or MR imaging alone for a wide range of disease conditions. This review highlights potential clinical applications in neurologic, cardiovascular, and musculoskeletal disease conditions, with special attention to applications in oncologic imaging.

Index **385**

PET CLINICS

FORTHCOMING ISSUES

October 2013
Novel Imaging Techniques in Neurodegenerative and Movement Disorders
Rathan Subramaniam, MD, and Jorge Barrio, PhD, *Editors*

January 2014
PET Imaging of Neuroendocrine Tumors
Stefano Fanti, MD, Christina Nanni, MD, and Richard Baum, MD, *Editors*

April 2014
FDG PET/CT Imaging: Normal Variations and Benign Findings
Mohsen Beheshti, MD, *Editor*

RECENT ISSUES

April 2013
PET Imaging of Brain Tumors
Sandip Basu, MBBS (Hons), DRM, DNB, and Wei Chen, MD, *Editors*

January 2013
Respiratory and Cardiac Gating in PET Imaging
Habib Zaidi, PhD, PD, and B. Kevin Teo, PhD, *Editors*

October 2012
PET Imaging of the Head and Neck
Min Yao, MD, PhD, and Peter F. Faulhaber, MD, *Editors*

PROGRAM OBJECTIVE:

The goal of the PET Clinics is to keep practicing radiologists and radiology residents up to date with current clinical practice in positron emission tomography by providing timely articles reviewing the state of the art in patient care.

TARGET AUDIENCE:

Practicing radiologists, radiology residents, and other health care professionals who provide patient care utilizing radiologic findings.

LEARNING OBJECTIVES

Upon completion of this activity, participants will be able to:

1. Review potential clinical applications of PET/MRI
2. Discuss chemical exchange saturation transfer MRI and its potential clinical applications
3. Recognize the potential impact on patient management with the use of diffusion MRI and fiber tractography.

ACCREDITATION

The Elsevier Office of Continuing Medical Education (EOCME) is accredited by the Accreditation Council for Continuing Medical Education (ACCME) to provide continuing medical education for physicians.

The EOCME designates this enduring material for a maximum of 15 *AMA PRA Category 1 Credit*(s)™. Physicians should claim only the credit commensurate with the extent of their participation in the activity.

All other health care professionals requesting continuing education credit for this enduring material will be issued a certificate of participation.

DISCLOSURE OF CONFLICTS OF INTEREST

The EOCME assesses conflict of interest with its instructors, faculty, planners, and other individuals who are in a position to control the content of CME activities. All relevant conflicts of interest that are identified are thoroughly vetted by EOCME for fair balance, scientific objectivity, and patient care recommendations. EOCME is committed to providing its learners with CME activities that promote improvements or quality in healthcare and not a specific proprietary business or a commercial interest.

The planning committee, staff, authors and editors listed below have identified no financial relationships or relationships to products or devices they or their spouse/life partner have with commercial interest related to the content of this CME activity:

Abass Alavi, MD, PhD (Hon), DSC (Hon); Alex Bhogal, PhD candidate; Matthew Blackledge, PhD; Adrianne Brigido; David R. Busch, PhD; Regine Choe, PhD; David J. Collins, PhD; Nicole Congleton; Bart de Keizer, MD, PhD; Jill B. De Vis, MD; Turgut Durduran, PhD; Jeroen Hendrikse, MD, PhD; Johannes Marinus Hoogduin, PhD; J. Martijn Jansma, PhD student; Dennis W.J. Klomp, PhD; Dow-Mu Koh, MD, MRCP, FRCR; Thomas C. Kwee, MD, PhD; Sandy Laverry; Alexander Leemans, PhD; Annemieke S. Littooij, MD; Peter R. Luijten, PhD; Jill McNair; Mahalakshmi Narayanan; Rutger A.J. Nievelstein, MD, PhD; Esben T. Petersen, PhD; Daniel Louis Polders, PhD; Jeroen C.W. Siero, PhD; Chantal M.W. Tax, PhD candidate; Drew A. Torigian, MD, MA; Nina Tunariu, MD; Anja G. van der Kolk, MD; Sjoerd B. Vos, PhD student; Jannie P. Wijnen, PhD; Arjun G. Yodh, PhD; Habib Zaidi, PhD, PD; and Jaco J.M. Zwanenburg, PhD.

UNAPPROVED/OFF-LABEL USE DISCLOSURE

The EOCME requires CME faculty to disclose to the participants:

1. When products or procedures being discussed are off-label, unlabelled, experimental, and/or investigational (not US Food and Drug Administration (FDA) approved); and
2. Any limitations on the information presented, such as data that are preliminary or that represent ongoing research, interim analyses, and/or unsupported opinions. Faculty may discuss information about pharmaceutical agents that is outside of FDA-approved labelling. This information is intended solely for CME and is not intended to promote off-label use of these medications. If you have any questions, contact the medical affairs department of the manufacturer for the most recent prescribing information.

TO ENROLL

To enroll in the PET Clinics Continuing Medical Education program, call customer service at 1-800-654-2452 or sign up online at http://www.theclinics.com/home/cme. The CME program is available to subscribers for an additional annual fee of USD 225.

METHOD OF PARTICIPATION

In order to claim credit, participants must complete the following:

1. Complete enrolment as indicated above.
2. Read the activity.
3. Complete the CME Test and Evaluation. Participants must achieve a score of 70% on the test. All CME Tests and Evaluations must be completed online.

CME INQUIRIES/SPECIAL NEEDS

For all CME inquiries or special needs, please contact elsevierCME@elsevier.com.

Preface
Evolving Medical Imaging Techniques

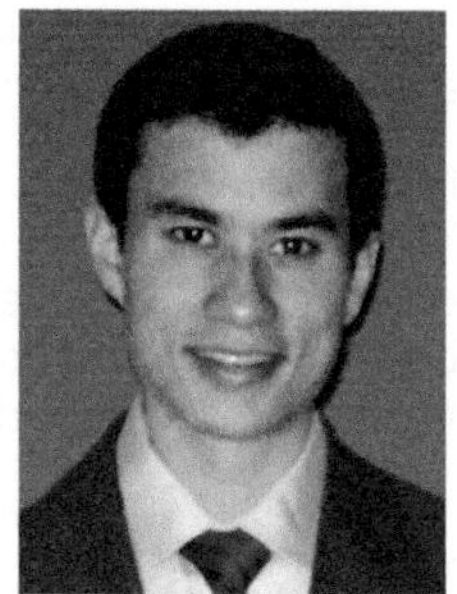

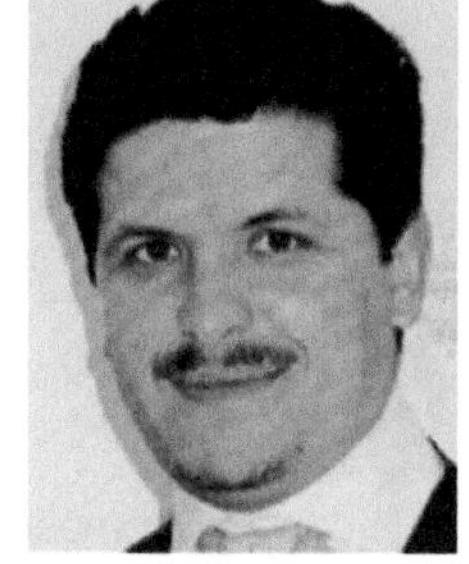

Thomas C. Kwee, MD, PhD Habib Zaidi, PhD, PD
Editors

Thanks to the recent entrance of hybrid PET/MR imaging systems into clinical practice, a new dimension in multimodality and multiparametric anato-molecular imaging has become available. PET/MR imaging provides unprecedented possibilities to study and improve the treatment of various diseases. The ultimate goal is to improve quality of life and outcome of patients, and this should always be kept in mind when using any new technology in the health sector. On another level, the beauty of PET/MR imaging will also enchant medical imaging specialists and clinicians from other specialties; if one image is worth more than a thousand words, one PET/MR image can be worth more than a million words. The introduction of PET/MR imaging will also bring nuclear medicine physicians and radiologists closer and work together with imaging scientists, technologists, and biomedical engineers as one powerful interdisciplinary team.

There is no doubt that the combination of both techniques provides more information than either one of them alone. However, to achieve the full potential of PET/MR imaging, the technique should be used wisely, and this requires detailed knowledge of both PET and MR imaging. The capabilities of PET as a molecular imaging modality are well established, while MR imaging in the setting of PET/MR imaging is often appreciated as a radiation-free modality that provides high soft tissue resolution. However, it would be unjustified and incorrect to regard MR imaging as a mere anatomical imaging modality. With MR imaging, both exquisite anatomical details and quantitative information on a variety of physiologic and metabolic processes can be obtained. The versatility of MR imaging is expected to be one of the key factors that can lead to the successful clinical implementation of PET/MR imaging. The basic knowledge of some important advanced functional MR imaging techniques that are already in clinical use or that will likely be in clinical use in the near future is therefore essential. In the first 7 articles of this issue, a selection of promising advanced MR imaging techniques (MR spectroscopy, chemical exchange saturation transfer MR imaging, diffusion-weighted MR imaging, diffusion tensor imaging, arterial spin labeling perfusion MR imaging, ultra-high-field MR imaging, and fMRI/BOLD) are reviewed by world leaders in these fields. The next article is dedicated to optical imaging, a topic that cannot be ignored when

PET Clin 8 (2013) xi–xii
http://dx.doi.org/10.1016/j.cpet.2013.04.005
1556-8598/13/$ – see front matter

reviewing evolving imaging technologies. In the last article, potential clinical applications of PET/MR imaging will be reviewed.

We would like to thank the contributing authors for their excellent articles that provide an invaluable source of frontline information for medical imaging specialists who are or will be using PET/MR imaging and related evolving technologies. We hope the readers will enjoy this issue, learn from it, and get inspired to apply the newly acquired knowledge to their clinical practice and research activities.

Thomas C. Kwee, MD, PhD
Department of Radiology and Nuclear Medicine
University Medical Center Utrecht
Heidelberglann 100
CX 3584
Utrecht, The Netherlands

Habib Zaidi, PhD, PD
Division of Nuclear Medicine and
Molecular Imaging
Geneva University Hospital
Geneva CH-1211, Switzerland

Geneva Neuroscience Center
Geneva University
Geneva CH-1211, Switzerland

Department of Nuclear Medicine and
Molecular Imaging
University Medical Center Groningen
University of Groningen
Groningen 9700 RB, Netherlands

E-mail addresses:
thomaskwee@gmail.com (T.C. Kwee)
habib.zaidi@hcuge.ch (H. Zaidi)

Advances in Magnetic Resonance Spectroscopy

Jannie P. Wijnen, PhD*, Dennis W.J. Klomp, PhD

KEYWORDS

• Magnetic resonance spectroscopy • Diagnosis • Metabolites • Chemical shift imaging
• Endogenous contrast

KEY POINTS

- Magnetic resonance spectroscopy (MRS), an insensitive technique, has been shown to be valuable for clinical use.
- MRS substantially benefits clinical diagnosis and treatment planning in various diseases.
- Because the advantages of MRS are clear, new and robust MRS techniques can be made available to all clinics.

INTRODUCTION

Magnetic resonance (MR) spectroscopy (MRS) is a noninvasive technique capable of assessing free small molecules (metabolites) in human tissue. It uses the magnetic properties of nuclei surrounded by electron clouds in molecules that produce a specific resonance frequency when placed in a strong magnetic field. For example, with MRS, tissue levels of glucose, glutamate, and creatine can be established, which provides information about the energy metabolism of the tissue. Therefore, in contrast with PET, MRS reveals multiple endogenous markers of metabolism within one measurement at similar spatial resolutions. These metabolite levels need to have a millimolar tissue concentration to be detectable with MRS. However, PET is a more sensitive technique and capable of imaging metabolites down to nanomolar concentrations. Nonetheless, MRS can be used to study a broad range of metabolites in a dynamic and longitudinal way and does not require any exogenous tracer.

MR SPECTROSCOPY

MR is based on the quantum mechanical property of nuclei called spin. The most commonly used nuclei for biomedical MRS are the spin 1/2 nuclei of hydrogen (^{1}H), phosphorous (^{31}P), and carbon (^{13}C), which naturally occur in the human body. Spin is related to the rotation of the nucleus around its own axis and, because the nucleus has an electric charge, the rotating charge creates a magnetic dipole. The orientation of the spins is normally random, but when placed in a magnetic field they rotate around the direction of the magnetic field with the Larmor frequency (precession). This resonance frequency depends on the type of nucleus and the magnetic field strength. Although this means that all hydrogen nuclei in a sample would have the same frequency, the electron clouds that surround the nucleus shields each nucleus from the main magnetic field with a unique shielding factor depending on the chemical environment of the nucleus. This shielding results in a slightly different effective magnetic field experienced by each nucleus in the molecule, providing the basis for MR spectroscopy. For instance, the methyl (CH_3) and methylene (CH_2) groups of a creatine molecule resonate at slightly different frequencies, providing a signal at 2 different positions in a ^{1}H MR spectrum, whereas the CH_3 group of choline provides a signal at another frequency.

The net magnetization of a spin population is aligned parallel to the main magnetic field (B_0). In

[a] Department of Radiology/Image Sciences Institute, University Medical Center Utrecht, P.O. Box 85500, Heidelberglaan 100 Q.S.459, Utrecht, GA 3508, The Netherlands
* Corresponding author.
E-mail address: jwijnen@umcutrecht.nl

PET Clin 8 (2013) 237–244
http://dx.doi.org/10.1016/j.cpet.2013.03.001

a typical MR experiment, the net magnetization is tilted from its original orientation (along B_0) to the transversal orientation by a radio frequency (RF) pulse at the Larmor frequency. The duration and the power of the RF pulse can be adjusted to orient the net magnetization precisely in a desired plane at the end of the pulse (excitation). After the RF pulse has been turned off, the magnetization is subject to relaxation processes that cause the spins to go back to equilibrium situation. Two types of relaxation are recognized that occur simultaneously: the recovery of the longitudinal magnetization along the direction of B_0 according to the relaxation time T1, and the decay of the transverse magnetization in the transverse plane, which occurs according to relaxation time T2. The precessing magnetization in the transverse plane induces an alternating voltage in the RF coil (antenna), which is placed around the tissue. The resulting oscillating signal in the time domain is then Fourier transformed to obtain the equivalent frequency domain signal. This frequency domain signal is the MR spectrum. The position on the X axis is characteristic for a specific molecule and the position of the Y axis is related to the number of molecules. Therefore, the concentration of specific metabolites in the tissue can be quantified by comparing the surface area under the signal with the area under a signal of a metabolite with a known concentration (often water).

Several techniques can be applied to map the spatial location of the signals in MRS. When a magnetic field gradient is applied on top of B_0, in combination with an RF pulse with a certain frequency and bandwidth, only spins in a single slice in space are excited (slice selection). By applying 3 slice selections orthogonal to each other, a single volume in space can be selected (**Fig. 1**A, B). Accurate localization is important in MRS to make sure that the MR spectrum that is obtained purely originates from the voxel of interest and not from tissue elsewhere. There are several potential artifacts associated with localization, but, with the proper techniques, these can be eliminated.

When an MR signal is obtained from a volume of interest in the human body, water is responsible for the largest signal content. Metabolite concentrations are usually in the range of 1 to 20 mM, whereas water in human tissue has a concentration on the order of 4000 mM (see **Fig. 1**C). This large concentration difference can cause problems and, to obtain reliable MR spectra of metabolites, the water signal needs to be suppressed. Various methods are available to suppress the signal of water enabling the study of metabolites.

Water suppression is not a problem when using MRS of other nuclei, such as ^{31}P and ^{13}C. For these nuclei signal can be directly obtained without the need of water suppression because these nuclei are not present in the water molecule. The downside is that both ^{31}P and ^{13}C have a lower abundance in the human body and, in addition, have an intrinsically lower MR sensitivity because of a lower gyromagnetic ratio.

CURRENT CLINICAL USE

All clinical MR scanners are equipped with basic MRS pulse sequences that can generate data with potentially sufficient quality to be used to study metabolism. In clinical research centers, more advanced MRS techniques are usually available, which results in improved data quality and sensitivity and specificity for metabolite detection. Either way, the detection and quantification of a wide range of metabolites has led to the characterization of disease progression, allowing the study of intervention by medication or surgery and allowing identification or categorization of diseases by observing specific metabolic markers.

For example, using pattern recognition algorithms on ^{1}H MR spectra, a wide range of brain tumor types can reliably be identified.[1–3] Furthermore, in brain tumor treatment, MRS is used to differentiate between tumor recurrence and radiation necrosis[4] and to guide treatment planning and follow-up.[5] MRS could also be a valuable tool in the determination of tumor aggressiveness.[6]

Pattern recognition was initially based on MR spectra from 1 voxel within the tumor, and therefore sensitive to errors caused by under sampling of a large heterogeneous tissue. With multivoxel MRS, MRS imaging (MRSI), or chemical shift imaging techniques (CSI) it is possible to map metabolite concentrations over a large area,[7] revealing heterogeneous distribution of metabolites in diseases. For instance, CSI has been used to find tumor margins in prostate and brain[8–10] (**Fig. 2**), and to guide radiotherapy planning.[11]

Because of its noninvasive nature, MRS is often preferred in pediatric patients with metabolic diseases. For example, in neonatal hypoxia, MRS can be used to estimate the damage to the brain by revealing the level of lactate and *N*-acetylaspartate[12] (NAA; NAA is representative of viable neurons) (**Fig. 3**). Furthermore, several inborn errors of metabolism have been characterized with MRS.[13]

Another example of clinical MRS is in epilepsy research; NAA has been identified as an important marker for the detection of foci of epileptic seizures,[14] whereas the cerebral levels of gamma-aminobutyric acid (GABA) and homocarnosine

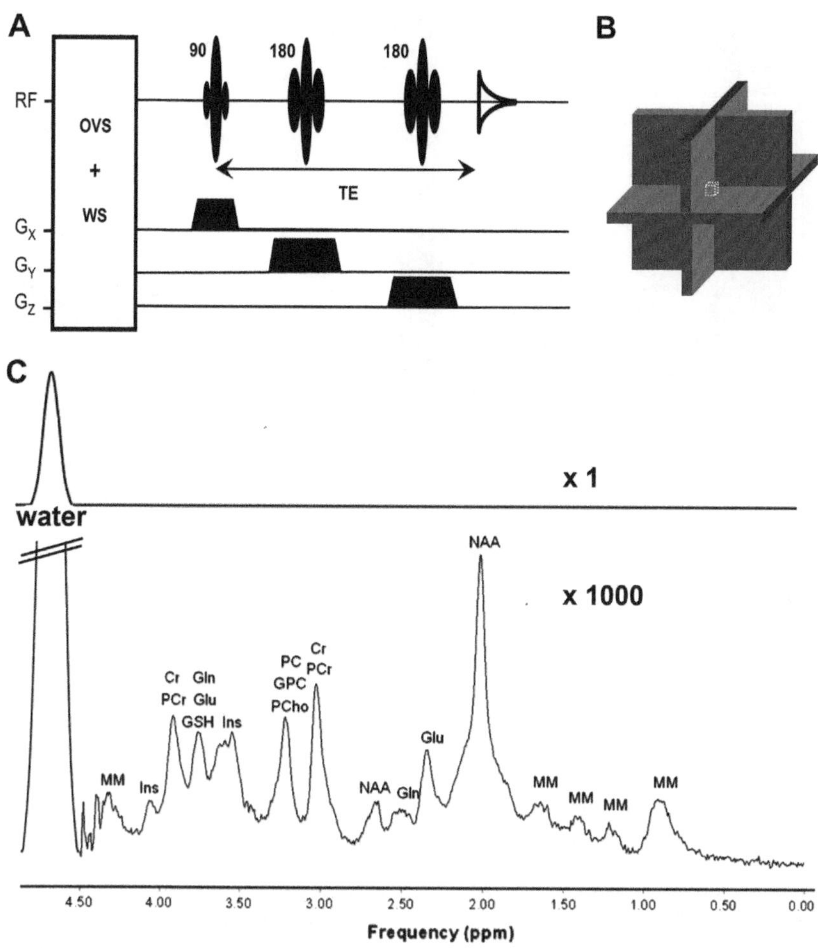

Fig. 1. (*A*) RF pulse scheme for point-resolved spectroscopy. A volume of interest is selected in a single shot by 3 RF pulses combined with 3 slice-selective gradients (*B*). ^{1}H MR spectrum of the human brain in which water is the largest signal. When zooming in 1000 times, the resonances of metabolites become visible (*C*). Cr, creatine; Gln, glutamine; Glu, glutamate; GSH, glutathione; GPC, glycerophosphocholine; Ins, myo-inositol; NAA, *N*-acetylaspartate; MM, macromolecule; PC, phosphocholine; PCr, phosphocreatine; OVS: outer volume suppression; TE: echo time; WS: water suppression.

have been correlated with the frequency of epileptic seizures.[15]

These examples are only a fraction of the clinical cases in which MRS is used for the detection of static metabolic concentrations. Despite this ability, detection of static metabolite concentrations alone provides only a partial description of metabolism. In vivo metabolism is largely characterized by dynamic processes, like enzyme-catalyzed chemical exchange, transfer of chemical groups throughout metabolic pathways, and, specific for MRS, relaxation processes. Using appropriate experimental techniques, MRS can be sensitized to a wide variety of dynamic processes, such as chemical exchange and diffusion. When MRS is combined with the infusion of exogenous compounds such as ^{13}C-glucose, it allows the in vivo detection of metabolic fluxes noninvasively. In contrast with PET, the ^{13}C-labeled nucleus not only remains detectable but its conversion into other molecules can be detected as well (**Fig. 4**).[16,17]

PEARLS AND PITFALLS

As discussed earlier, the most important advantage of MRS is its ability to study endogenous markers in diseases in a noninvasive way. There is no need for contrast agents or metabolic substrates to obtain metabolic information, but these can be used when studying metabolic conversions. However, experiments involving administration of metabolic substrates are not straightforward regarding acquisition and data analysis, some expertise is needed to make these experiments succeed. This requirement reveals one of the pitfalls of MRS and is the reason why currently

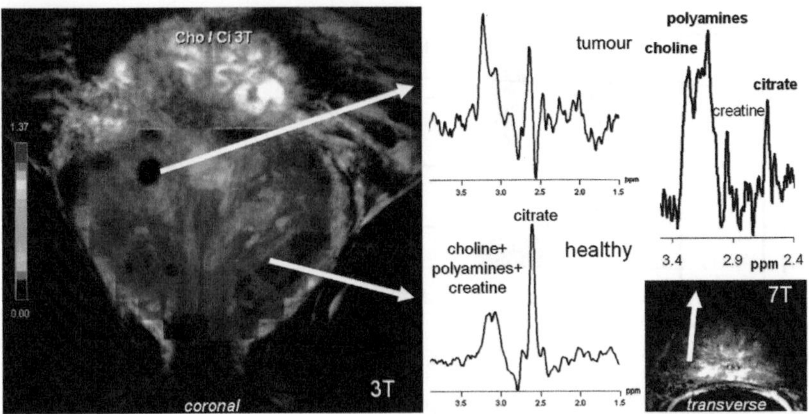

Fig. 2. Three-dimensional ^{1}H MRSI of the prostate at 3 T. The ratio of choline (Cho) to citrate (Ci) is mapped over the prostate and overlaid on an MR image. In the tumor, the Cho/Ci ratio is higher than in the healthy prostate. At 7 T, ^{1}H MRS of the prostate becomes more specific (*right* side of figure); here the resonances around 3.2 ppm can be separated into signal of choline, polyamines, and creatine, whereas these three are hard to distinguish from each other in the MR spectrum obtained at 3 T. (*Data from* Scheenen TW, Heijmink SW, Roell SA, et al. Threedimensional proton MR spectroscopy of human prostate at 3 T without endorectal coil: feasibility. Radiology 2007;245(2):507–16.)

MRS is mostly used in research settings. MRS protocols still require disease-specific optimization and technicians need to be trained to perform extra preparation steps that may not be automatically performed by the scanner without interaction by the user. Furthermore, the interpretation of MRS data is not as straightforward as the most commonly used MR imaging data, so the radiologist also needs to be trained to read MR spectra.

WHAT THE REFERRING PHYSICIAN NEEDS TO KNOW

For the referring physician it is important to know which metabolites can be detected with MRS and with what reliability.[18] When metabolites are detected reliably, the referring physician needs to know how metabolites are related to diseases and how to interpret the data.

Particularly in the ^{1}H MR spectrum, all metabolite resonances overlap and modeling of each metabolite individually is needed to extract the metabolite-specific pattern and translate it into concentrations. For metabolites that have high tissue concentration, such as NAA and creatine in the brain, this is easy, but for metabolites such as glutamate and glucose this is more difficult, particularly at low magnetic field strength. At higher magnetic field strength, the chemical shift dispersion is increased, which means that the

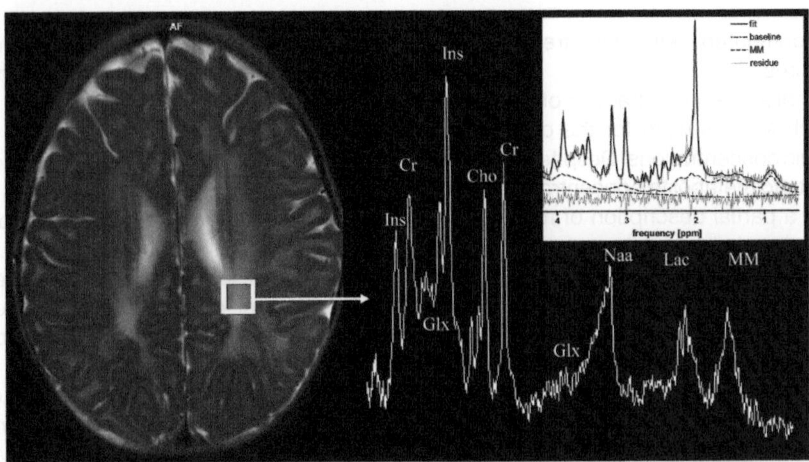

Fig. 3. ^{1}H MR spectrum of white matter in the brain of a 2-year-old child with Sandhoff disease[43] compared with the ^{1}H MR spectrum of normal white matter (*inset*). Note that the signal of NAA is severely decreased and that the signal of myo-inositol is increased in the diseased brain.

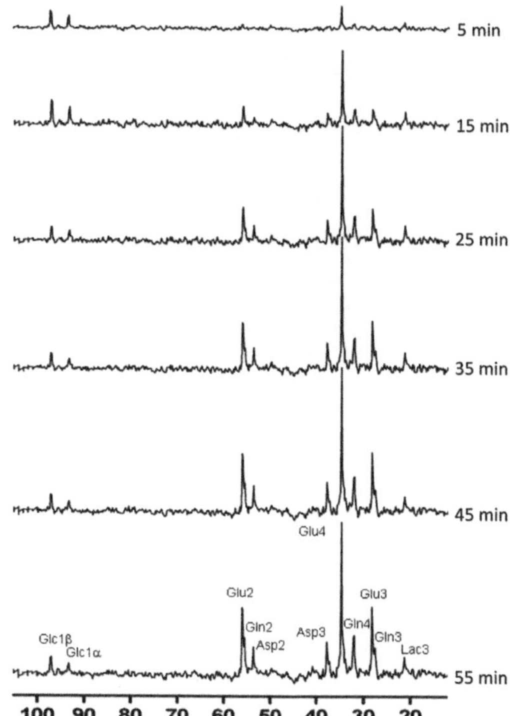

Fig. 4. Series of ^{13}C-MR spectra of the normal brain after administration of ^{13}C-enriched glucose. Five minutes after the bolus injection of ^{13}C-glucose, only resonances of glucose and glutamate can be observed (*top*). When continuing the glucose infusion while maintaining a stable blood glucose level, the incorporation of ^{13}C label into other intermediates of the tricarboxylic acid (TCA) cycle can be followed over time. The numbers refer to the position of the ^{13}C label in the molecule. Asp, aspartate; Glc, glucose; Lac, lactate.

individual resonances are further apart (increased spectral resolution) and easier to distinguish from each other. For example, signals from glutamate are not accurately assessable at 1.5 T, still have substantial overlap at 3 T, but become almost completely nonoverlapping at 7 T, which is an example of the more robust and accurate detection of metabolites at high fields.[19,20]

NEW TECHNIQUES AND POTENTIAL FOR MRS

More Signal, Smaller Volumes

Although MRS is an older technique than MR imaging, its applicability in clinics has been lagging behind, mainly because of long scan times and low spatial resolution. However, with recent technological developments, single-shot MRS techniques have been reported,[21–25] and nominal spatial resolutions can be 3.6 mm isotropic.[26] Spectroscopic imaging is no longer time consuming when using acceleration techniques that have shown their applicability in MRI, like Sensitivity Encoding or Echo Planar Imaging,[27–29] furthermore, spectroscopic imaging benefits from inherent internal referencing of metabolite levels within the same subject.

Whereas single-voxel methods had to rely on absolute quantification, the transition to spectroscopic imaging at resolutions that meet pathologic sizes relaxes the essence of quantification. As in MR imaging, MR techniques can consequently be used that, although dependent on relaxation effects, boost signal/noise ratio (SNR) and hence translate into increased spatial resolutions.[30] The SNR and spectral resolution gains at ultra high fields in particular make the transition to high-resolution imaging of metabolite levels feasible.

For well-defined areas in organs or diseases, single-voxel MRS also provides new areas of interest. First, a single-shot (subsecond) MR spectrum can be obtained that, when combined in stimulation paradigms like those used in functional MR imaging, can reveal metabolic alterations related to activity (ie, increased lactate and glutamate levels.[31] Also, with the increased SNR, metabolite signals that are generally overlapped by other highly concentrated metabolites can be extracted from the MRS data using editing techniques. These techniques use the specific MR properties of the metabolite of interest to uniquely manipulate its signal without affecting the overlapping signals, which, after subtraction, reveals metabolite levels that have not (or hardly) been detectable before. With such spectral editing techniques, metabolites like GABA and lactate can be detected, which are otherwise obscured by the signals of creatine, lipids, and macromolecules.[32–35]

The increased SNR is crucial in the detection of MRS at nuclei other than ^{1}H, such as ^{31}P and ^{13}C. However, because these nuclei are often coupled to ^{1}H, the ^{1}H polarization can be transferred to these nuclei. With these techniques, the high magnetization of ^{1}H is used to boost the magnetization of ^{31}P or ^{13}C nuclei. By manipulating the magnetization in the right way, magnetization can be transferred from, for instance, ^{1}H to ^{31}P. The signal is still detected via the ^{31}P nuclei but at higher SNR. Although these pulse sequences require dedicated MR hardware, the boost in SNR is essential when translating these studies to the clinic at acceptable spatial and temporal resolutions (**Fig. 5**).[36]

Better Localization

Accurate localization of the MR spectra is important to avoid misinterpretation of the data. When

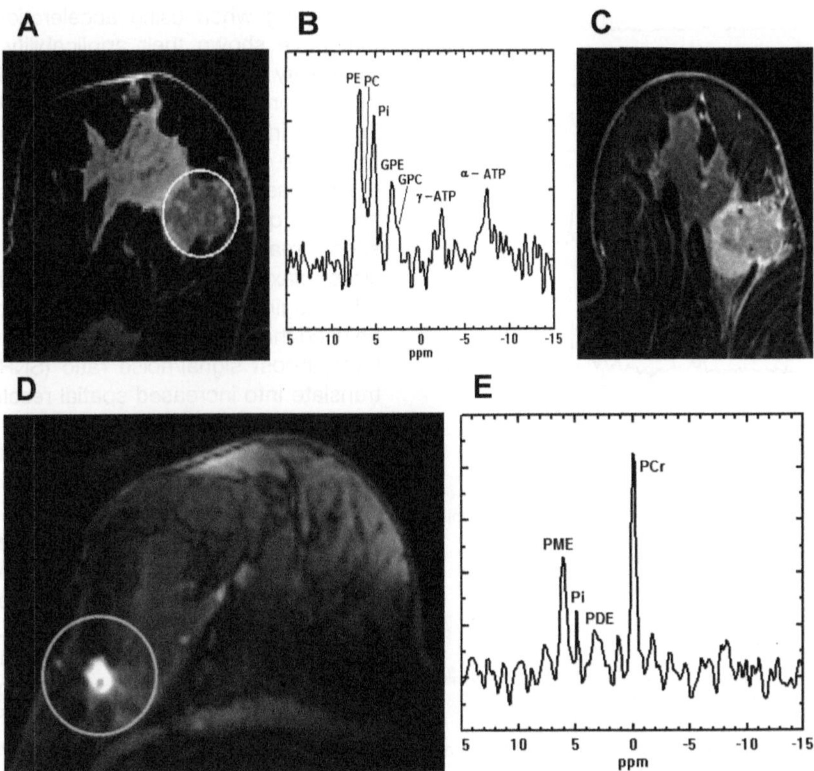

Fig. 5. MR imaging and ^{31}P MR spectroscopy in breast cancer. (*A–C*) Invasive ductal carcinoma with 3.2-cm diameter. (*A*) 7-T T1-weighted image without contrast agent, with the tumor mass encircled; (*B*) ^{31}P MR spectrum of a voxel containing the tumor mass showing enhanced intensities of the phosphomonoesters phosphoethanolamine (PE) and phosphocholine (PC) compared with the phosphodiesters glycerophosphoethanolamine (GPE) and glycerophosphocholine (GPC); (*C*) 3-T T1-weighted image after administering gadolinium-based contrast agent. (*D*) Ductulolobular carcinoma with 0.9-cm diameter. 7-T contrast-enhanced image showing the high contrast available at 7 T highlighting tumor mass; (*E*) ^{31}P spectrum of a voxel containing the tumor mass, showing enhanced phosphomonoester (PME) intensity compared with the phosphodiester (PDE) intensity, even at a small tumor volume of only 2 mL. Note that the PCr signal is caused by voxel bleeding from the underlying pectoralis muscle. Pi: inorganic phosphate.

proper localization fails, signals from outside the volume of interest cause artifacts that obscure the data. For a long time, MRS localization used conventional RF pulses that assumed uniform and strong magnetic fields throughout the sample; however, susceptibility differences between tissues cause nonuniformities in the static magnetic field. Furthermore, at high field strength, the RF field is not strong and becomes nonuniform as well. However, adiabatic RF pulses have been incorporated into MRS sequences (such as semi-localization by adiabatic selective refocusing[23,24]) that are insensitive to the magnetic field distortions, and can operate at weak RF fields.

Another technical improvement is available for reducing magnetic field distortions. High-order shim coils, up to fifth order, can be purchased that can counteract the natural field nonuniformities caused by susceptibility transitions in tissues. Moreover, it is well recognized that the main magnetic field varies over time as well because of physiologic processes in the human body, such as breathing and cardiac motion. Navigator techniques have consequently been incorporated that can either correct the acquired data for related frequency shifts in the MR spectra before averaging, or even in real time correct the magnetic field based on acquired field information.[37] Better shimming improves spectral resolution but also water suppression and localization.

All technical improvements mentioned earlier enable a more robust and more reliable MRS acquisition and therefore benefit the clinical application of MRS. With good localization, metabolic information from specific anatomic structures can be obtained, which increases the specificity of MRS as a diagnostic tool.

Nonproton MRS

Another potential of MRS is that different types of metabolism can be studied via other nuclei than protons. For example, with ^{31}P MRS the energy metabolism can be studied via the levels of phosphocreatine and adenosine triphosphates (ATPs). With recent advances in high-field MRS, particularly, MRS of other nuclei than protons is gaining interest because it benefits from the increased SNR, because background signals (such as water in ^{1}H MRS) are orders of magnitude less. Also, signal resonances are further apart, particularly in the ^{31}P MR spectrum, and therefore the MR spectrum is less sensitive to B_0 inhomogeneity. The ^{31}P nucleus has a lower intrinsic SNR than ^{1}H, but at 7 T the SNR is increased and ^{31}P CSI can be done at spatial resolutions that become clinically relevant. It was recently shown that the spatial resolution is sufficient to detect the MR spectra of gray matter and white matter.[38]

Because specific resonances can be saturated, the magnetization of the saturated metabolite can be passed to other resonances via chemical conversion. This process allows the assessment of chemical exchange rates without the use of any contrast agent.[39]

The development of technology that applies dynamic nuclear polarization to generate hyperpolarized ^{13}C-labeled metabolic substrates has changed the clinical potential of ^{13}C MRS. Hyperpolarized substrates generate a strong MR signal boosting the SNR more than 10,000-fold. Preclinical studies have shown the potential of ^{13}C MRS of hyperpolarized substrates, for example in cancer imaging and imaging of heart disease.[40–42]

SUMMARY

Although MRS is an insensitive technique, particularly at low magnetic field strength, several applications have been shown to be valuable for clinical use. Despite it taking several years to reach the high level of technology that is available today, enabling reliable and robust MRS acquisition, the translation of anatomic imaging to metabolic imaging has already started. MRS benefits clinical diagnosis and treatment planning in various diseases. Because the advantages of MRS are clear, new and robust MRS techniques can be made available to all clinics.

REFERENCES

1. Julia-Sape M, Acosta D, Mier M, et al. A multi-centre, web-accessible and quality control-checked database of in vivo MR spectra of brain tumour patients. MAGMA 2006;19(1):22–33.
2. Perez-Ruiz A, Julia-Sape M, Mercadal G, et al. The INTERPRET Decision-Support System version 3.0 for evaluation of magnetic resonance spectroscopy data from human brain tumours and other abnormal brain masses. BMC Bioinformatics 2010;11:581.
3. Tate AR, Underwood J, Acosta DM, et al. Development of a decision support system for diagnosis and grading of brain tumours using in vivo magnetic resonance single voxel spectra. NMR Biomed 2006; 19(4):411–34.
4. Chernov MF, Hayashi M, Izawa M, et al. Multivoxel proton MRS for differentiation of radiation-induced necrosis and tumor recurrence after gamma knife radiosurgery for brain metastases. Brain Tumor Pathol 2006;23(1):19–27.
5. Nelson SJ, Graves E, Pirzkall A, et al. In vivo molecular imaging for planning radiation therapy of gliomas: an application of 1H MRSI. J Magn Reson Imaging 2002;16(4):464–76.
6. Kobus T, Hambrock T, Hulsbergen-van de Kaa CA, et al. In vivo assessment of prostate cancer aggressiveness using magnetic resonance spectroscopic imaging at 3 T with an endorectal coil. Eur Urol 2011;60(5):1074–80.
7. Maudsley AA, Domenig C, Govind V, et al. Mapping of brain metabolite distributions by volumetric proton MR spectroscopic imaging (MRSI). Magn Reson Med 2009;61(3):548–59.
8. Nelson SJ. Multivoxel magnetic resonance spectroscopy of brain tumors. Mol Cancer Ther 2003;2(5): 497–507.
9. Scheenen TW, Futterer J, Weiland E, et al. Discriminating cancer from noncancer tissue in the prostate by 3-dimensional proton magnetic resonance spectroscopic imaging: a prospective multicenter validation study. Invest Radiol 2011;46(1):25–33.
10. Futterer JJ, Heijmink SW, Scheenen TW, et al. Prostate cancer localization with dynamic contrast-enhanced MR imaging and proton MR spectroscopic imaging. Radiology 2006;241(2):449–58.
11. Payne GS, Leach MO. Applications of magnetic resonance spectroscopy in radiotherapy treatment planning. Br J Radiol 2006;79(Spec No 1):S16–26.
12. de Vries LS, Groenendaal F. Patterns of neonatal hypoxic-ischaemic brain injury. Neuroradiology 2010;52(6):555–66.
13. Engelke UF, Moolenaar SH, Hoenderop SM, et al. Handbook of 1H-NMR spectroscopy in inborn errors of metabolism: body fluid NMR spectroscopy and in vivo MR spectroscopy. Heilbronn (Germany): SPS Verlagsgesellschaft; 2007.
14. Hetherington HP, Pan JW, Spencer DD. 1H and 31P spectroscopy and bioenergetics in the lateralization of seizures in temporal lobe epilepsy. J Magn Reson Imaging 2002;16(4):477–83.
15. Petroff OA, Mattson RH, Behar KL, et al. Vigabatrin increases human brain homocarnosine and

improves seizure control. Ann Neurol 1998;44(6): 948–52.
16. de Graaf RA, Mason GF, Patel AB, et al. In vivo 1H-[13C]-NMR spectroscopy of cerebral metabolism. NMR Biomed 2003;16(6–7):339–57.
17. Wijnen JP, Van der Graaf M, Scheenen TW, et al. In vivo 13C magnetic resonance spectroscopy of a human brain tumor after application of 13C-1-enriched glucose. Magn Reson Imaging 2010; 28(5):690–7.
18. Wijnen J, van Asten J, Klomp D, et al. Short echo time 1H MRSI of the human brain at 3T with adiabatic slice-selective refocusing pulses; reproducibility and variance in a dual centre setting. J Magn Reson Imaging 2010;31(1):61–70.
19. Emir UE, Auerbach EJ, Van De Moortele PF, et al. Regional neurochemical profiles in the human brain measured by (1) H MRS at 7 T using local B(1) shimming. NMR Biomed 2011;25(1):152–60.
20. Pfeuffer J, Tkac I, Provencher SW, et al. Toward an in vivo neurochemical profile: quantification of 18 metabolites in short-echo-time (1)H NMR spectra of the rat brain. J Magn Reson 1999;141(1):104–20.
21. Bottomley PA. Spatial localization in NMR spectroscopy in vivo. Ann N Y Acad Sci 1987;508:333–48.
22. Frahm J, Merboldt KD, Hanicke W. Localized proton spectroscopy using stimulated echoes. J Magn Reson 1987;72:502–8.
23. Garwood M, DelaBarre L. The return of the frequency sweep: designing adiabatic pulses for contemporary NMR. J Magn Reson 2001;153(2): 155–77.
24. Scheenen TW, Klomp DW, Wijnen JP, et al. Short echo time 1H-MRSI of the human brain at 3T with minimal chemical shift displacement errors using adiabatic refocusing pulses. Magn Reson Med 2008;59(1):1–6.
25. Slotboom J, Mehlkopf AF, Bovee WM. A single-shot localization pulse sequence suited for coils with inhomogeneous RF fields using adiabatic slice-selective RF pulses. J Magn Reson 1991;95:396–404.
26. Scheenen TW, Heerschap A, Klomp DW. Towards 1H-MRSI of the human brain at 7T with slice-selective adiabatic refocusing pulses. MAGMA 2008;21(1–2):95–101.
27. Lin FH, Tsai SY, Otazo R, et al. Sensitivity-encoded (SENSE) proton echo-planar spectroscopic imaging (PEPSI) in the human brain. Magn Reson Med 2007; 57(2):249–57.
28. Posse S, Dager SR, Richards TL, et al. In vivo measurement of regional brain metabolic response to hyperventilation using magnetic resonance: proton echo planar spectroscopic imaging (PEPSI). Magn Reson Med 1997;37(6):858–65.
29. Posse S, Otazo R, Dager SR, et al. MR spectroscopic imaging: principles and recent advances. J Magn Reson Imaging 2012. http://dx.doi.org/10.1002/jmri.23945.
30. Boer VO, Siero JC, Hoogduin H, et al. High-field MRS of the human brain at short TE and TR. NMR Biomed 2011;24(9):1081–8.
31. Lin Y, Stephenson MC, Xin L, et al. Investigating the metabolic changes due to visual stimulation using functional proton magnetic resonance spectroscopy at 7 T. J Cereb Blood Flow Metab 2012;32(8): 1484–95.
32. Andreychenko A, Boer VO, Arteaga de Castro CS, et al. Efficient spectral editing at 7 T: GABA detection with MEGA-sLASER. Magn Reson Med 2012; 68(4):1018–25.
33. Smith MA, Koutcher JA, Zakian KL. J-difference lactate editing at 3.0 Tesla in the presence of strong lipids. J Magn Reson Imaging 2008;28(6): 1492–8.
34. Boer VO, Luijten PR, Klomp DW. Refocused double-quantum editing for lactate detection at 7 T. Magn Reson Med 2013;69(1):1–6.
35. Pan JW, Duckrow RB, Spencer DD, et al. Selective homonuclear polarization transfer for spectroscopic imaging of GABA at 7T. Magn Reson Med 2012; 69(2):310–6.
36. Wijnen JP, Scheenen TW, Klomp DW, et al. 31P magnetic resonance spectroscopic imaging with polarisation transfer of phosphomono- and diesters at 3 T in the human brain: relation with age and spatial differences. NMR Biomed 2010;23(8):968–76.
37. Boer VO, van de Bank BL, van Vliet G, et al. Direct B0 field monitoring and real-time B0 field updating in the human breast at 7 Tesla. Magn Reson Med 2012;67(2):586–91.
38. Zhu XH, Qiao H, Du F, et al. Quantitative imaging of energy expenditure in human brain. Neuroimage 2012;60(4):2107–17.
39. Du F, Zhu XH, Qiao H, et al. Efficient in vivo 31P magnetization transfer approach for noninvasively determining multiple kinetic parameters and metabolic fluxes of ATP metabolism in the human brain. Magn Reson Med 2007;57(1):103–14.
40. Brindle KM, Bohndiek SE, Gallagher FA, et al. Tumor imaging using hyperpolarized 13C magnetic resonance spectroscopy. Magn Reson Med 2011; 66(2):505–19.
41. Malloy CR, Merritt ME, Sherry AD. Could 13C MRI assist clinical decision-making for patients with heart disease? NMR Biomed 2011;24(8):973–9.
42. Kurhanewicz J, Bok R, Nelson SJ, et al. Current and potential applications of clinical 13C MR spectroscopy. J Nucl Med 2008;49(3):341–4.
43. Klomp DW, van der Graaf M, Willemsen MA, et al. Transmit/receive headcoil for optimal 1H MR spectroscopy of the brain in paediatric patients at 3T. MAGMA 2004;17(1):1–4.

Chemical Exchange Saturation Transfer MR Imaging

Potential Clinical Applications

Daniel Louis Polders, PhD[a],
Johannes Marinus Hoogduin, PhD[a,b,*]

KEYWORDS

- Chemical exchange saturation transfer (CEST) • Magnetization transfer (MT)
- Amide proton transfer (APT)

KEY POINTS

- Chemical exchange saturation transfer (CEST) is a frequency-specific implementation of magnetization transfer measurements. This makes the measurement sensitive to the exchange of protons belonging to specific molecules with labile proton groups.
- As the exchange rates depend strongly on the type of target molecule, the measurement can (and should) be optimized for each specific CEST application.
- There are several endogenous targets for CEST, such as protons in amides, glycogen, and glycosaminoglycans. In addition, novel exogenous CEST agents with tailored exchange rates and chemical shifts can provide specific contrasts without the use of gadolinium-based chelates.

INTRODUCTION

Chemical exchange saturation transfer (CEST) is an exciting new application of magnetic resonance (MR) imaging that aims to obtain metabolic imaging information in a completely noninvasive manner. The type of information (sensitizing the images for specific metabolic compounds), as well as the terms used in CEST experiments (ie, "saturation frequency offsets") might hint at a strong overlap with MR spectroscopy or spectroscopic imaging (MRSI). However, this is not the case. Although both methods sensitize at specific frequencies, the metabolites that are visible in MRSI experiments are generally invisible in CEST experiments, and vice versa. As such, the methods contain complementary information.

In terms of the method of acquisition, CEST is a variation of a rather old MR imaging technique, that of magnetization transfer (MT). In the past, the effect of an off-resonance saturation prepulse on the main water signal was contributed to all mechanisms that allowed magnetization to transfer toward the bulk water pool. Basic MR imaging experiments have identified molecules with labile protons (protons that are in chemical exchange with the bulk water pool). By using frequency-specific saturation, it is now possible to specifically saturate protons resonating at these chemical shifts, thereby also selecting specific groups of molecules. This increase in specificity has led to a deepening of our understanding of the exchange mechanisms that play a role in in vivo MT, and has also led to the optimization of saturation experiments aimed at these specific molecules. Several endogenous CEST agents with specific clinical applications have been identified, and it is expected that more will follow (**Table 1**).

BACKGROUND

One important observation in MR imaging is that most of the measured signal comes from protons in liquid form (ie, bulk water or adipose tissue);

[a] Imaging Division, Department of Radiology, UMCU, Heidelberglaan 100, 3584 CX, Utrecht, The Netherlands;
[b] Brain Division, UMCU, Heidelberglaan 100, 3584 CX, Utrecht, The Netherlands
* Corresponding author.
E-mail address: j.m.hoogduin-2@umcutrecht.nl

PET Clin 8 (2013) 245–257
http://dx.doi.org/10.1016/j.cpet.2013.04.001

Table 1
Endogenous CEST agents and their clinical applications

Molecule	Chemical Shift (Relative to the Bulk Water Resonance)	Origin	Clinical Application
Amides	+3.5 ppm	Present in the backbone structure of proteins, therefore expected to be increasingly detectable wherever proteins are degraded (exposing more of the backbone to the bulk water pool)	Detection of tumors and changes in pH
Glycosaminoglycans	+0.9–1.9 ppm	Polysaccharide present in cartilage	Detection of cartilage diseases
Glycogen	+0.5–1.5 ppm	Glycogen is a primary form of glucose storage in liver and muscle tissue	Detection of metabolic disorders influencing energy storage and retrieval
Glutamate	+3 ppm	Excitatory neurotransmitter	Glutamate is associated with several neurologic disorders, including amyotrophic lateral sclerosis, and Alzheimer disease
Urea	+1 ppm	Primary nitrogen-containing substance in urine	Renal function
Mio-inositol	+0.2–1.56 ppm	Sugarlike brain metabolite, located in glial cells where it functions as an osmolyte	Mio-inositol is a glial marker; changes in its concentration occur in brain tumors, multiple sclerosis, and Alzheimer disease

An increasing number of endogenous CEST agents can be targeted in a CEST measurement. The table shows the most important ones, including their origin and clinical relevance.

however, there are many more protons present in more rigid forms, which are generally not observed in MR imaging methods. For example, many protons are part of lipid bilayers, structural and larger globular proteins, and so forth. These protons are covalently bound to slowly moving structures, and have very limited motional freedom. This results in quick dephasing of the MR signal or short T2 relaxation times. Also, not all bulk water can be considered truly liquid because much of it is located in hydration layers around these macromolecules. The bound water fraction is of specific interest because it can be visualized, albeit indirectly, using conventional magnetization transfer measurements.

When looking in the spectral domain, a short T2 is equal to a broad resonance peak. In "free" bulk water, the motion of the protons causes narrowing of the resonance peak. The width of this peak is mostly determined by variations in the B0 field. This is in the order of a few hundred hertz or less in the human brain at 7 T. In the case of the bound water pool, however, T2 effects cause the resonance spectrum to become as wide as tens of thousands of hertz. It was shown as early as in 1989 that applying radiofrequency (RF) pulses off-resonance at a few thousand hertz from the water resonance has a suppressing effect on the acquired signal from the water pool.[1] Thus, the magnetization that was applied off-resonance is somehow transferred to the bulk water pool. Several mechanisms for this magnetization transfer effect have been suggested, such as the exchange of water from the bound water pool to the bulk water pool (a relatively slow process), spin-diffusion from bound water protons to bulk water protons (much faster), and chemical exchange from exchanging moieties on molecules with labile (nonpermanently bound) protons.

Magnetization Transfer by Chemical Exchange

Probing the mechanism of magnetization transfer by chemical exchange has sparked much interest in the past 20 years, starting with its translation from nuclear magnetic resonance (NMR) to MR imaging experiments in 1990 by Wolff and Balaban.[2] It was hypothesized that specific exchanging moieties at endogenous molecules display a specific resonance frequency, just as in MR spectroscopy. These exchanging groups are rarely observed in spectroscopy, precisely because of the continuous exchange of these groups with the bulk water pool.

In a CEST experiment, the MR imaging signal is sensitized for chemical exchange using saturation pulses at specific radiation power levels and off-resonance frequencies tuned to saturate specific moieties of labile protons at known molecules. This is different from the previously described magnetization transfer techniques, in which the saturation pulse was optimized to maximize all magnetization transfer effects. For instance, proteins and peptides contain amide groups, which in turn have a labile proton (the amide proton). From in vitro experiments, the resonance frequency and exchange rate have been determined to be +3.5 ppm (from the water resonance) and about 28 Hz at pH 7, respectively.[3]

From exchange theory, it is known that the exchange rate of labile protons is governed by the environment of the molecule, especially the acidity (pH) and temperature. By sensitizing the MR imaging experiment to the exchange of a known type of labile protons, CEST experiments promise to offer a window into these fundamental physical properties, as well as the relative amount of these labile protons. In case of large proteins in their natural confirmation (ie, folding of the amino acid chain), not all of the amide protons are at the outside of the protein structure, so not all of them are expected to contribute much to the exchange process. If by disease, however, a protein becomes partly broken down or incorrectly folded, more amide protons are expected to become exposed and thus "visible" in a CEST experiment.

IMAGING PROTOCOLS: MEASURING CEST

A central concept in CEST measurements is that of the Z-spectrum (**Box 1**). Designing an MR imaging–CEST measurement begins with the realization that the classic saturation-based magnetization transfer method has a strong frequency dependency.

Box 1
Magnetization transfer among pools, Z-spectra, and asymmetry analysis

Consider a simplified 2-pool system, in which a small fraction of protons on a specific type of molecule (solute/pool B) is in continuous exchange with the bulk water pool (solvent/pool A). By applying RF radiation at resonance frequency specific for this pool, the bulk water pool can be saturated. Repeating a saturation experiment at several frequencies yields the Z-spectrum. The Z-spectrum was generally considered symmetric around the water resonance, leading to the asymmetry analysis to calculate the effect due to CEST. More recent studies have shown that this is likely an oversimplification.

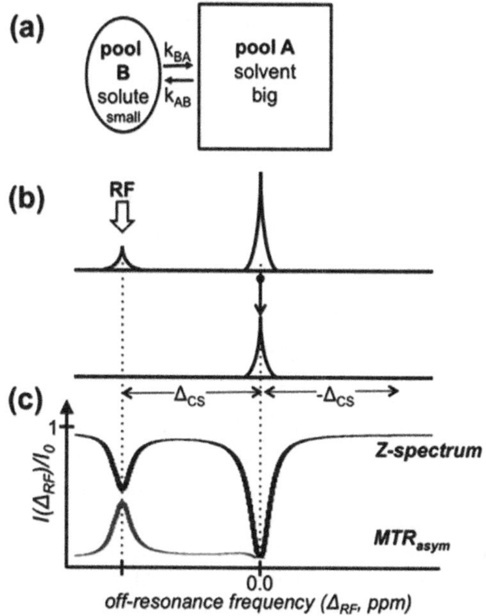

Schematic representation of CEST experiment. (a) Pool A (solvent) is in exchange with pool B (solute). (b) Pools A and B have distinct chemical shifts, with the difference of Δ_{CS}. RF is applied on-resonance with pool B, resulting in saturation transfer and signal decrease of pool A. (c) Z-spectrum: normalized water intensity (I/I_0) versus off-resonance frequency of the saturation RF (Δ_{RF}). Water resonance is assigned 0 ppm value. MTR_{asym}, Z-spectrum asymmetry versus RF off-resonance value.

From Vinogradov E, Sherry AD, Lenkinski RE. CEST: from basic principles to applications, challenges and opportunities. J Magn Reson 2013;229:155–72. http://dx.doi.org/10.1016/j.jmr.2012.11.024; with permission.

When a saturation transfer experiment is repeated multiple times with varying saturation frequencies, a Z-spectrum is obtained, illustrating the frequency dependency of magnetization transfer measurements. The overall shape of the Z-spectrum is dominated by conventional magnetization transfer and direct water saturation. This results in a wide v-shape with its minimum on the water frequency. These 2 saturation effects are generally considered more or less symmetric around this frequency, although there is some evidence that this might not be the case.[4] In addition to these large-scale effects, which span many hundreds of ppm, there are also asymmetric effects working on a smaller frequency range. These result from chemical exchange of protons originating from molecules where they have a substantial chemical shift. By performing a saturation experiment at this shifted frequency, there is signal attenuation due to (1) direct saturation of the water pool, (2) conventional magnetization transfer, and (3) saturation transfer due to chemical exchange. By comparing this signal with the saturation effects measured at the frequency opposite from the water resonance, an approach called asymmetry analysis, it is possible to separate the chemical exchange effect from the other contributions.

There are many ways to design a saturation experiment and many of the current methods are reviewed by Van Zijl and Yadav,[5] and more recently by Vinogradov and colleagues.[6]

In a nutshell, there are 3 strategies to employ saturation to the system. (1) Applying a long (seconds) saturation pulse followed by as much read out (either imaging or spectroscopy) as possible. In practice, RF amplifiers have not been built to deliver such long pulses while maintaining power, so the pulses are separated into multiple smaller pulses or pulse-trains. (2) Applying only short saturation pulses, interleaved with partial read-out segments, aiming to achieve a steady-state condition during the acquisition. (3) Applying a short saturation pulse and measuring only a transient CEST effect, which is less than the steady-state magnitude.

Once a saturation scheme is selected, the saturation duration and amplitude need to be optimized to the exchanging protons of the intended CEST agent. Agents that have a high exchange rate (ie, protons have only a short residence time on the agent) need to be saturated with a stronger saturation pulse, to fully inverse the spins (maximum saturation). The drawback of this is that higher amplitude will also increase concomitant MT effects via other mechanisms than chemical exchange.

After optimizing both saturation duration and amplitude, the intended frequencies need to be set. In many clinical settings it is not feasible to collect a densely sampled Z-spectrum over a broad frequency range because of scan time limitations. Instead, one might compromise with a selection of relevant off-resonance frequencies of interest. Typical scan times depend on the number of off-resonance frequencies included and can be between 3 and 30 minutes. Image resolution depends on the application ranging from below 1 $\times$ 1 mm^2 in-plane for cartilage imaging to several millimeters in the brain. Slice thickness is on the order of several millimeters.

Postprocessing

B0 and B1 inhomogeneities

Even after shimming using higher-order shim gradients, there will be some residual variations in the B0 field, which will effectively shift the acquired Z-spectra. To interpret or quantify CEST images, this needs to be corrected for. One way to do this is to use additional B0 information by acquiring a separate B0 map and shift the measured Z-spectra by the same amount as the offset. Another approach is to deduce the B0 information by finding the minimum in a sufficiently sampled Z-spectrum using the water saturation shift referencing (WASSR) method.[7] In any case, it holds that if only a limited number of points of the Z-spectra are acquired, it is important to include some room for correction because of B0 inhomogeneity.

Similarly, the amount of saturation depends strongly on the amplitude of the B1 field. Furthermore, the different mechanisms of saturation transfer have different, nonlinear, dependencies on the B1 field, and correction for variations of B1 cannot be a simple scaling with the B1 amplitude.[8,9]

Quantifying CEST

As discussed previously, CEST studies have used asymmetry analysis to quantify the saturation effect due to chemical exchange. It has become clear that there are additional saturation effects often located at the opposite site from the water resonance, probably nuclear Overhauser effects (NOE), that severely hamper asymmetry analysis. This effect is especially pronounced in amide proton transfer (APT) imaging at high field (**Fig. 1**). To overcome this issue, other approaches to model the Z-spectrum have been proposed, such as fitting the spectrum to a Lorentz curve,[10] or by approximating the curve by a straight line in a small region around the expected CEST effect.[11] Another, maybe more correct approach is to fully

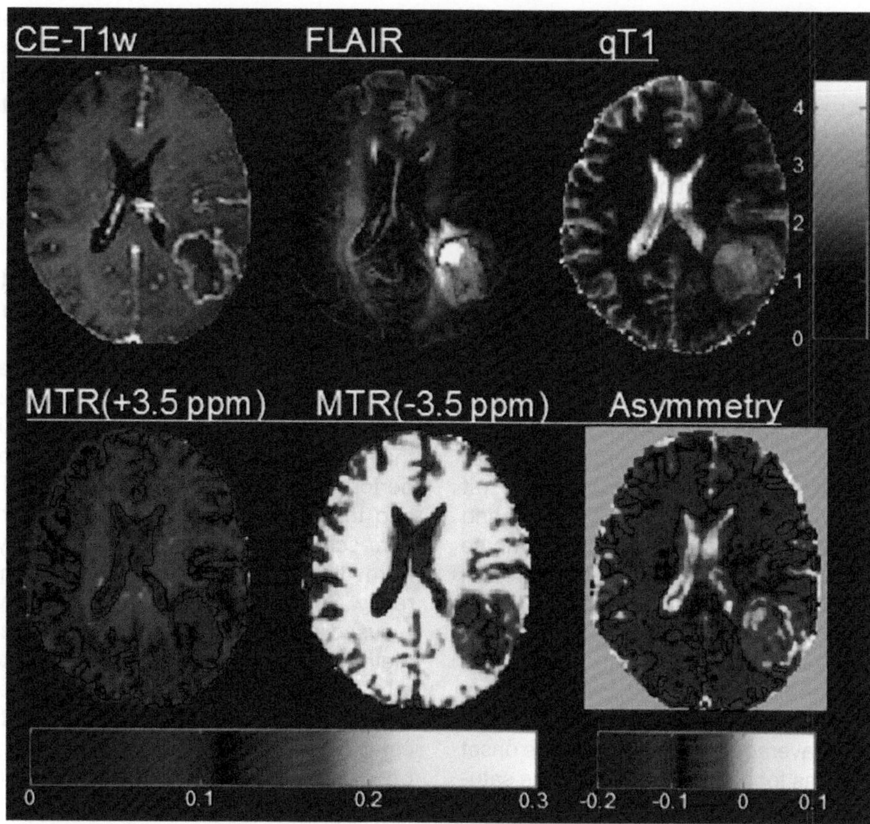

Fig. 1. Overview of a tumor case, showing the T1-weighted images after contrast injection, FLAIR, quantitative T1 map, MTR at +3.5 ppm and −3.5 ppm, and the asymmetry score.

model the system using a multipool model and modified Bloch equations.[12,13]

As can be concluded, modeling of CEST and concomitant effects and their dependencies on scanner parameters is a quickly developing field. Many groups are focusing on this aspect of CEST imaging, and it remains to be seen what approach will be robust enough to be brought into clinical practice.[14–18] However, consensus on this topic is essential for further clinical application of this technique.

CEST AND HIGH-FIELD MR IMAGING

There are advantages to performing CEST measurements at 7 T or higher field strength and they are analogous to those found in spectroscopy. The spectral dispersion of resonances in hertz increases with the field strength, while the bandwidth of RF pulses remains dependent mainly on the duration and pulse shapes used (irrespective of resonance frequency). This means that it becomes easier to selectively saturate a narrow bandwidth centered on the group of interest. Currently, not much is known of the clinical relevance of the different exchanging protons near the water resonance, but a higher specificity of the saturation process will simplify the interpretation of CEST effects.

An additional advantage is the increase in T1 relaxation time. As CEST experiments depend on the build-up of saturation, which is often not achieved in a single saturation pulse, it is of importance to consider that the saturation effect decays with T1. Therefore, longer T1 values allow for the build-up of more saturation, effectively increasing the sensitivity of the measurement.

Of course the technical limitations of ultra-high field MR imaging, especially with regard to the inhomogeneity of the RF field and specific absorption rate (SAR) constraints, make the implementation of an efficient CEST measurement a challenge on its own. It is expected that CEST sequences that deposit less SAR, such as the pulsed steady-state method, might be more suitable for CEST measurements at higher field strengths.[10]

Initial results of CEST measurements at 7 T[19,20] have observed larger differences between gray and white matter than earlier observed at lower field strengths and have shown that the method could be well-suited for the characterization of white matter pathology.

CURRENT APPLICATIONS OF ENDOGENOUS CEST CONTRAST IN HUMANS

The literature on the application of CEST imaging in human volunteers and patients using endogenous contrast is summarized in **Table 2**.

APT

The pH sensitivity of the APT contrast approximately 3.5 ppm downfield of the water resonance, was first reported by Zhou and colleagues[3] in 2003. Since then, the APT-based pH-weighted MR imaging (pHWI) has been used to characterize the acute phase of ischemic stroke in a rat model.[41–43] Combined with diffusion and perfusion-weighted imaging, pHWI in the acute phase of ischemic stroke might have the potential to predict the tissue outcome[44] in a later phase. Imaging humans in the early phase of stroke is complicated. This might explain why the method has not been used in humans thus far. The only study[21] reporting on APT in human stroke included 4 patients at an average of 2.5 days after the onset of stroke and was focused on optimizing the saturation power. Other hurdles on the way to clinical application are discussed in a recent article by Zhou and van Zijl.[45]

The use of APT imaging to detect tumors is based on the increased concentration of intracellular proteins and peptides in malignant versus normal tissue. This was first shown in rats by Zhou and colleagues.[46] After this, APT-weighted imaging was applied in the study of human brain tumors. Jones and colleagues[22] reported on the potential to separate tumor tissue and peritumoral edema. The use of APT to detect heterogeneity in high-grade tumors was confirmed in more recent studies.[21,23,24] An example of APT contrast in a tumor case is shown in **Fig. 1**. The next step on the way to a clinically valuable method will be the differentiation between tumor recurrence and radiation necrosis. This has recently been shown in a rat model.[47] Once this differentiation capability is shown in humans, it is expected to have clinical implications. Thus far there is only 1 case report showing the effect of radiation necrosis after the treatment of an arteriovenous malformation on APT imaging.[29]

The potential of APT imaging has also been explored for monitoring chemotherapy response in 3 patients with breast cancer.[28] These initial results show an increase in APT in the nonresponder and a decrease in the partial and complete responders. APT imaging was also successfully applied to differentiate between cancer and benign tissue in prostate cancer.[27]

The application of APT imaging in patients with neurodegenerative diseases is still in its infancy. In a study on developing APT imaging at 7 T on volunteers,[20] 4 patients with multiple sclerosis were included. Differences in APT scores between healthy volunteers and patients, as well as between different lesions within patients, were observed. Whether this reflects a different chemical composition of the tissue remains to be seen and requires studies with more patients.

Looking at the CEST sequence parameters, such as saturation period and power used in the APT studies reported (see **Table 2**), it is clear that there is currently no consensus on how to perform APT studies. Because the APT contrast, and thus quantification, depends on the saturation scheme,[8] the reported APT asymmetries from different studies cannot be compared directly. Some of the studies on human volunteers focused on optimizing the saturation scheme or method,[16,19,21,26] whereas others looked at the reproducibility of the results.[28] The definition of a standard robust APT sequence with a well-established APT ratio in healthy volunteers will be of crucial importance for the spread of this promising technique.

glycoCEST

Glycogen is a polysaccharide that is used in energy storage in the human body. It is primarily produced and stored in cells located in the liver and muscles. When cells require energy, glycogen is converted into glucose and subsequently metabolized. The CEST method that focuses on detecting glycogen is called glycoCEST. In principle, glycoCEST can be used to detect abnormalities in glycogen production and storage and could, for example, be of interest in studies of diabetes and obesity. The contrast was introduced by van Zijl and colleagues[48] and demonstrated in phantoms and perfused ex vivo mouse livers. The exchanging hydroxyl protons of glycogen have a chemical shift in close proximity to the water resonance (0.5–1.5 ppm downfield shift relative to water), which complicates in vivo detection due to residual B0 inhomogeneities. Kim and colleagues[7] introduced the WASSR method to correct for these B0 variations. Using the WASSR method, they were able to demonstrate the glycoCEST contrast in the calf muscle of 4 healthy volunteers. In another study,[30] using gagCEST (focused on hydroxyl protons in the 0.9–1.9 ppm range downfield of water; see the next section) to study lumbar intervertebral discs in humans, the glycoCEST

Table 2
Overview of studies exploiting endogenous CEST contrasts in humans

Contrast	Area of Application	No. Pat	No. Vol	Saturation Time, ms	Saturation Power, μT	Field	Reference
APT	Brain tumors Stroke Brain	8 4	 4	500	1, 2, 4 Range 0.5–4	3T	21
APT	Brain tumors Brain	10	 3	3000	3	3T	22
APT	Brain tumors	12		500	3	3T	23
APT	Brain tumors	9		500	4	3T	24
APT	Brain tumors Brain	8	 4	500	2	3T	25
APT/NOE	Brain		7	40 × 98.6	Range 0.2–4.7	7T	16
APT	Brain		4	3000	0.78	3T	26
APT	Prostate	13		16 × 31	3.8	3T	27
APT	Breast tumors Breast	3	 10	35 × 25	0.5	3T	28
APT	Radiation necrosis after arteriovenous malformation treatment	1		Not reported	Not reported	7T	29
APT	Brain multiple sclerosis Healthy brain	4	 10	1000	3.5		20
APT	Healthy brain		4	20 × 3.3 +others	3.79	7T	19
glycoCEST	Calf muscle		4	500	0.75	3T	7
glycoCEST gagCEST	Muscle lower back Intervertebral disc lumbar spine		12	400	0.75	3T	30
gagCEST	Knee cartilage		1	320	1	3T	31
gagCEST	Knee cartilage after autologous osteochondral transplantation	9		1000	0.8 (CW equivalent)	7T	32
gagCEST	Intervertebral disc lumbar spine	16		500	1.5 (CW equivalent)	3T	33
gagCEST	Knee cartilage		3	5 Gaussian-shaped pulses	1.5	3T	34
gagCEST	Knee cartilage		5	500	2.2 (rms)	3T/7T	35
gagCEST	Knee cartilage; cartilage repair surgery	12		Series of Gaussian-shaped pulses	0.8 (CW equivalent)	7T	36
gluCEST	Brain		3	1000	3.6	7T	37
gluCEST	Brain		4	1000	3.6	7T	38
MICEST	Brain		5	6000	1.76	7T	39
ureaCEST	Kidney		5	20 × 175 ms sinc FWHM 43 ms	Not clear 240 W	1.5T	40

Studies published before February 2013 are included. Conference proceedings are not reported.

Abbreviations: APT, amide proton transfer; CEST, chemical exchange saturation transfer; Contrast, Type of CEST effect studied; CW, continuous wave; FWHM, full width at half maximum; gagCEST, CEST method that focuses on detecting glycosaminoglycan; gluCEST, CEST method that focuses on detecting glutamate; glycoCEST, CEST method that focuses on detecting glycogen; MICEST, CEST method that focuses on detecting mio-inositol; No. Pat/No. Vol, Number of patients/healthy volunteers in the study; NOE, nuclear Overhauser effect; ureaCEST, CEST method that focuses on detecting urea.

contrast was observed in muscles in the lower back in 12 volunteers. The in vivo application to liver seems a primary target for glycoCEST, but has yet to be addressed in healthy volunteers or patients.

gagCEST

Glycosaminoglycans are a main component of cartilage tissue. With hydroxyl protons resonating in the 0.9 to 1.9 ppm range downfield of water protons, they overlap with the glycogen groups described previously. Nonetheless, as the coincidence of cartilage and muscle tissue can be de deduced from anatomy, it still is a promising endogenous contrast agent for CEST imaging. Since the introduction of the so-called gagCEST contrast in the publication by Ling and colleagues,[31] the method rapidly found its way to study knee cartilage in both volunteers[31,34,35] and patients after knee surgery.[32,36] The latter 2 studies were performed at 7 T and showed good correlation between ^{23}Na imaging and gagCEST contrast (**Fig. 2**) and indicated gagCEST as a potential biomarker for cartilage evaluation. However, Krusche and colleagues[32] could not demonstrate a relationship between clinical outcome and gagCEST asymmetry. A similar result was obtained when the method was applied to study lumbar intervertebral discs in both volunteers[30] and patients with low-back pain.[33] The latter study concluded that gagCEST asymmetry can assess glycosaminoglycan loss but that there is only a moderate correlation with grade of morphologic degeneration. Given the limited number of volunteers and patients studied so far, it is too early to come to a definite conclusion about the clinical applicability of gagCEST. As with the APT studies, it is clear from **Table 2** that a uniform saturation scheme is still to be defined.

gluCEST

Glutamate is an excitatory neurotransmitter and, as such, plays an important role in signal processing in the brain. The use of CEST to image the amine protons of glutamate was recently published by Cai and colleagues.[37] Extensive modeling, imaging, and spectroscopy were performed in both phantoms and animals to demonstrate that the human in vivo gluCEST contrast at 7 T was specifically originating from glutamate and not from other brain metabolites. To give an example, glutamate was injected in an in vivo rat tumor model and an increase in gluCEST contrast was shown. This signal increase was confirmed with spectroscopy. A key step in the postprocessing of the gluCEST images is the correction for B1-inhomogeneities, which is essential at higher field strengths, such as at 7 T. On the other hand, the ultra-high field strength is required to obtain sufficient signal, given the chemical shift and exchange rate of glutamate. The B1-correction method was published in a separate report by Singh and colleagues.[38] Without B1-correction, the gluCEST contrast between gray and white matter is less pronounced. If these findings can be reproduced by other groups and in more volunteers,

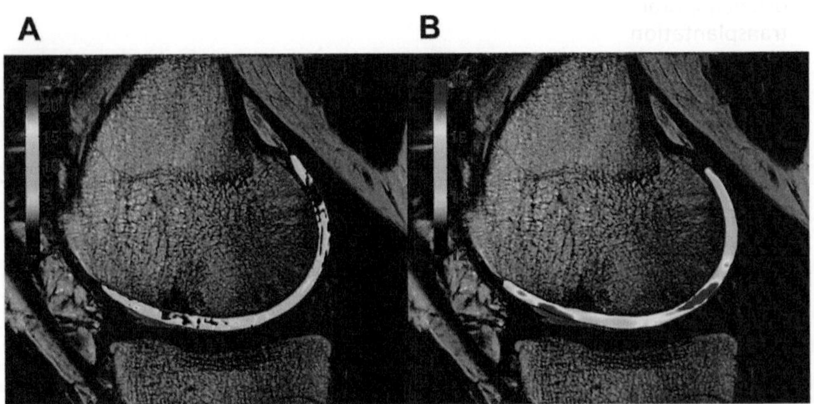

Fig. 2. Correlation between gagCEST and ^{23}Na imaging in a patient after autologous osteochondral transplantation. On the left (*A*) gagCEST asymmetry percentage. On the right (*B*) ^{23}Na signal-to-noise ratio. Both overlaid on a proton density–weighted image. In both overlays, lower values mean less glycosaminoglycan content in the cartilage. The gagCEST results show a pattern comparable to the ^{23}Na images. Scan time was about halved for the gagCEST acquisition: 15 minutes versus 32 minutes for the ^{23}Na image. (*From* Krusche-Mandl I, Schmitt B, Zak L, et al. Long-term results 8 years after autologous osteochondral transplantation: 7 T gagCEST and sodium magnetic resonance imaging with morphologic and clinical correlation. Osteoarthritis Cartilage 2012;20(5):357–63. http://dx.doi.org/10.1016/j.joca.2012.01.020; with permission.)

a powerful method to image glutamate will become available, which might have an impact on the (early) diagnosis and treatment monitoring of neurodegenerative diseases. As a first step toward a clinical application, it was shown by the same group[49] that gluCEST asymmetry is reduced in a mouse model of Alzheimer disease when compared with wild-type mice.

MICEST

Another important metabolite in the brain is mio-inositol (MI), which functions as an osmolyte. MI is thought to play a role in many brain disorders with both increased and decreased levels, as shown by spectroscopy. Just before the publication on glutamate,[37] as discussed previously, MICEST[39] asymmetry was demonstrated in human volunteers. Both studies were performed by the same group and have a similar setup, but use a different saturation scheme to select the brain metabolite of interest. In line with results from spectroscopy, a higher MICEST asymmetry was found in white matter when compared with gray matter. In a follow-up study,[50] increased levels of MICEST asymmetry were detected in the brains of a mouse model of Alzheimer disease when compared with age-matched wild-type mouse controls (**Fig. 3**). Again, these are very promising results, which might have an impact on diagnosis and treatment monitoring of neurodegenerative diseases, if reproduced in a larger cohort of both volunteers and patients.

UreaCEST

Already in 1998, the CEST pioneers in the group of Balaban[51] reported on the possibility to observe urea using the chemical exchange. In a later study,[40] ureaCEST was demonstrated in vivo by imaging human kidneys at 1.5 T. Although the investigators point out the potential clinical application of their work to patients with kidney failure, no additional studies using ureaCEST were published. Application of ureaCEST to visualize renal function or pathology in downstream organs, such as ureter or bladder, remains an unexplored field.

EXOGENOUS CEST AGENTS

Another category of CEST contrasts is enabled by the exogenous CEST agents. As they are fully designed to maximize chemical exchange while minimizing overlap with normal tissue resonances, these particles and aggregates can display CEST

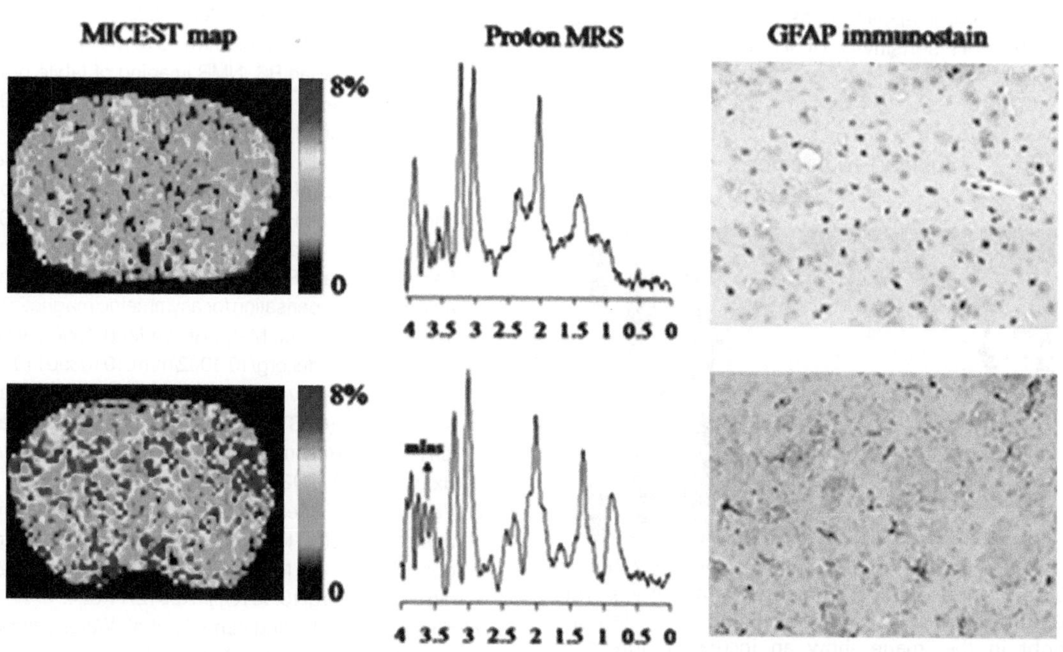

Fig. 3. Comparison between a wild-type (*top row*) and an Alzheimer mouse (*bottom row*). From left to right: MICEST images, spectra, and histology. The Alzheimer mouse shows an increased level of MICEST asymmetry compared with the wild-type mouse (*left column*). This finding is confirmed by spectroscopy (*central column*) and the immunostain (*right column*). (*From* Haris M, Singh A, Cai K, et al. MICEST: a potential tool for non-invasive detection of molecular changes in Alzheimer's disease. J Neurosci Methods 2013;212(1):87–93. http://dx.doi.org/10.1016/j.jneumeth.2012.09.025; with permission.)

enhancements many orders of magnitude larger than the endogenous CEST agents. Their application is currently preclinical and beyond the scope of this article and we indicate only a small selection of studies here. For much more on the topic, the reader is referred to the review by Zhou and Van Zijl[52] to get an overview of the possibilities that these compounds can enable.

One of the exciting paths is the use of biodegradable exogenous contrast agents, as was recently done by Chan and colleagues.[53] D-glucose was infused in mice to study cancerous tissue. GlucoCEST was used to detect signal enhancement in the tumor tissue during infusion (**Fig. 4**).

Also, in so-called "multicolor" molecular MR imaging, bio-organic or biodegradable substances are used. In this case, the substances, each with a different off-resonance relative to water, are loaded into liposomes. Each of them can be imaged by hitting the right off-resonance and displayed with its own color (hence the term "multicolor"). This was recently presented by Liu and colleagues,[54] who used diaCEST liposomes for lymphatic imaging in mice.

Yet another possibility is the use of existing contrast agents for CEST imaging.[55] An example is the use of iopamidol, normally used as a CT contrast agent, in ureaCEST.[56,57] In these studies, iopamidol was applied to assess kidney failure, using the pH sensitivity of iopamidol in a mouse model.

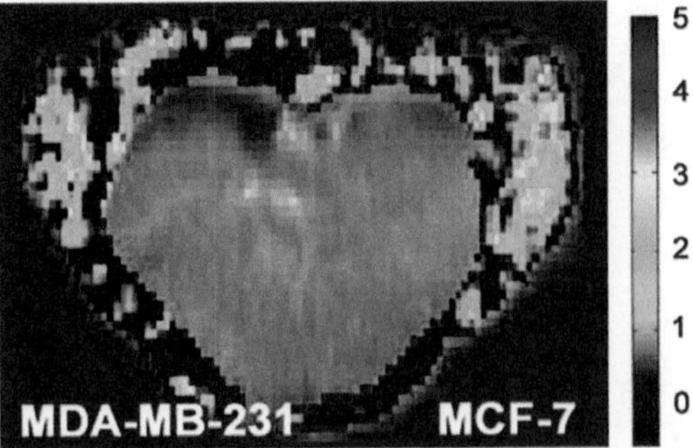

Fig. 4. GlucoCEST signal enhancement in 2 human breast cancer cell lines implanted in a mouse during D-glucose infusion. Both the cell line on the left and right in the image show an increased uptake of D-glucose, reflecting the increased metabolism in these cells. (*From* Chan KW, McMahon MT, Kato Y, et al. Natural D-glucose as a biodegradable MRI contrast agent for detecting cancer. Magn Reson Med 2012;68(6):1764–73. http://dx.doi.org/10.1002/mrm.24520; with permission.)

SUMMARY

CEST measurements hold great promise as the next step in magnetization transfer imaging and possibly allow for in vivo quantification of many clinically relevant parameters, including pH, temperature, and amide concentration.

Currently, development is in full progress, with the first clinical studies showing small-scale but promising results. The biggest hurdle to take will be the agreement on a method for robust quantification. As the specifications of the sequence parameters greatly influence the amount of saturation and thus the observed contrast, it is essential that a common framework is agreed on to compare CEST results from different centers. Similar problems have plagued the clinical implementation of quantitative magnetization transfer and diffusion MR imaging. Although the former has never seen broad clinical use, the latter is now widely used.

When further optimization of the sequences and modeling of the signal is completed, we believe that validation studies will show that CEST is a valuable tool to add to the MR imaging toolbox.

REFERENCES

1. Wolff SD, Balaban RS. Magnetization transfer contrast (MTC) and tissue water proton relaxation in vivo. Magn Reson Med 1989;10(1):135–44. http://dx.doi.org/10.1002/mrm.1910100113.
2. Wolff SD, Balaban RS. NMR imaging of labile proton exchange. J Magn Reson 1990;86(1):164–9. http://dx.doi.org/10.1016/0022-2364(90)90220-4.
3. Zhou J, Payen JF, Wilson DA, et al. Using the amide proton signals of intracellular proteins and peptides to detect pH effects in MRI. Nat Med 2003; 9(8):1085–90. http://dx.doi.org/10.1038/nm907.
4. Pekar J, Jezzard P, Roberts DA, et al. Perfusion imaging with compensation for asymmetric magnetization transfer effects. Magn Reson Med 1996;35(1): 70–9. http://dx.doi.org/10.1002/mrm.1910350110.
5. Van Zijl PC, Yadav NN. Chemical exchange saturation transfer (CEST): what is in a name and what isn't? Magn Reson Med 2011;65(4):927–48. http://dx.doi.org/10.1002/mrm.22761.
6. Vinogradov E, Sherry AD, Lenkinski RE. CEST: from basic principles to applications, challenges and opportunities. J Magn Reson 2013;229:155–72. http://dx.doi.org/10.1016/j.jmr.2012.11.024.
7. Kim M, Gillen J, Landman BA, et al. Water saturation shift referencing (WASSR) for chemical exchange saturation transfer (CEST) experiments. Magn Reson Med 2009;61(6):1441–50. http://dx.doi.org/10.1002/mrm.21873.
8. Sun PZ, van Zijl PC, Zhou J. Optimization of the irradiation power in chemical exchange dependent

saturation transfer experiments. J Magn Reson 2005;175(2):193–200. http://dx.doi.org/10.1016/j.jmr.2005.04.005.
9. Sun PZ, Farrar CT, Sorensen AG. Correction for artifacts induced by B0 and B1 field inhomogeneities in pH-sensitive chemical exchange saturation transfer (CEST) imaging. Magn Reson Med 2007;58(6):1207–15. http://dx.doi.org/10.1002/mrm.21398.
10. Jones CK, Polders D, Hua J, et al. In vivo three-dimensional whole-brain pulsed steady-state chemical exchange saturation transfer at 7 T. Magn Reson Med 2012;67(6):1579–89. http://dx.doi.org/10.1002/mrm.23141.
11. Jin T, Wang P, Zong X, et al. MR imaging of the amide-proton transfer effect and the pH-insensitive nuclear Overhauser effect at 9.4 T. Magn Reson Med 2012. http://dx.doi.org/10.1002/mrm.24315.
12. Li AX, Hudson RH, Barrett JW, et al. Four-pool modeling of proton exchange processes in biological systems in the presence of MRI-paramagnetic chemical exchange saturation transfer (PARACEST) agents. Magn Reson Med 2008;60(5):1197–206. http://dx.doi.org/10.1002/mrm.21752.
13. Woessner DE, Zhang S, Merritt ME, et al. Numerical solution of the Bloch equations provides insights into the optimum design of PARACEST agents for MRI. Magn Reson Med 2005;53(4):790–9. http://dx.doi.org/10.1002/mrm.20408.
14. Hua J, Jones CK, Blakeley J, et al. Quantitative description of the asymmetry in magnetization transfer effects around the water resonance in the human brain. Magn Reson Med 2007;58(4):786–93. http://dx.doi.org/10.1002/mrm.21387.
15. Sun PZ, Zhou J, Huang J, et al. Simplified quantitative description of amide proton transfer (APT) imaging during acute ischemia. Magn Reson Med 2007;57(2):405–10. http://dx.doi.org/10.1002/mrm.21151.
16. Liu D, Zhou J, Xue R, et al. Quantitative characterization of nuclear Overhauser enhancement and amide proton transfer effects in the human brain at 7 tesla. Magn Reson Med 2012. http://dx.doi.org/10.1002/mrm.24560.
17. Zaiß M, Schmitt B, Bachert P. Quantitative separation of CEST effect from magnetization transfer and spillover effects by Lorentzian-line-fit analysis of z-spectra. J Magn Reson 2011;211(2):149–55. http://dx.doi.org/10.1016/j.jmr.2011.05.001.
18. Zhou J, Wilson DA, Sun PZ, et al. Quantitative description of proton exchange processes between water and endogenous and exogenous agents for WEX, CEST, and APT experiments. Magn Reson Med 2004;51(5):945–52. http://dx.doi.org/10.1002/mrm.20048.
19. Mougin OE, Coxon RC, Pitiot A, et al. Magnetization transfer phenomenon in the human brain at 7 T. Neuroimage 2010;49(1):272–81. http://dx.doi.org/10.1016/j.neuroimage.2009.08.022.
20. Dula AN, Asche EM, Landman BA, et al. Development of chemical exchange saturation transfer (CEST) at 7T. Magn Reson Med 2011;66(3):831–8. http://dx.doi.org/10.1002/mrm.22862.
21. Zhao X, Wen Z, Huang F, et al. Saturation power dependence of amide proton transfer image contrasts in human brain tumors and strokes at 3 T. Magn Reson Med 2011;66(4):1033–41. http://dx.doi.org/10.1002/mrm.22891.
22. Jones CK, Schlosser MJ, Zijl V, et al. Amide proton transfer imaging of human brain tumors at 3T. Magn Reson Med 2006;56(3):585–92. http://dx.doi.org/10.1002/mrm.20989.
23. Wen Z, Hu S, Huang F, et al. MR imaging of high-grade brain tumors using endogenous protein and peptide-based contrast. Neuroimage 2010;51(2):616–22. http://dx.doi.org/10.1016/j.neuroimage.2010.02.050.
24. Zhou J, Blakeley JO, Hua J, et al. Practical data acquisition method for human brain tumor amide proton transfer (APT) imaging. Magn Reson Med 2008;60(4):842–9. http://dx.doi.org/10.1002/mrm.21712.
25. Zhao X, Wen Z, Zhang G, et al. Three-dimensional turbo-spin-echo amide proton transfer MR imaging at 3-Tesla and its application to high-grade human brain tumors. Mol Imaging Biol 2013;15(1):114–22. http://dx.doi.org/10.1007/s11307-012-0563-1.
26. Scheidegger R, Vinogradov E, Alsop DC. Amide proton transfer imaging with improved robustness to magnetic field inhomogeneity and magnetization transfer asymmetry using saturation with frequency alternating RF irradiation. Magn Reson Med 2011;66(5):1275–85. http://dx.doi.org/10.1002/mrm.22912.
27. Jia G, Abaza R, Williams JD, et al. Amide proton transfer MR imaging of prostate cancer: a preliminary study. J Magn Reson Imaging 2011;33(3):647–54. http://dx.doi.org/10.1002/jmri.22480.
28. Dula AN, Arlinghaus LR, Dortch RD, et al. Amide proton transfer imaging of the breast at 3 T: establishing reproducibility and possible feasibility assessing chemotherapy response. Magn Reson Med 2012. http://dx.doi.org/10.1002/mrm.24450.
29. Gerigk L, Schmitt B, Stieltjes B, et al. 7 tesla imaging of cerebral radiation necrosis after arteriovenous malformations treatment using amide proton transfer (APT) imaging. J Magn Reson Imaging 2012;35(5):1207–9. http://dx.doi.org/10.1002/jmri.23534.
30. Kim M, Chan Q, Anthony MP, et al. Assessment of glycosaminoglycan distribution in human lumbar intervertebral discs using chemical exchange

saturation transfer at 3 T: feasibility and initial experience. NMR Biomed 2011;24(9):1137–44. http://dx.doi.org/10.1002/nbm.1671.
31. Ling W, Eliav U, Navon G, et al. Chemical exchange saturation transfer by intermolecular double-quantum coherence. J Magn Reson 2008; 194(1):29–32. http://dx.doi.org/10.1016/j.jmr.2008.05.026.
32. Krusche-Mandl I, Schmitt B, Zak L, et al. Long-term results 8 years after autologous osteochondral transplantation: 7 T gagCEST and sodium magnetic resonance imaging with morphological and clinical correlation. Osteoarthr Cartil 2012;20(5):357–63. http://dx.doi.org/10.1016/j.joca.2012.01.020.
33. Haneder S, Apprich SR, Schmitt B, et al. Assessment of glycosaminoglycan content in intervertebral discs using chemical exchange saturation transfer at 3.0 Tesla: preliminary results in patients with low-back pain. Eur Radiol 2012. http://dx.doi.org/10.1007/s00330-012-2660-6.
34. Varma G, Lenkinski RE, Vinogradov E. Keyhole chemical exchange saturation transfer. Magn Reson Med 2012. http://dx.doi.org/10.1002/mrm.23310.
35. Singh A, Haris M, Cai K, et al. Chemical exchange saturation transfer magnetic resonance imaging of human knee cartilage at 3 T and 7 T. Magn Reson Med 2012;68(2):588–94. http://dx.doi.org/10.1002/mrm.23250.
36. Schmitt B, Zbýň Š, Stelzeneder D, et al. Cartilage quality assessment by using glycosaminoglycan chemical exchange saturation transfer and 23Na MR Imaging at 7 T. Radiology 2011;260(1):257–64. http://dx.doi.org/10.1148/radiol.11101841.
37. Cai K, Haris M, Singh A, et al. Magnetic resonance imaging of glutamate. Nat Med 2012;18(2):302–6. http://dx.doi.org/10.1038/nm.2615.
38. Singh A, Cai K, Haris M, et al. On B1 inhomogeneity correction of in vivo human brain glutamate chemical exchange saturation transfer contrast at 7T. Magn Reson Med 2012. http://dx.doi.org/10.1002/mrm.24290.
39. Haris M, Cai K, Singh A, et al. In vivo mapping of brain myo-inositol. Neuroimage 2011;54(3):2079–85. http://dx.doi.org/10.1016/j.neuroimage.2010.10.017.
40. Dagher AP, Aletras A, Choyke P, et al. Imaging of urea using chemical exchange-dependent saturation transfer at 1.5T. J Magn Reson Imaging 2000;12(5):745–8. pii:10.1002/1522-2586(200011)12:5<745::AID-JMRI12>3.0.CO;2-H.
41. Sun PZ, Cheung JS, Wang E, et al. Association between pH-weighted endogenous amide proton chemical exchange saturation transfer MRI and tissue lactic acidosis during acute ischemic stroke. J Cereb Blood Flow Metab 2011;31(8):1743–50. http://dx.doi.org/10.1038/jcbfm.2011.23.
42. Jokivarsi KT, Gröhn HI, Gröhn OH, et al. Proton transfer ratio, lactate, and intracellular pH in acute cerebral ischemia. Magn Reson Med 2007;57(4):647–53. http://dx.doi.org/10.1002/mrm.21181.
43. Sun PZ, Zhou J, Sun W, et al. Detection of the ischemic penumbra using pH-weighted MRI. J Cereb Blood Flow Metab 2007;27(6):1129–36. http://dx.doi.org/10.1038/sj.jcbfm.9600424.
44. Jokivarsi KT, Hiltunen Y, Tuunanen PI, et al. Correlating tissue outcome with quantitative multiparametric MRI of acute cerebral ischemia in rats. J Cereb Blood Flow Metab 2010;30(2):415–27. http://dx.doi.org/10.1038/jcbfm.2009.236.
45. Zhou J, van Zijl PC. Defining an acidosis-based ischemic penumbra from pH-weighted MRI. Transl Stroke Res 2011;3(1):76–83. http://dx.doi.org/10.1007/s12975-011-0110-4.
46. Zhou J, Lal B, Wilson DA, et al. Amide proton transfer (APT) contrast for imaging of brain tumors. Magn Reson Med 2003;50(6):1120–6. http://dx.doi.org/10.1002/mrm.10651.
47. Zhou J, Tryggestad E, Wen Z, et al. Differentiation between glioma and radiation necrosis using molecular magnetic resonance imaging of endogenous proteins and peptides. Nat Med 2011;17(1):130–4. http://dx.doi.org/10.1038/nm.2268.
48. van Zijl PC, Jones CK, Ren J, et al. MRI detection of glycogen in vivo by using chemical exchange saturation transfer imaging (glycoCEST). Proc Natl Acad Sci U S A 2007;104(11):4359–64. http://dx.doi.org/10.1073/pnas.0700281104.
49. Haris M, Nath K, Cai K, et al. Imaging of glutamate neurotransmitter alterations in Alzheimer's disease. NMR Biomed 2012. http://dx.doi.org/10.1002/nbm.2875.
50. Haris M, Singh A, Cai K, et al. MICEST: a potential tool for non-invasive detection of molecular changes in Alzheimer's disease. J Neurosci Methods 2013;212(1):87–93. http://dx.doi.org/10.1016/j.jneumeth.2012.09.025.
51. Guivel-Scharen V, Sinnwell T, Wolff SD, et al. Detection of proton chemical exchange between metabolites and water in biological tissues. J Magn Reson 1998;133(1):36–45. http://dx.doi.org/10.1006/jmre.1998.1440.
52. Zhou J, van Zijl PC. Chemical exchange saturation transfer imaging and spectroscopy. Prog Nucl Mag Res Sp 2006;48(2–3):109–36. http://dx.doi.org/10.1016/j.pnmrs.2006.01.001.
53. Chan KW, McMahon MT, Kato Y, et al. Natural D-glucose as a biodegradable MRI contrast agent for detecting cancer. Magn Reson Med 2012;68(6):1764–73. http://dx.doi.org/10.1002/mrm.24520.
54. Liu G, Moake M, Har-el Y, et al. In vivo multicolor molecular MR imaging using diamagnetic chemical exchange saturation transfer liposomes. Magn

Reson Med 2012;67(4):1106–13. http://dx.doi.org/10.1002/mrm.23100.
55. Aime S, Calabi L, Biondi L, et al. Iopamidol: exploring the potential use of a well-established x-ray contrast agent for MRI. Magn Reson Med 2005;53(4):830–4. http://dx.doi.org/10.1002/mrm.20441.
56. Longo DL, Dastrù W, Digilio G, et al. Iopamidol as a responsive MRI-chemical exchange saturation transfer contrast agent for pH mapping of kidneys: in vivo studies in mice at 7 T. Magn Reson Med 2011;65(1):202–11. http://dx.doi.org/10.1002/mrm.22608.
57. Longo DL, Busato A, Lanzardo S, et al. Imaging the pH evolution of an acute kidney injury model by means of iopamidol, a MRI-CEST pH-responsive contrast agent. Magn Reson Med 2012. http://dx.doi.org/10.1002/mrm.24513.

Competing Technology for PET/Computed Tomography

Diffusion-weighted Magnetic Resonance Imaging

Dow-Mu Koh, MD, MRCP, FRCR[a,*],
Nina Tunariu, MRCP, FRCR[a],
Matthew Blackledge, BSc, MSc, PhD[b],
David J. Collins, BA, CPhys, MInstP[b]

KEYWORDS

• PET • Computed tomography • Magnetic resonance imaging • Diffusion-weighted imaging

KEY POINTS

- Diffusion-weighted magnetic resonance (MR) imaging uses an endogenous contrast based on differences in water mobility within tissues. Tumor tissues have impeded water mobility, which facilitates their detection and characterization.
- Whole-body diffusion-weighted MR imaging results in images that superficially resemble PET imaging.
- Whole-body diffusion-weighted MR imaging is being widely investigated in oncology for tumor staging, disease characterization, and for the assessment of treatment response.

INTRODUCTION

PET/computed tomography (CT) is now established as a standard of care for the management of oncology patients. The most widely used radiotracer, ^{18}F-fluorodeoxyglucose (^{18}F-FDG), a glucose analogue, localizes within tumor cells, which exhibit an increased rate of glucose metabolism. ^{18}F-FDG-PET has a high sensitivity for tumors of various histologic subtypes, and has been applied extensively for tissue characterization, disease staging, and the assessment of tumor response. The standardized uptake value (SUV), a quantitative index that normalizes tracer activity to body weight, has been also shown to be of prognostic significance in several tumor types.[1,2] One of the key advantages of radionuclear PET studies using ^{18}FDG-PET is the high target-to-background image contrast, which enables tumors to be clearly visualized as increased tracer activity against low background activity. The images are typically displayed using an inverted gray scale, with increased tracer activity depicted as darker areas on imaging. By using radial maximum-intensity projections (MIPs), whole-body (WB) images are produced that can be assessed at a glance for disease evaluation.

This article discusses a competing technology, namely diffusion-weighted (DW) magnetic resonance (MR) imaging (DW-MR imaging). The basis of image contrast in DW-MR imaging is the difference in the mobility of water molecules within tissues.[3] The technique relies on an endogenous contrast mechanism; enhancement by the administration of exogenous contrast medium is not required. The technique is quick to perform and images can be acquired from the skull base to the midthigh level, analogous to PET-CT, in 30 to 60 minutes.[4] By postprocessing of the acquired images,

[a] Department of Radiology, Royal Marsden Hospital, Downs Road, Sutton, Surrey SM2 5PT, UK; [b] CRUK EPSRC Imaging Centre, Institute of Cancer Research, Sutton, SM2 5NG, UK
* Corresponding author.
E-mail address: dowmukoh@icr.ac.uk

PET Clin 8 (2013) 259–277
http://dx.doi.org/10.1016/j.cpet.2013.03.002
1556-8598/13/$ – see front matter

they can be displayed using an inverted gray scale to resemble PET imaging, or can be ascribed an appropriate color scale and fused with morphologic MR images (T1 or T2 weighted). Furthermore, using radial MIPs can also produce images that superficially resemble those obtained by PET/CT. In the early days of developing the technique, WB-DW MR imaging was given the term MR-PETography by some investigators. However, this is a misnomer because WB-DW imaging does not depend on radionuclear tracer uptake, although it may provide similar or analogous diagnostic information. The technique has attracted significant attention among MR researchers, and is currently being widely evaluated in oncology as a complementary or competitive imaging modality[5] for the assessment of patients with cancer (**Fig. 1**).

This article, examines the biological underpinning of imaging the DW-MR imaging technique, the impetus for the development of WB-DW imaging, as well as the current clinical evidence for its deployment in oncologic imaging. The similarities and differences between WB-DW imaging are compared and contrasted. In addition, the potential of combining WB-DW imaging with the information from radionuclear and PET imaging in a multimodality imaging paradigm is presented.

DW-MR IMAGING: BIOLOGICAL CORRELATES

DW imaging is a technique that is sensitive to the mobility of water in tissues. In tissues, the apparent diffusion of water is impeded to different extents in the intracellular space, extracellular space, and also the intravascular compartments. In simple terms, cellular tissues (for example, tumors) impede water diffusion to a greater extent compared with normal tissues, which facilitates their detection by the technique.

The apparent water diffusion in tissues reflects cellular density, the tortuosity of the extracellular space, cell membrane integrity, interactions with macromolecules, fluid homeostasis, and microcapillary perfusion.[3,6] On modern clinical MR systems, body DW-MR imaging is usually performed by incorporating a sequence of diffusion-sensitizing gradients into a standard T2-weighted imaging protocol. The strength of the diffusion weighting can be varied by changing the b-values on the scanner, which can easily be altered by the operator.

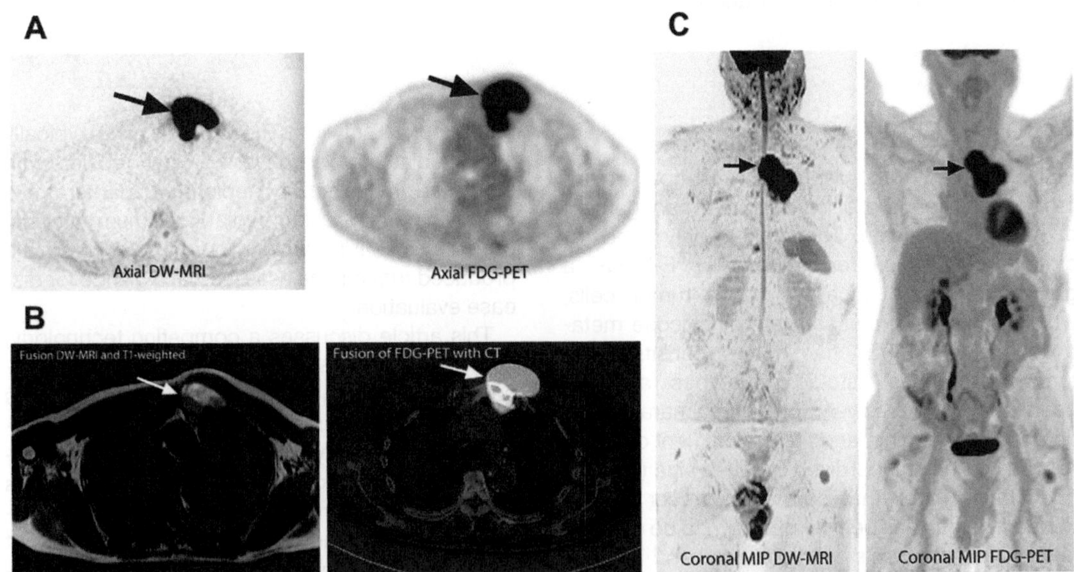

Fig. 1. Comparative DW-MR and ^{18}F-FDG-PET images obtained in an elderly man with metastatic prostate cancer. (*A*) Axial images, (*B*) axial fusion images, and (*C*) coronal MIP images of DW-MR imaging and ^{18}F-FDG-PET studies. Images are displayed using inverted gray scale, in which impeded diffusion or increased tracer activity appear darker against the background. (*A*) On axial DW-MR imaging and ^{18}F-FDG-PET imaging, disease in the sternum, which extends into the left chest wall is seen as an area of impeded diffusion and increased tracer activity (*arrows*). (*B*) Fusion axial DW-MR imaging with corresponding T1-weighted image and ^{18}F-FDG-PET with corresponding CT image help to localize the area of disease to anatomic features (*arrows*). (*C*) Coronal MIP images show abnormality in the sternum (*arrows*) using both techniques but also differences in normal background signal. On DW-MR imaging, note the normal impeded diffusion in brain, cervical nodes, parotid glands, spleen, testes, kidneys, and spinal cord. By contrast, note the normal tracer activity visible on ^{18}F-FDG-PET imaging within the myocardium, bowel, liver, muscle, urinary tract, and vascular tree.

Two or more b-values are generally used, because disease detection and characterization are based on the relative attenuation of tissue signal intensity with increasing b-value. The b-values have a unit of s/mm^2 and the range applied for clinical evaluation typically ranges between 0 and 1000 s/mm^2.

In general, signal from highly mobile intravascular water molecules are rapidly attenuated by applying a small diffusion weighting or b-value. Free fluids (eg, fluid within the gallbladder and simple cysts) also show greater signal attenuation with increasing b-value compared with soft tissue. By contrast, water molecules associated with highly cellular tissues (eg, tumors) show less signal attenuation at higher b-value compared with normal background tissue, thus enhancing their detection (**Fig. 2**). On this basis, DW-MR imaging has been used to improve disease detection across the body.

One of the key advantages of using DW-MR imaging is that it is also a quantitative imaging technique. By evaluating the exponential relationship between the measured tissue signal intensity and the b-value, it is possible to calculate the apparent diffusion coefficient (ADC) of tissue, which is derived from the slope of the line that describes their relationship. The ADC value reflects tissue water diffusivity, is generally lower in tumor tissues compared with normal tissue, and has the unit of mm^2/s. Effective treatment of tumors results in an increase in ADC value, because of treatment-induced reduction in tumor cellularity, loss of cell membrane integrity, tumor necrosis, and apoptosis. In several studies conducted in various tumors across the body, ADC has shown moderate to good measurement reproducibility.[7–11] In a well-conducted DW-MR imaging study using

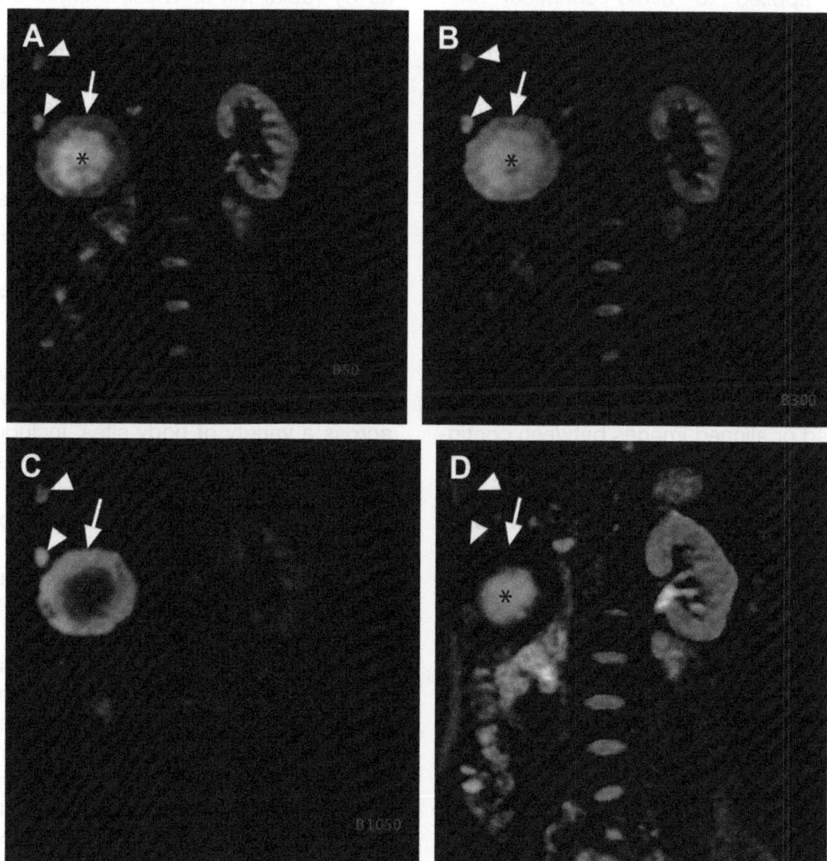

Fig. 2. Differential signal attenuation between solid and necrotic cystic components in renal cell carcinoma with increasing diffusion-weightings (b-values). Coronal oblique DW-MR images obtained at b-values of (*A*) 50 s/mm^2, (*B*) 300 s/mm^2 and (*C*) 1050 s/mm^2. Note tumor arising from the upper pole of the right kidney (*arrows*). With increasing b-values, cellular tumor rim shows relative preservation of high signal intensity, whereas the central necrotic/cystic region (*asterisk*) shows progressive signal loss. (*D*) The quantitative apparent diffusion coefficient (ADC) map calculated by slope of signal attenuation of each image voxel shows high ADC values within the necrotic/cystic area, indicating high water diffusivity, compared with low ADC values returned from the cellular rim. Note coincidental findings of 2 metastases within the right lobe of the liver (*arrowheads*).

a free-breathing imaging protocol, it is realistic to expect an ADC measurement reproducibility of between 10% and 30%, suggesting that the quantitative ADC parameters could be applied with confidence for tissue characterization and the assessment of treatment response. Measurement reproducibility tends to be better in normal tissue compared with tumor tissues.[12] Thus, it is important to establish measurement reproducibility in pathologic disease so that the appropriate threshold can be applied when considering interval change.

TECHNICAL CONSIDERATION

DW-MR imaging can be performed using most state-of-the-art 1.5 T or 3.0 T MR scanners. Imaging is usually performed with the patient in quiet respiration, using a spin-echo echo-planar imaging technique.[13] Fat signal suppression schemes are always applied to avoid chemical shift ghosting artifacts at fat-water interfaces.

At present, DW-MR imaging studies in the body seem to be more robust when performed at 1.5 T compared with imaging at 3.0 T.[4] This is because, at 3.0 T, there is often greater local magnetic field inhomogeneity, which can lead to nonuniform fat suppression and, hence, chemical shift ghosting artifacts. In one study,[14] WB-DW imaging at 3.0 T resulted in better lesion/bone contrast ratio but greater susceptibility-induced image distortion, signal intensity losses, and also motion blurring artifacts. Furthermore, significant frequency shifts between individual imaging stations at the higher field strength of 3.0 T can make it difficult to obtain well-registered or aligned images between contiguous body sections.[4] However, the use of dual-source parallel radiofrequency excitation[15] and combinatorial fat suppression (eg, slice-selective gradient reversal and short-tau inversion recovery [STIR])[16,17] have been shown to improve image quality at 3.0 T.

In recent years, there has been a convergence of MR imaging technologies available on different vendor imaging platforms, to the extent that hardware setup for DW-MR imaging examinations are similar between MR systems. To maximize MR signal collection, surface MR coils are usually deployed over the parts of the body to be evaluated, which, in the case of WB-DW imaging, extends from the skull vertex to the midthigh level. This extent of imaging coverage is analogous to that achieved using PET/CT.

For WB-DW imaging, each body section (typically over a 20-cm to 25-cm craniocaudal direction) is acquired separately, and the extent of coverage requires 5 to 6 contiguous body sections to be imaged, depending on the height of the individual. Each imaging station typically takes 4 to 6 minutes to acquire, and is usually performed in the axial plane, although coronal acquisitions are favored by some clinicians. For WB studies, imaging is typically performed using 2 b-values between 0 and 1000 s/mm^2 (eg, 50 and 900 s/mm^2). At each imaging station, conventional morphologic T1-weighted and/or T2-weighted MR images are usually also acquired using the same image section thickness and imaging field of view, which facilitates image fusion of the b-value and anatomic images.

Although DW-MR imaging can be performed with ease, the technique is prone to imaging artifacts that can significantly degrade image quality. For this reason, it is important to engage the help of an expert radiographer or physicist to ensure that the highest quality images are attained. Once acquired, the high b-value images can be displayed by using multiplanar reformats, as well as by radial MIPs. These images are often displayed using an inverted gray scale, resulting in image series that superficially resemble PET-CT imaging. Although there are superficial similarities between WB-DW imaging and ^{18}FDG-PET examinations, there are also key differences. The similarities and differences are summarized in **Table 1**. A typical imaging protocol used for image acquisition at field strength of 1.5 T is shown in **Table 2**.

DEVELOPMENT AND CLINICAL APPLICATIONS OF DW-MR IMAGING

There is now a growing body of evidence that DW-MR imaging improves disease detection across a variety of body sites, including the liver, pancreas, breast, peritoneum, prostate gland, cervix, uterus, and bone marrow.[3] However, as technology improves, it is becoming possible to acquire DW-MR images over several contiguous body sections in a short time, which has stimulated the development of WB-DW imaging. There is now substantial interest in evaluating and establishing the role of WB-DW imaging for disease staging, assessment of treatment response, and assessing disease relapse in the patient with cancer.[18]

Interest in WB-DW imaging has grown because enabling technology has improved the speed of image acquisition and the ability to display and view such large and complex data sets on modern imaging workstations. Slightly more than a decade ago, WB-MR imaging examinations performed without DW-MR imaging using conventional T1-weighted and fat-suppressed T2-weighted sequences typically took 60 minutes or more to acquire. Once the images were acquired, there was the practical issue of viewing all the images generated on hard copy films, before the widespread availability of

Table 1
Similarities and differences between ^{18}FDG-PET/CT and WB-DW imaging

	^{18}FDG-PET/CT	WB-DW Imaging
Similarities	Body imaging usually performed from skull base to midthigh level Images displayed using inverted gray scale and MIPs obtained in different planes Functional images can be fused with anatomic images Tumors show increased signal on imaging Disease response may be observed as decreased signal Studies have shown improved disease detection and characterization using these techniques. May be used to assess tumor response	
Differences	Disease detection related to increased glycolysis in tumors	Disease detection related to increased tissue cellularity leading to impeded water diffusion
	Requires the injection of a radiotracer	Based on an endogenous MR contrast
	Normal tracer uptake can be seen in brown fat, brain, myocardium, gastrointestinal tract, muscle, salivary glands, and kidneys. Tracer excretion into ureters and urinary bladder	Normal impeded diffusion seen in brain, lymph nodes, spinal cord, spleen, testes, ovaries, and red marrow
	The semiquantitative index of SUV is derived for disease assessment	The ADC is measured as a quantitative index of water diffusivity
	Exposure to ionizing radiation	Technique free from ionizing radiation

imaging workstations. Technological hardware and software innovations have enabled high-quality DW-MR images to be acquired in a short time (30–60 minutes) and the processing power of modern picture archive and communication systems (PACS) with specialized image-viewing software means that WB-DW images can be displayed and read with ease.

Two other reasons could be suggested for the development of WB-DW imaging. First, the possible detrimental effects of ionizing radiation with repeated CT examinations are being recognized in patients with cancer (especially children). As such, there is greater awareness in adopting imaging technologies, if possible, that are free from potentially harmful ionizing radiation. Second, in patients suspected of metastatic bone disease, the uncertainty in the availability of technetium-labeled radiotracer for bone scintigraphy means that there is a desire to develop alternative technologies that may provide similar diagnostic information. Because DW-MR imaging seems to be highly sensitive for the detection of focal marrow deposits or bone marrow infiltration,[19] WB-DW imaging is a diagnostic test that can be applied for this purpose.

Table 2
An imaging protocol that could be used to acquire WB DW images on a 1.5-T MR system

WB-DW MR Imaging with Background Signal Suppression (Free Breathing)	
Field of view (cm)	38–40
Matrix size	150 × 256
TR (ms)	14,000
TE (ms)	72
Echo-planar imaging factor	150
Parallel imaging factor	2
No. of signals averaged	4
Section thickness (mm)	5
Direction of motion probing gradients	3 scan trace
Receiver bandwidth	1800
Fat Suppression	STIR (T1 = 180 ms)
b-values (s/mm^2)	Typically 50 and 800–1000

Abbreviations: TE, echo time; TR, recovery time.

ONCOLOGIC APPLICATIONS OF WB-DW IMAGING

There is now a substantial body of medical literature that supports the use of DW-MR imaging in oncology. When the technique is applied to specific regions in the body, DW-MR imaging has been shown to improve disease detection, aid lesion characterization, and can be used to monitor therapeutic effects. Although WB DW-MR imaging is new, there is already published evidence revealing its usefulness in the patient with cancer.

Cancer Detection

Detection of metastatic bone disease

Technetium-labeled radionuclear bone scan has inherent limitations, because disease confined to the bone marrow not invoking substantial bone turnover produces false-negative results (**Fig. 3**). By comparison, WB-DW imaging is at least equivalent, if not superior, to radionuclide bone scan for the detection of metastatic bone disease in patients with prostate cancer,[19] with good interobserver agreement.[20]

Bone metastases replacing normal bone marrow appear as areas of high signal-impeded diffusion against the signal-suppressed yellow bone marrow on WB-DW imaging. However, in the younger population in which normal active red marrow is expected, diffuse marrow infiltration by disease could be obscured or masked by the normal hypercellular red marrow, because both disease and normal red marrow show varying degrees of impeded diffusion on DW-MR imaging.

Studies in lung cancer,[21] prostate cancer,[19,22] and breast cancer[23] have found that WB-DW

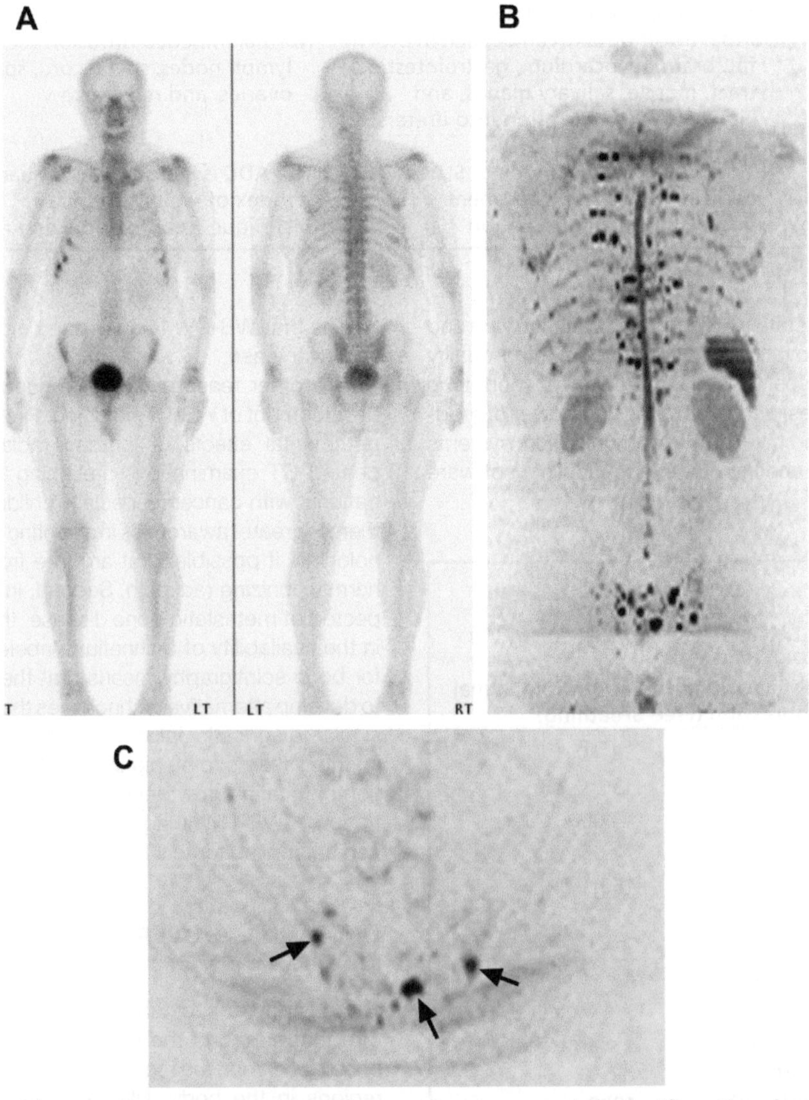

Fig. 3. A man with prostate cancer presenting with increasing serum prostate-specific antigen levels. (*A*) Technetium bone scan (anterior and posterior views) show some tracer uptake in the right anterior lower ribs, which was thought to be nonspecific. (*B*) Coronal inverted gray-scale MIP image shows multiple foci of impeded water diffusion throughout the axial skeleton, including multiple ribs and the pelvis. (*C*) Inverted gray-scale axial DW-MR image obtained through the pelvis shows several foci (*arrows*) of impeded diffusion localized to the bone marrow, typical of bone metastases.

imaging has a high diagnostic accuracy in identifying metastatic bone disease. In one study, discrepancy between WB-DW imaging and bone scintigraphy was greatest in the pelvis, coccyx, and sternum; sites where bone scintigraphy is known to have inherent limitations and where WB-DW imaging detected more disease.[20] In another study,[22] WB-DW imaging was reportedly better in showing the extent of malignant bone metastases in patients with more than 10 lesions compared with skeletal radiotracer scintigraphy. However, no statistical difference was found for diagnostic sensitivity for patients with fewer than 5 bony lesions. A recent study compared ^{18}NaF PET/CT with WB-DW imaging for the detection of bone metastases in 49 patients with high-risk prostate cancer.[24] WB-DW imaging had higher specificity but lower sensitivity than ^{18}NaF PET/CT on a lesion-by-lesion basis.

In patients with multiple myeloma, focal marrow infiltrations appear as areas of impeded diffusion. Sommer and colleagues[25] reported that the signal intensity of lesions was higher on WB-DW imaging in patients with high serum concentrations of the M-component of serum paraproteins. Furthermore, the ADC values of these lesions were lower than those in patients showing a lower M-component serum concentration.[25]

The DW-MR imaging signal of bone disease has been reported to vary with histology. Compared with STIR imaging, metastases arising from prostate cancer and multiple myeloma were usually more prominent (higher signal/background ratio) on DW-MR imaging compared with those arising from breast cancer.[26]

Nevertheless, there are potential pitfalls and challenges in using WB-DW imaging for metastatic bone disease. First, even though many sclerotic bone metastases are visible on DW-MR imaging, densely sclerotic bone disease may not show significant impeded diffusion and could be missed (**Fig. 4**). For this reason, when using the technique to evaluate metastatic bone disease, particularly in cancers that are known to result in densely sclerotic lesions (eg, breast and prostate cancers), WB-DW imaging should not be interpreted alone but should be combined with T1-weighted and/or CT imaging so as to avoid mistakes. In one study, T1-weighted imaging performed better in identifying sclerotic metastases (defined as >600 Hounsfield units on CT), whereas WB-DW imaging was better for the detection nonsclerotic lesions (<300 Hounsfield units on CT).[27] Second, there is a nonlinear relationship between the measured signal intensity and the ADC values.[28] This is because the normal adult marrow contains fat, whose signal is suppressed on the fat-suppressed DW-MR imaging and is associated with low ADC values. With increasing marrow infiltration, there is paradoxically an increase in the ADC value accompanied by increase in the diffusion signal. For this reason, the ADC values of marrow disorders are frequently higher than that of normal background bone marrow.[29] Further increase in disease burden may lead to higher diffusion signal but a decrease in the ADC value. Because metastatic disease involving the bone marrow is affected by the presence of yellow marrow (fat), red marrow, and malignant cells, the proportions of these within each voxel affect the diffusion signal and the ADC values. Thus, research is being undertaken to further clarify the relationship between biological tumor response and the changes in the diffusion signal and ADC at DW-MR imaging. The diagnostic performance of WB-DW imaging for the evaluation of metastatic bone disease is summarized in **Table 3**.

Peritoneal disease

There is now compelling evidence to show that using DW-MR imaging in the abdomen and pelvis improves the detection of peritoneal disease.[34] In

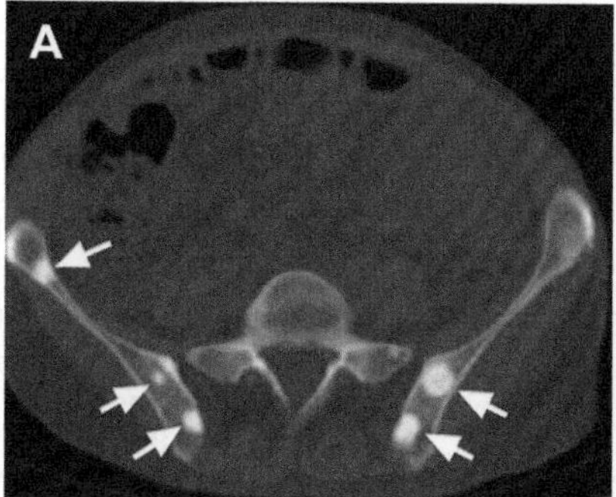

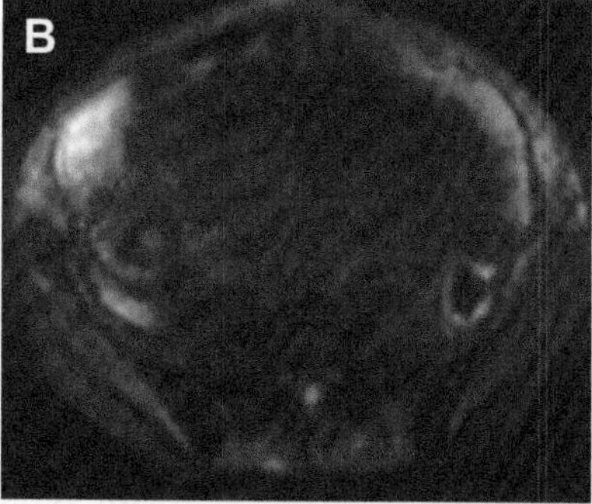

Fig. 4. A man with metastatic prostate cancer. (*A*) Axial CT image through the pelvis shows multiple sclerotic bone metastases (*arrows*). (*B*) These lesions do not show significant impeded diffusion or high signal intensity on the (b = 900 s/mm^2) DW image.

Table 3
Summary of WB-DW imaging studies evaluating skeletal disease in oncology patients

Study (Year)	No. of Patients	WB Technique	Comparison	Findings
Stecco et al,[20] 2012	23	DW-MR imaging	Bone scintigraphy	DW-MR imaging showed high sensitivity (80%) and specificity (98%) in detecting skeletal metastases
Mosavi et al,[24] 2012	49	DW-MR imaging	NaF PET/CT	WB-DW imaging showed a higher specificity but lower sensitivity compared with NaF PET/CT
Leucovet et al,[19] 2012	100	DW-MR imaging	CT, bone scintigraphy, skeletal radiographs	WB-DW imaging showed higher sensitivity (98%–100%) in detecting prostate bone metastases compared with bone scintigraphy and radiography (86%)
Fischer et al,[30] 2011	68	T2W and DW-MR imaging	^{18}FDG-PET-CT	High detection rate and PPV using DW-MR imaging with T2W imaging evaluated side by side (72%, 89%) or by fusion (74%, 91%)
Sommer et al,[25] 2011	81	DW-MR imaging, T1W and T2W	T1W and T2W	High serum concentration of M-protein in patients with multiple myeloma was associated with lower ADC values
Gutzeit et al,[22] 2010	36	DW-MR imaging	^{18}FDG-PET-CT	DW-MR imaging had higher sensitivity (97%) than PET-CT (91%) for patients with >10 skeletal lesions
Nakanishi et al,[31] 2007	30	DW-MR imaging, STIR, T1W	Bone scintigraphy, CT	DW-MR imaging with STIR and T1 weighting resulted in higher sensitivity (96%) and PPV (98%) than bone scintigraphy or WB-MR imaging without DW-MR imaging
Xu et al,[32] 2008	45	DW-MR imaging	Bone scintigraphy	DW-MR imaging showed diagnostic sensitivity and PPV comparable with bone scintigraphy
Takenaka et al,[21] 2009	115	DW-MR imaging, T1W, STIR	^{18}FDG-PET-CT, ^{99}Tc bone scintigraphy	Specificity and accuracy of WB-MR imaging with DW-MR imaging was significantly better than scintigraphy for bone metastases
Ohno et al,[33] 2008	203	DW-MR imaging, T1W, STIR	^{18}FDG-PET-CT	Accuracy of WB-MR imaging with DW-MR imaging (Az 0.87) was similar to PET-CT (Az 0.89)

Abbreviations: PPV, positive predictive value; T1W, T1 weighted; T2W, T2 weighted; TE, echo time; TR, recovery time; ^{99}Tc, ^{99}Technetium.

patients with ovarian cancers, DW-MR imaging may be performed from the level of the diaphragm down into the pelvis to aid disease detection in the peritoneal cavity. Early experience with the technique reveals a high (>90%) diagnostic sensitivity and specificity for the detection of small-volume peritoneal disease (**Fig. 5**),[35] appearing as foci of impeded diffusion on the b-value images.

In several studies, DW-MR imaging of the abdomen and pelvis seems comparable with ^{18}F-FDG-PET/CT for peritoneal disease detection. Satoh and colleagues[36] reported that, on a lesion-by-lesion basis, the diagnostic sensitivity for peritoneal disease was 84% for imaging with DW-MR imaging and 89% for ^{18}F-FDG-PET/CT. However, the positive predictive value was lower for DW-MR imaging compared with ^{18}F-FDG-PET/CT (72% vs 93%).[36] More recently, in a study comparing ^{18}F-FDG-PET/CT with DW-MR imaging[37] for staging of gastrointestinal malignancy, a diagnostic accuracy of 80% was achieved using PET/CT and 83% for DW-MR imaging, suggesting both techniques were equally sensitive, even though subcentimeter lesions may be missed by both techniques. In a surgical series,[38] preoperative abdominal and pelvic DW-MR imaging accurately predicted the peritoneal cancer index, which corroborated the volume of disease found at surgery.

However, because the normal bowel wall and contents of the bowel can return varying degrees of high signal intensity, the radiologist should be familiar with these normal appearances to avoid false-positive results. As technology evolves, it may be possible to perform DW-MR imaging at higher spatial resolution, which may aid the identification of small peritoneal nodules, thus further improving the diagnostic performance of the technique in this disease setting.

Other tumors

Studies have shown the sensitivity of WB-DW imaging in assessing patients with multiple myeloma and malignant melanoma. In a study of 35 patients with malignant melanoma,[39] the sensitivity and specificity of WB-DW imaging were 82% and 97%, compared with 73% and 93% for ^{18}F-FDG-PET/CT. In this disease cohort, WB-DW imaging was more accurate than PET/CT for the diagnosis of liver, bone, subcutaneous, and intraperitoneal disease.[39] In another study evaluating patients presenting with metastatic disease for which the primary tumor was unknown,[40] DW-MR imaging was a useful technique that could help to localize the primary malignancy. In patients with colorectal cancer,[41] WB-DW imaging had a high sensitivity (81%) for localizing metastatic disease in these patients.

Cancer Staging

Lymphoma

Several studies have evaluated the role of WB-DW imaging for staging patients with lymphoma.[42–48] In assessing nodal and extranodal disease using WB-DW imaging, good interobserver agreement (kappa = 0.68) was reported in one study.[49]

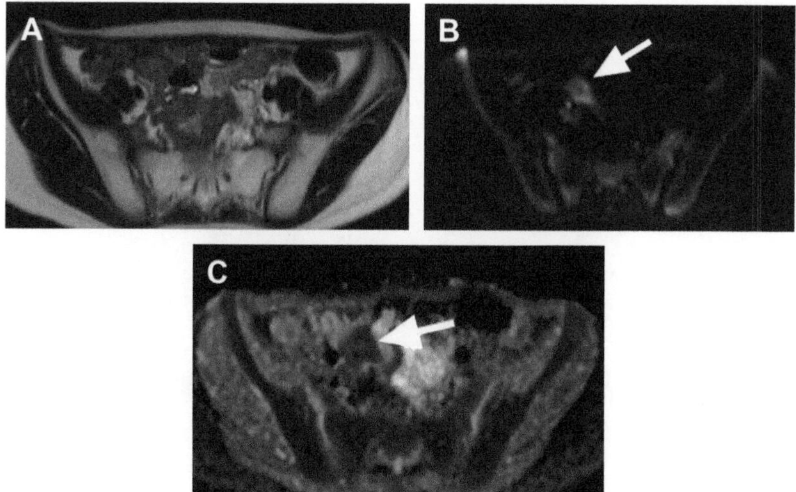

Fig. 5. A 20-year-old woman with immature ovarian teratoma and peritoneal gliomatosis. (*A*) Axial T2-weighted image shows no convincing peritoneal abnormality. (*B*) DW-MR imaging (b = 900 s/mm^2) shows a nodule of impeded diffusion (*arrow*) in right lower abdomen. (*C*) The abnormality returns a low ADC value (*arrow*). Imaging appearances are in keeping with a peritoneal implant, which showed interval tumor growth on follow-up imaging (not shown).

Compared with contrast enhanced CT, Kwee and colleagues[47] found that staging results using WB-MR with DW imaging were equal to CT in 75% (21/28), higher in 25% (7/28), and lower in 0% (0/28) of patients. WB-DW imaging has also been compared with ^{18}F-FDG-PET/CT for disease staging. Diseased lymph nodes have reportedly lower ADC compared with normal lymph nodes, but there is significant overlap. For this reason, some studies comparing PET imaging with WB-DW imaging have included size criteria ($\geq$1 cm) as the basis to determine involvement.[42,50] In one study,[42] WB-DW imaging results matched PET-CT findings in 94% of patients when nodal disease was assessed as such on a per-region basis (**Fig. 6**). Combining visual ADC analysis with size measurement increased the diagnostic specificity using WB-DW imaging.

In another study,[48] WB-DW imaging was as accurate as ^{18}F-FDG-PET/CT for the initial staging in a mixed population of patients with Hodgkin disease and non-Hodgkin lymphoma. Concordance between WB-DW imaging and ^{18}F-FDG-PET/CT for disease identification was as high as 90%.[48] In a further study of 22 patients with lymphoma, the Ann Arbor staging of disease using WB-DW imaging was concordant with PET-CT in 77%, whereas understaging occurred in 0%, and overstaging in 23%.[49] Overstaging and low diagnostic specificity in some studies could relate to these studies relying on the nodal signal intensity on the high b-value images alone, without considering their ADC characteristics. Overdependence on the DW-MR imaging signal could lead to erroneous classification because normal lymph nodes also show impeded diffusion on WB-DW imaging and be mistaken for disease.

Although lymphomatous nodes have been found to return lower ADC values compared with normal lymph nodes,[42,50–52] no significant difference was found in the ADC values between indolent and aggressive forms of lymphoma.[52] In one study, Wu and colleagues[53] evaluated ^{18}F-FDG-PET/CT with DW-MR imaging and found no

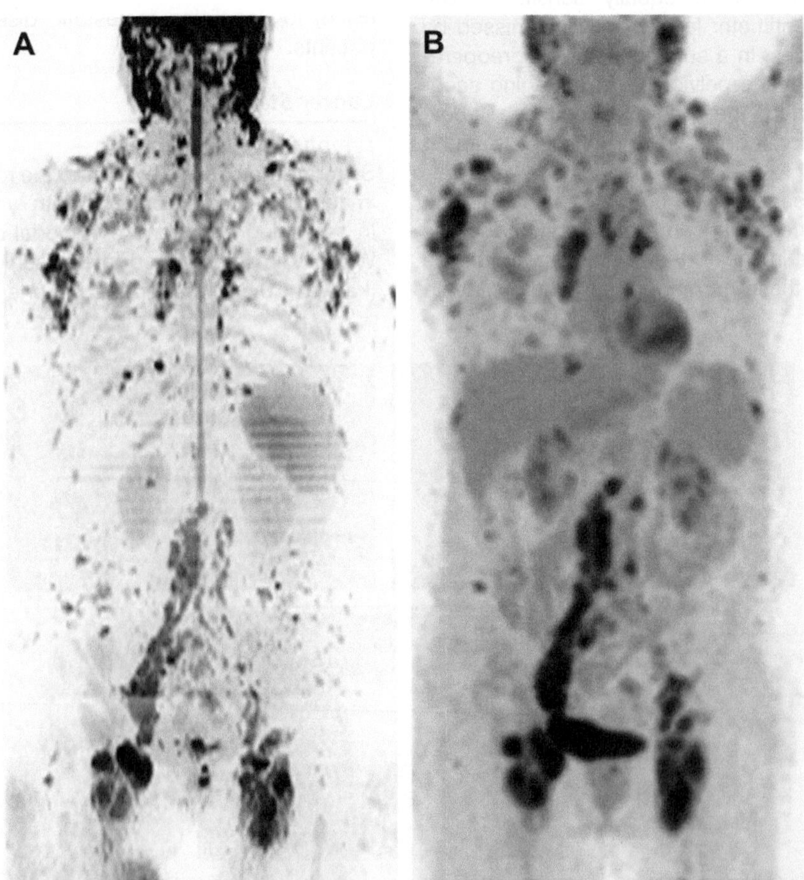

Fig. 6. A comparison of (*A*) WB-DW imaging (b = 900 s/mm^2) and (*B*) WB–^{18}F-FDG-PET in a middle-aged woman with non-Hodgkin lymphoma. Images are MIP along the coronal plane displayed using inverted gray scale. Note the correspondence of nodal disease in mediastinum, axillae, neck, and retroperitoneum depicted by each imaging technique.

correlation between the mean SUV (SUV_{mean}) and the ADC value.

One study performed at the higher field strength of 3.0 T showed that the addition of DW-MR imaging to a conventional WB-MR imaging study improved the diagnostic accuracy for disease staging in patients with lymphoma.[44] With the addition of DW-MR imaging to conventional MR imaging, an increase in the number of true-positive lesions and decrease in number of false-negative lesions[44] was achieved. WB-DW imaging also increased disease conspicuity compared with conventional imaging.

When assessing bone marrow involvement in lymphoma, the diagnostic accuracy of WB-DW imaging remains uncertain. In one study, WB-DW imaging had a diagnostic sensitivity of only 46% for the detection of marrow involvement compared with bone marrow biopsy.[45] However, in another study, WB-DW imaging was better than blind bone marrow biopsy in showing the presence of disease in the bone marrow.[54] Hence, further research in this area would be welcome.

With regard to showing the distribution of disease across the body, small lymph nodes in the mediastinum may potentially be missed on WB-DW imaging because of cardiac and respiratory motion. However, this theoretic limitation has not been a major issue in reported series. With regard to extranodal disease, WB-DW imaging seems to have a high sensitivity for detecting disease in the liver. However, lesions in the brain or the lungs may be missed because small pulmonary nodules (<5 mm) may be beyond what the resolution of the technique can confidently detect, especially in the presence of respiratory motion. The normal brain also shows impeded diffusion and may not reveal subtle cerebral involvement.

Non–small cell lung cancer

Several studies have evaluated the potential of WB-DW imaging for non–small cell lung cancer. In a large study by Ohno and colleagues,[33] the combination of DW-MR imaging with conventional STIR and T1-weighted sequences resulted in a diagnostic accuracy for staging that was similar to ^{18}F-FDG-PET/CT. Sommer and colleagues[55] reported T-staging accuracy of 63% for WB-DW imaging and 56% for ^{18}F-FDG-PET/CT; N-staging accuracy of 66% for WB-DW imaging and 71% for ^{18}F-FDG-PET/CT. They concluded that WB-DW imaging with conventional MR imaging was comparable with ^{18}F-FDG-PET/CT for the staging of non–small cell lung cancer.[55] However, in another study,[56] a higher diagnostic accuracy was reported for nodal staging using ^{18}F-FDG-PET/CT (97%) compared with WB-DW imaging because assessment of neck nodes and small metastatic lung nodules was more difficult using WB-DW imaging. In a study of 115 consecutive patients with non–small cell lung cancer,[21] the specificity and diagnostic accuracy of WB-DW imaging (on its own or combined with conventional MR imaging) were significantly higher compared with ^{18}F-FDG-PET/CT for the detection of metastatic bone disease.

Breast cancer

DW-MR imaging has been found to aid cancer detection in the breast. In a study at 3.0 T of 93 women with 101 breast lesions,[57] the addition of DW-MR imaging to T1-weighted contrast-enhanced imaging improved disease detection compared with conventional imaging on its own. In one recent study,[58] the addition of DW-MR imaging to the assessment of breast dynamic contrast-enhanced MR images significantly reduced the number of false-positives that may occur with reading of the contrast-enhanced MR imaging on its own, thereby potentially reducing the number of tissue biopsies performed.

The ADC of benign breast lesions is reportedly higher than that of malignant breast lesions,[59–61] and the ADC value of malignant tumors seems to be related to tumor biology. In one study,[62] the median ADC was higher in Estrogen-receptor (ER)-positive tumors compared with ER-negative tumors. In another study[63] evaluating DW-MR imaging with contrast-enhanced MR imaging, the ADC value was significantly higher for lesions showing persistent contrast enhancement at dynamic contrast-enhanced MR imaging, compared with those that showed predominantly washout or plateau pattern of contrast uptake, again suggesting a possible link between ADC and tumor biological behavior (**Fig. 7**).

When WB-DW imaging was applied to patients with breast cancers,[23] WB-DW imaging had a diagnostic sensitivity, specificity, accuracy, positive predictive value, and negative predictive value as follows: 91%, 72%, 76%, 50%, and 96%. By comparison, the corresponding results for ^{18}F-FDG-PET/CT were 94%, 99%, 98%, 97%, and 98%. The lower specificity and accuracy using WB-DW imaging could in part be ascribed to using only the high b-value images for disease assessment, which can lead to false-positive results.

The Assessment of Treatment Response

One of the continuing challenges of oncologic imaging is the early and accurate assessment of treatment response. The issue is particularly problematic for metastatic bone disease because there is no widely accepted method to determine whether disease in bone is responding to treatment;

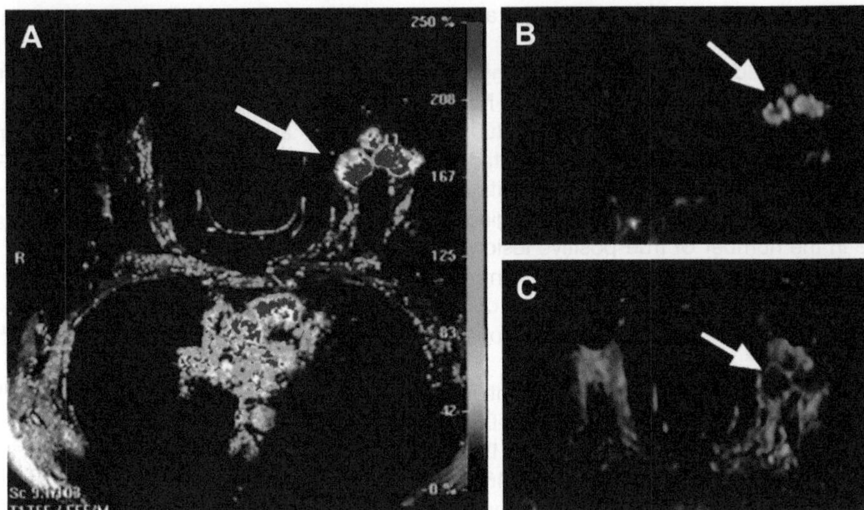

Fig. 7. Breast cancer. (*A*) Relative enhancement map showing multicentric disease (*arrow*) in the left breast, which shows increased enhancement compared with normal parenchyma. (*B*) The disease shows impeded diffusion on DW-MR imaging (b = 800 s/mm^2) (*arrow*), as well as (*C*) reduced ADC (*arrow*) on the ADC map. (*Courtesy of* Dr Elizabeth O'Flynn, Institute of Cancer Research and Royal Marsden Hospital, United Kingdom.)

disease confined to the bone marrow is not measurable on conventional CT or MR imaging.[64] Radionuclide bone scintigraphy may be used to diagnose bone metastases, but cannot be used to indicate treatment response. However, unequivocal emergence of 2 or more new bone lesions on scintigraphy at follow-up indicates disease progression. There is some evidence that PET/CT using ^{18}FDG or ^{18}NaF could be used to assess therapeutic response in specific clinical settings.[65] However, these studies necessarily incur a radiation burden and should be applied judiciously.

Studies have already shown across different cancer types that the tumor ADC increases in responders to chemotherapy, radiotherapy, embolization, molecular targeted treatment, or a combination of these.[66,67] Furthermore, such ADC change may be detected at 1 to 4 weeks from the commencement of therapy.[67] Thus, ADC is being investigated as a response biomarker in patients with metastatic bone disease and the initial results seem promising.

In patients with treatment-naive prostate cancer presenting with bone metastases, the mean ADC of metastases significantly increased at 1, 2, and 3 months after starting androgen blockade treatment, which was corroborated with a reduction in serum prostate-specific antigen (PSA) levels.[68] However, in another study,[69] the mean ADC increased in both responders and nonresponders to treatment, highlighting the potential complexity of ADC changes in bones in relation to treatment, especially in the presence of partially responding disease.

Nevertheless, it seems that, with effective treatment, a substantial increase in the ADC values will be observed (**Fig. 8**). For example, in a study evaluating WB-DW imaging in patients with multiple myeloma,[70] responders showed a 64% increase in the mean ADC value, whereas the mean ADC was decreased by 8% in nonresponders. The ADC changes were accompanied by a 45% decrease in serum paraprotein measurements in responders and a 22% increase in nonresponders. The mean ADC of myeloma disease was also reported to significantly increase in another study[29] among responders, but was unchanged in those who showed stable or progressive disease. Thus, using the ADC value could enable tumor response in bones to be classified as responders and nonresponders, which represents a significant step forward for the assessment of metastatic bone disease. Wider validation studies should be undertaken to further develop and qualify the ADC measurement as a response biomarker in bone disease.

In patients with lymphoma, effective treatment results in normalization of nodal size. However, the ADC value of nodes has also been found to increase following treatment. In a WB-DW imaging study,[50] residual nodes after completion of chemotherapy showed increase in their mean ADC values. Of these, only about 23% of these showed residual tracer activity on ^{18}FDG-PET/CT examination. However, combing ADC measurement with size measurement criteria (>1 cm) could reduce the incidence of false-positive results after therapy. Hence, further work is required to improve the characterization of the residual nodal

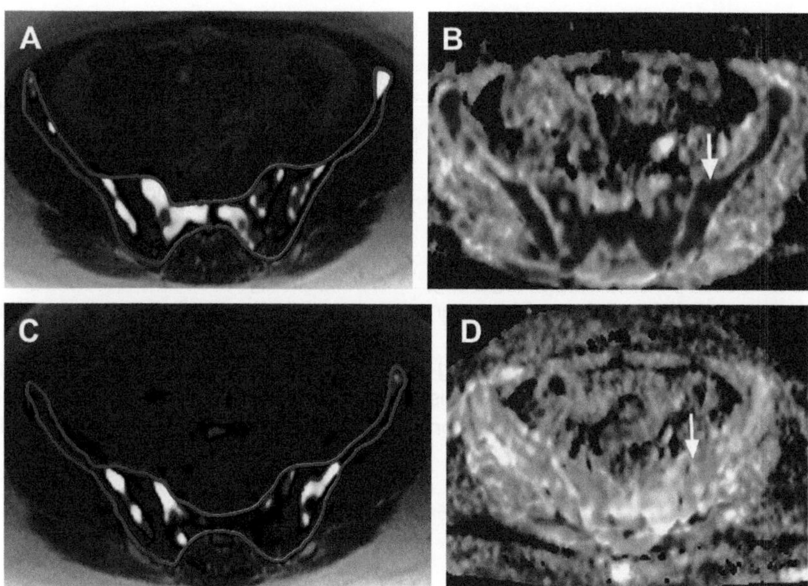

Fig. 8. Treatment response in metastatic bone disease. Fused anatomic T1-weighted (*gray scale*) with DW-MR (*color*) images obtained (*A*) before and (*C*) after treatment. The pelvic bone is outlined in red. Corresponding ADC map (*B* and *D*). Note that pelvic bone (*arrow*) appears dark on the ADC map and returns a mean ADC value of 1.00×10^{-3} mm^2/s before treatment. Following therapy using a novel agent, the bone (*arrow*) appears light on the ADC map and returns a mean ADC value of 1.90×10^{-3} mm^2/s, in keeping with therapeutic effects.

masses after chemotherapy as benign or malignant. In another study, an increase of ADC values could be observed as early as 1 week following the commencement of treatment[71] in nodes that were responding to treatment, suggesting that ADC could be an early indicator of response before a change in nodal size.

In studies focused on specific tumor types, the ADC value has also been shown to have prognostic importance. In a variety of tumors including colorectal cancer,[72] breast,[73] and lung cancers,[74] a high pretreatment ADC value has been associated with a poorer response to chemotherapy treatment.[3] More recently, in a study of non–small cell lung cancer, patients with tumors showing mean ADC value equal to or greater/less than 2.1×10^{-3} mm^2/s showed significantly different progression-free and overall survival, with survival being better in the group with lower ADC values.[74] In a study in patients with lymphoma,[75] the pretreatment ADC was significantly lower in patients who showed adequate response compared with those who showed inadequate response using a multivariate model.

A MULTIPARAMETRIC IMAGING PARADIGM

Because WB-DW imaging and ^{18}F-FDG-PET imaging have different biological underpinnings, the two techniques may seem to be in competition, but they can also be combined to enhance diagnosis. Multiparametric or multiplex imaging points the way to future imaging paradigms, in which the careful assessment of synchronously acquired imaging data or careful registration of metachronous imaging data could help to further understand the complexity and heterogeneity of tumors, thus providing greater insights into tumor growth behavior, drug sensitivity, and the development of therapeutic resistance in vivo.

With the advent of synchronous PET-MR imaging scanners, it is now possible to acquire PET and MR imaging at the same time. A recent study on a synchronous PET-MR imaging scanner has shown that the hardware setup for PET acquisition on a synchronous PET-MR imaging scanner does not interfere with the acquisition of the DW images nor does it adversely affect the quantification of the ADC values.[76] In this regard, early studies are being adopted on PET-MR imaging scanners to combine the unique functional information derived using each technique.

FURTHER DEVELOPMENTS

For WB-DW imaging to be widely adopted in clinical practice, the work flow of processing and reading these studies should be streamlined to facilitate reporting. More sophisticated viewing tools are being developed to enable these complex data sets to be viewed with ease and also compared and corroborated with conventional

MR images and data sets from other imaging modalities. In anticipation of the requirements for multimodal or multiplex imaging, image-viewing platforms should be developed to simultaneously display multimodal data that are spatially registered, so that intratumor and intertumor differences can be appraised by comparing parametric imaging maps that reflect different aspects of tumor biology. In this way, noninvasive imaging can be used to better understand tumor heterogeneity and observe tumor evolution within and between tumors with treatment.

By the applying the computed DW (cDW) imaging technique[77] on DW-MR imaging data sets, it is possible to maximize background suppression and potentially improve contrast between disease and normal tissue. Using cDW imaging, calculated images of a higher b-value (eg, b = 2000 s/mm^2) can be obtained from images acquired at lower b-values (b = 0 and 1000 s/mm^2). Using this technique, the computed cDW image may help to improve the diagnostic specificity by suppressing signal from benign or normal tissues that can mimic disease. Promising results have been shown using this technique for the evaluation of metastatic bone disease and primary prostate tumors.

By applying a semiautomatic segmentation process on the WB-DW imaging data, it is possible to obtain a diffusion volume, which describes the

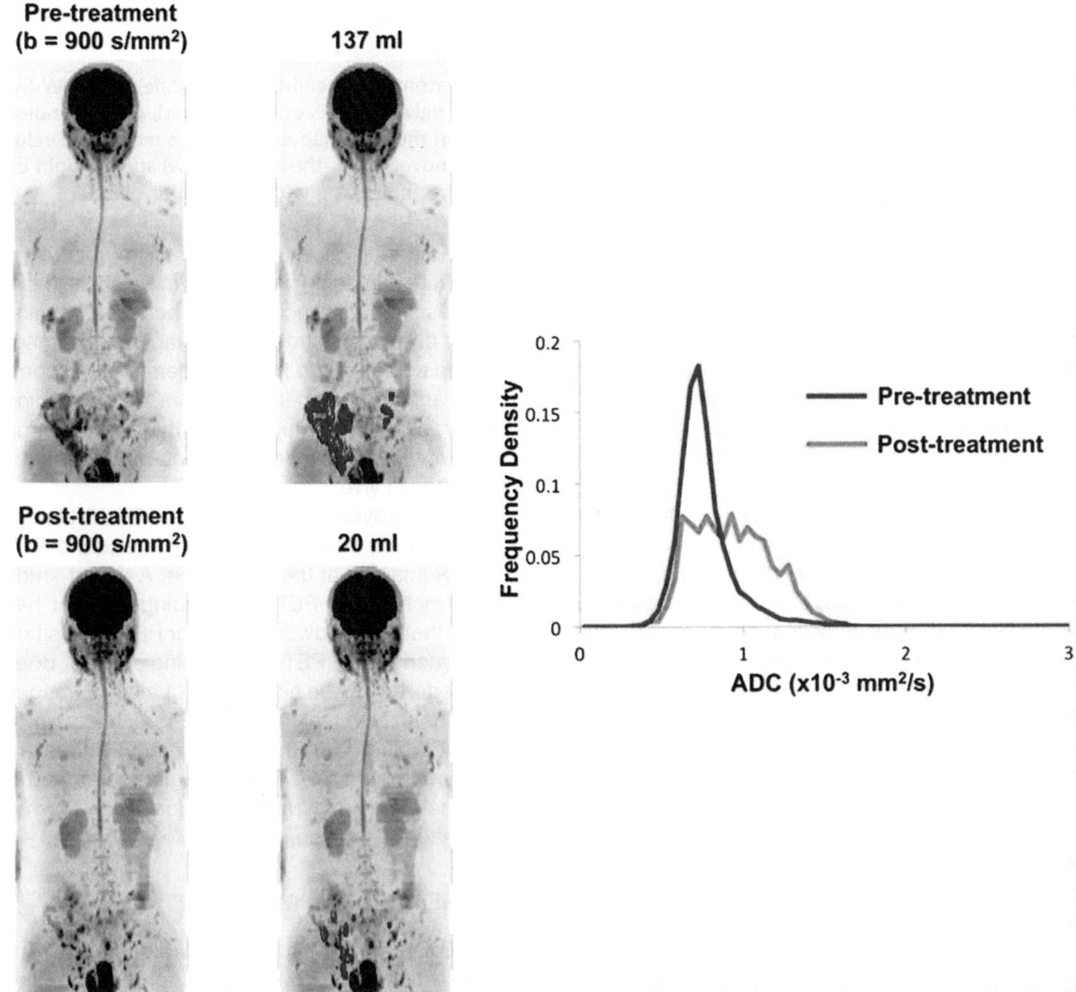

Fig. 9. Diffusion tumour volume and global tumour ADC. An example of tumour segmentation from WBDWI in patient with metastatic prostate cancer. Note reduction in intensity and number of 'hotspots' over the right hemipelvis after treatment. Using semi-automatic segmentation technique, tumour regions were coloured red and used to derive tumour total diffusion volume (tDV) and global ADC (gADC). This patient responded to treatment. Tumour volume was reduced with an increase in median ADC and right shift of the ADC histogram after therapy.

tumor volume across the body, as well as the global mean or median ADC value that is associated with this volume, and provides the opportunity to investigate these quantitative parameters as potential response or predictive biomarkers (**Fig. 9**). Furthermore, it may also be possible to use DW images as a basis to segment PET imaging data,[78] which could be used to provide SUV statistics that reflect tumor activity across the body and also potentially enhance SUV quantification (**Fig. 10**).

One of the problems of adapting WB-DW imaging for clinical use is that different studies in the literature seem to use different diagnostic criteria to determine the presence or absence of disease. Many of these studies use subjective scoring, which relies on observing lesion signal intensity on the high b-value images. However, studies using lower b-values (eg, b = 600 s/mm^2) may encounter reduced specificity because of poorer contrast between the lesion and background, and also because of the difficulty in distinguishing between benign and malignant abnormalities in this b-value range, without taking into account the lesion ADC values. Thus, future studies should help to define more objective criteria, which should combine morphologic imaging, b-value images (with or without the use of cDW imaging), and ADC maps to add confidence to the radiological assessment and for the assessment of treatment response.

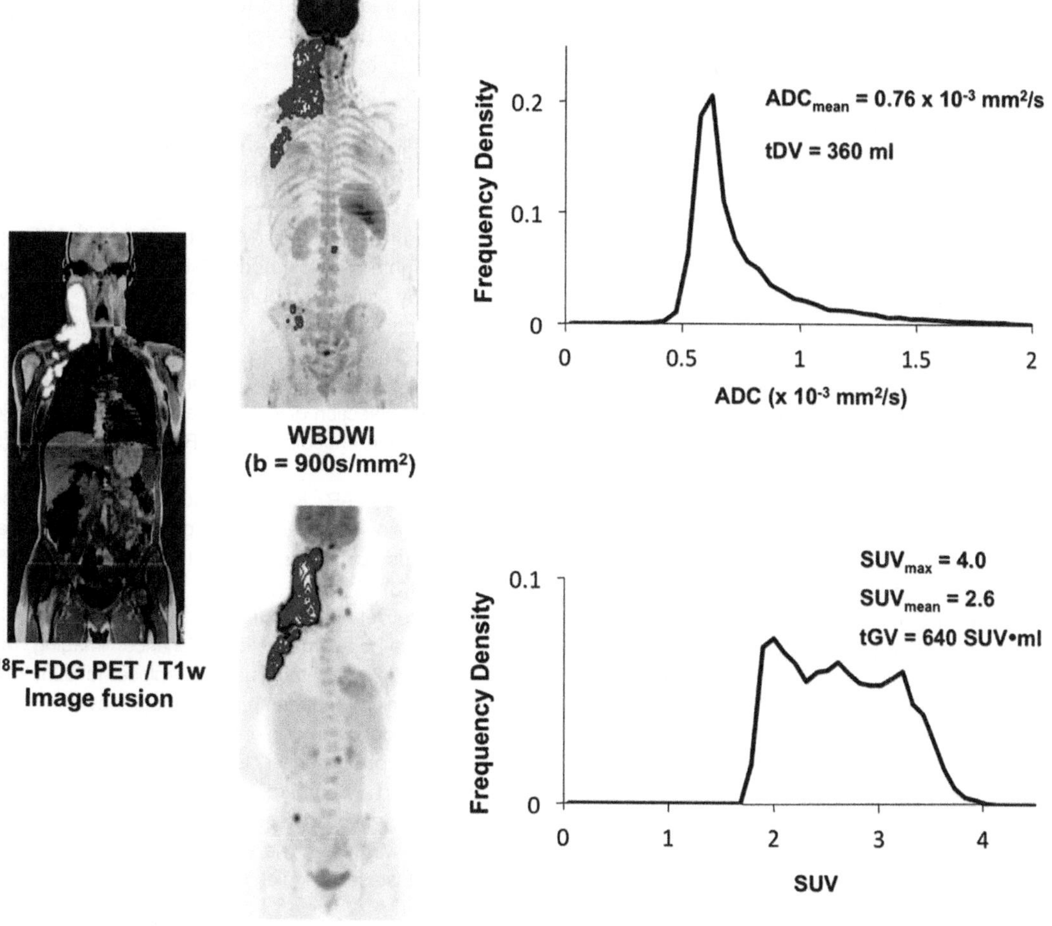

Fig. 10. Registration of PET and WB-DW imaging data enables multiparametric evaluation of disease burden. In this patient with lymphoma, disease volume segmented from WB-DW imaging was applied for segmentation of PET data, allowing evaluation of quantitative indices such as SUV_{max}, SUV_{mean}, and total glycolytic volume (tGV) along with other statistics attainable from SUV histograms (*bottom right*). Combination of these parameters with WB-DW imaging–derived parameters (*top right*) could in future allow better multiparametric comparison of PET and WB-DW imaging data.

ACKNOWLEDGEMENT

CRUK & EPSRC Cancer Imaging Centre in association with MRC and Dept of Health C1060/A10334 & NHS funding to the NIHR Biomedical Research Centre and the Clinical Research Facility in Imaging.

REFERENCES

1. Berghmans T, Dusart M, Paesmans M, et al. Primary tumor standardized uptake value (SUV_{max}) measured on fluorodeoxyglucose positron emission tomography (FDG-PET) is of prognostic value for survival in non-small cell lung cancer (NSCLC): a systematic review and meta-analysis (MA) by the European Lung Cancer Working Party for the IASLC Lung Cancer Staging Project. J Thorac Oncol 2008;3(1):6–12.
2. Dickinson M, Hoyt R, Roberts AW, et al. Improved survival for relapsed diffuse large B cell lymphoma is predicted by a negative pre-transplant FDG-PET scan following salvage chemotherapy. Br J Haematol 2010;150(1):39–45.
3. Koh DM, Collins DJ. Diffusion-weighted MRI in the body: applications and challenges in oncology. AJR Am J Roentgenol 2007;188(6):1622–35.
4. Koh DM, Blackledge M, Padhani AR, et al. Whole-body diffusion-weighted MRI: tips, tricks, and pitfalls. AJR Am J Roentgenol 2012;199(2):252–62.
5. Kwee TC, Takahara T, Ochiai R, et al. Complementary roles of whole-body diffusion-weighted MRI and 18F-FDG PET: the state of the art and potential applications. J Nucl Med 2010;51(10):1549–58.
6. Padhani AR, Liu G, Koh DM, et al. Diffusion-weighted magnetic resonance imaging as a cancer biomarker: consensus and recommendations. Neoplasia 2009;11(2):102–25.
7. Kwee TC, Takahara T, Koh DM, et al. Comparison and reproducibility of ADC measurements in breathhold, respiratory triggered, and free-breathing diffusion-weighted MR imaging of the liver. J Magn Reson Imaging 2008;28(5):1141–8.
8. Malyarenko D, Galban CJ, Londy FJ, et al. Multisystem repeatability and reproducibility of apparent diffusion coefficient measurement using an ice-water phantom. J Magn Reson Imaging 2012. [Epub ahead of print].
9. Kim SY, Lee SS, Byun JH, et al. Malignant hepatic tumors: short-term reproducibility of apparent diffusion coefficients with breath-hold and respiratory-triggered diffusion-weighted MR imaging. Radiology 2010;255(3):815–23.
10. Koh DM, Blackledge M, Collins DJ, et al. Reproducibility and changes in the apparent diffusion coefficients of solid tumours treated with combretastatin A4 phosphate and bevacizumab in a two-centre phase I clinical trial. Eur Radiol 2009;19(11):2728–38.
11. Braithwaite AC, Dale BM, Boll DT, et al. Short- and midterm reproducibility of apparent diffusion coefficient measurements at 3.0-T diffusion-weighted imaging of the abdomen. Radiology 2009;250(2):459–65.
12. Andreou A, Koh DM, Collins DJ, et al. Measurement reproducibility of perfusion fraction and pseudodiffusion coefficient derived by intravoxel incoherent motion diffusion-weighted MR imaging in normal liver and metastases. Eur Radiol 2013;23(2):428–34.
13. Koh DM, Takahara T, Imai Y, et al. Practical aspects of assessing tumors using clinical diffusion-weighted imaging in the body. Magn Reson Med Sci 2008;6(4):211–24.
14. Murtz P, Krautmacher C, Traber F, et al. Diffusion-weighted whole-body MR imaging with background body signal suppression: a feasibility study at 3.0 Tesla. Eur Radiol 2007;17(12):3031–7.
15. Murtz P, Kaschner M, Traber F, et al. Evaluation of dual-source parallel RF excitation for diffusion-weighted whole-body MR imaging with background body signal suppression at 3.0 T. Eur J Radiol 2012;81(11):3614–23.
16. Murtz P, Kaschner M, Traber F, et al. Diffusion-weighted whole-body MRI with background body signal suppression: technical improvements at 3.0 T. J Magn Reson Imaging 2012;35(2):456–61.
17. Nagy Z, Weiskopf N. Efficient fat suppression by slice-selection gradient reversal in twice-refocused diffusion encoding. Magn Reson Med 2008;60(5):1256–60.
18. Padhani AR, Koh DM, Collins DJ. Whole-body diffusion-weighted MR imaging in cancer: current status and research directions. Radiology 2011;261(3):700–18.
19. Lecouvet FE, El Mouedden J, Collette L, et al. Can whole-body magnetic resonance imaging with diffusion-weighted imaging replace Tc 99m bone scanning and computed tomography for single-step detection of metastases in patients with high-risk prostate cancer? Eur Urol 2012;62(1):68–75.
20. Stecco A, Lombardi M, Leva L, et al. Diagnostic accuracy and agreement between whole-body diffusion MRI and bone scintigraphy in detecting bone metastases. Radiol Med 2012. [Epub ahead of print].
21. Takenaka D, Ohno Y, Matsumoto K, et al. Detection of bone metastases in non-small cell lung cancer patients: comparison of whole-body diffusion-weighted imaging (DWI), whole-body MR imaging without and with DWI, whole-body FDG-PET/CT, and bone scintigraphy. J Magn Reson Imaging 2009;30(2):298–308.

22. Gutzeit A, Doert A, Froehlich JM, et al. Comparison of diffusion-weighted whole body MRI and skeletal scintigraphy for the detection of bone metastases in patients with prostate or breast carcinoma. Skeletal Radiol 2010;39(4):333–43.
23. Heusner TA, Kuemmel S, Koeninger A, et al. Diagnostic value of diffusion-weighted magnetic resonance imaging (DWI) compared to FDG PET/CT for whole-body breast cancer staging. Eur J Nucl Med Mol Imaging 2010;37(6):1077–86.
24. Mosavi F, Johansson S, Sandberg DT, et al. Whole-body diffusion-weighted MRI compared with (18)F-NaF PET/CT for detection of bone metastases in patients with high-risk prostate carcinoma. AJR Am J Roentgenol 2012;199(5): 1114–20.
25. Sommer G, Klarhofer M, Lenz C, et al. Signal characteristics of focal bone marrow lesions in patients with multiple myeloma using whole body T1w-TSE, T2w-STIR and diffusion-weighted imaging with background suppression. Eur Radiol 2011;21(4): 857–62.
26. Pearce T, Philip S, Brown J, et al. Bone metastases from prostate, breast and multiple myeloma: differences in lesion conspicuity at short-tau inversion recovery and diffusion-weighted MRI. Br J Radiol 2012;85(1016):1102–6.
27. Eiber M, Holzapfel K, Ganter C, et al. Whole-body MRI including diffusion-weighted imaging (DWI) for patients with recurring prostate cancer: technical feasibility and assessment of lesion conspicuity in DWI. J Magn Reson Imaging 2011;33(5): 1160–70.
28. Padhani AR, van Ree K, Collins DJ, et al. Assessing the relation between bone marrow signal intensity and apparent diffusion coefficient in diffusion-weighted MRI. AJR Am J Roentgenol 2013;200(1): 163–70.
29. Messiou C, Giles S, Collins DJ, et al. Assessing response of myeloma bone disease with diffusion-weighted MRI. Br J Radiol 2012;85(1020): e1198–203.
30. Fischer MA, Nanz D, Hany T, et al. Diagnostic accuracy of whole-body MRI/DWI image fusion for detection of malignant tumours: a comparison with PET/CT. Eur Radiol 2011;21(2):246–55.
31. Nakanishi K, Kobayashi M, Nakaguchi K, et al. Whole-body MRI for detecting metastatic bone tumor: diagnostic value of diffusion-weighted images. Magn Reson Med Sci 2007;6(3):147–55.
32. Xu X, Ma L, Zhang JS, et al. Feasibility of whole body diffusion weighted imaging in detecting bone metastasis on 3.0T MR scanner. Chin Med Sci J 2008;23(3):151–7.
33. Ohno Y, Koyama H, Onishi Y, et al. Non-small cell lung cancer: whole-body MR examination for M-stage assessment–utility for whole-body diffusion-weighted imaging compared with integrated FDG PET/CT. Radiology 2008;248(2): 643–54.
34. Levy A, Medjhoul A, Caramella C, et al. Interest of diffusion-weighted echo-planar MR imaging and apparent diffusion coefficient mapping in gynecological malignancies: a review. J Magn Reson Imaging 2011;33(5):1020–7.
35. Fujii S, Matsusue E, Kanasaki Y, et al. Detection of peritoneal dissemination in gynecological malignancy: evaluation by diffusion-weighted MR imaging. Eur Radiol 2008;18(1):18–23.
36. Satoh Y, Ichikawa T, Motosugi U, et al. Diagnosis of peritoneal dissemination: comparison of 18F-FDG PET/CT, diffusion-weighted MRI, and contrast-enhanced MDCT. AJR Am J Roentgenol 2011; 196(2):447–53.
37. Soussan M, Des Guetz G, Barrau V, et al. Comparison of FDG-PET/CT and MR with diffusion-weighted imaging for assessing peritoneal carcinomatosis from gastrointestinal malignancy. Eur Radiol 2012;22(7):1479–87.
38. Low RN, Barone RM. Combined diffusion-weighted and gadolinium-enhanced MRI can accurately predict the peritoneal cancer index preoperatively in patients being considered for cytoreductive surgical procedures. Ann Surg Oncol 2012;19(5): 1394–401.
39. Laurent V, Trausch G, Bruot O, et al. Comparative study of two whole-body imaging techniques in the case of melanoma metastases: advantages of multi-contrast MRI examination including a diffusion-weighted sequence in comparison with PET-CT. Eur J Radiol 2010;75(3):376–83.
40. Gu TF, Xiao XL, Sun F, et al. Diagnostic value of whole body diffusion weighted imaging for screening primary tumors of patients with metastases. Chin Med Sci J 2008;23(3):145–50.
41. Lambregts DM, Maas M, Cappendijk VC, et al. Whole-body diffusion-weighted magnetic resonance imaging: current evidence in oncology and potential role in colorectal cancer staging. Eur J Cancer 2011;47(14):2107–16.
42. Lin C, Luciani A, Itti E, et al. Whole-body diffusion-weighted magnetic resonance imaging with apparent diffusion coefficient mapping for staging patients with diffuse large B-cell lymphoma. Eur Radiol 2010;20(8):2027–38.
43. Lin C, Itti E, Luciani A, et al. Whole-body diffusion-weighted imaging in lymphoma. Cancer Imaging 2010;10(Spec no A):S172–8.
44. Gu J, Chan T, Zhang J, et al. Whole-body diffusion-weighted imaging: the added value to whole-body MRI at initial diagnosis of lymphoma. AJR Am J Roentgenol 2011;197(3):W384–91.
45. Kwee TC, Fijnheer R, Ludwig I, et al. Whole-body magnetic resonance imaging, including

diffusion-weighted imaging, for diagnosing bone marrow involvement in malignant lymphoma. Br J Haematol 2010;149(4):628–30.
46. Kwee TC, Takahara T, Vermoolen MA, et al. Whole-body diffusion-weighted imaging for staging malignant lymphoma in children. Pediatr Radiol 2010; 40(10):1592–602 [quiz: 720–1].
47. Kwee TC, van Ufford HM, Beek FJ, et al. Whole-body MRI, including diffusion-weighted imaging, for the initial staging of malignant lymphoma: comparison to computed tomography. Invest Radiol 2009;44(10):683–90.
48. Abdulqadhr G, Molin D, Astrom G, et al. Whole-body diffusion-weighted imaging compared with FDG-PET/CT in staging of lymphoma patients. Acta Radiol 2011;52(2):173–80.
49. van Ufford HM, Kwee TC, Beek FJ, et al. Newly diagnosed lymphoma: initial results with whole-body T1-weighted, STIR, and diffusion-weighted MRI compared with 18F-FDG PET/CT. AJR Am J Roentgenol 2011;196(3):662–9.
50. Lin C, Itti E, Luciani A, et al. Whole-body diffusion-weighted imaging with apparent diffusion coefficient mapping for treatment response assessment in patients with diffuse large B-cell lymphoma: pilot study. Invest Radiol 2011;46(5):341–9.
51. Li S, Xue HD, Li J, et al. Application of whole body diffusion weighted MR imaging for diagnosis and staging of malignant lymphoma. Chin Med Sci J 2008;23(3):138–44.
52. Kwee TC, Ludwig I, Uiterwaal CS, et al. ADC measurements in the evaluation of lymph nodes in patients with non-Hodgkin lymphoma: feasibility study. MAGMA 2011;24(1):1–8.
53. Wu X, Korkola P, Pertovaara H, et al. No correlation between glucose metabolism and apparent diffusion coefficient in diffuse large B-cell lymphoma: a PET/CT and DW-MRI study. Eur J Radiol 2011; 79(2):e117–21.
54. Ribrag V, Vanel D, Leboulleux S, et al. Prospective study of bone marrow infiltration in aggressive lymphoma by three independent methods: whole-body MRI, PET/CT and bone marrow biopsy. Eur J Radiol 2008;66(2):325–31.
55. Sommer G, Wiese M, Winter L, et al. Preoperative staging of non-small-cell lung cancer: comparison of whole-body diffusion-weighted magnetic resonance imaging and 18F-fluorodeoxyglucose-positron emission tomography/computed tomography. Eur Radiol 2012;22(12):2859–67.
56. Chen W, Jian W, Li HT, et al. Whole-body diffusion-weighted imaging vs. FDG-PET for the detection of non-small-cell lung cancer. How do they measure up? Magn Reson Imaging 2010; 28(5):613–20.
57. Ei Khouli RH, Jacobs MA, Mezban SD, et al. Diffusion-weighted imaging improves the diagnostic accuracy of conventional 3.0-T breast MR imaging. Radiology 2010;256(1):64–73.
58. Parsian S, Rahbar H, Allison KH, et al. Nonmalignant breast lesions: ADCs of benign and high-risk subtypes assessed as false-positive at dynamic enhanced MR imaging. Radiology 2012;265(3): 696–706.
59. Guo Y, Cai YQ, Cai ZL, et al. Differentiation of clinically benign and malignant breast lesions using diffusion-weighted imaging. J Magn Reson Imaging 2002;16(2):172–8.
60. Hatakenaka M, Soeda H, Yabuuchi H, et al. Apparent diffusion coefficients of breast tumors: clinical application. Magn Reson Med Sci 2008; 7(1):23–9.
61. Partridge SC, Mullins CD, Kurland BF, et al. Apparent diffusion coefficient values for discriminating benign and malignant breast MRI lesions: effects of lesion type and size. AJR Am J Roentgenol 2010;194(6):1664–73.
62. Martincich L, Deantoni V, Bertotto I, et al. Correlations between diffusion-weighted imaging and breast cancer biomarkers. Eur Radiol 2012;22(7): 1519–28.
63. Partridge SC, Rahbar H, Murthy R, et al. Improved diagnostic accuracy of breast MRI through combined apparent diffusion coefficients and dynamic contrast-enhanced kinetics. Magn Reson Med 2011;65(6):1759–67.
64. Costelloe CM, Chuang HH, Madewell JE, et al. Cancer response criteria and bone metastases: RECIST 1.1, MDA and PERCIST. J Cancer 2010; 1:80–92.
65. Cook G Jr, Parker C, Chua S, et al. 18F-fluoride PET: changes in uptake as a method to assess response in bone metastases from castrate-resistant prostate cancer patients treated with 223Ra-chloride (Alpharadin). EJNMMI Res 2011;1(1):4.
66. Padhani AR, Koh DM. Diffusion MR imaging for monitoring of treatment response. Magn Reson Imaging Clin N Am 2011;19(1):181–209.
67. Afaq A, Andreou A, Koh DM. Diffusion-weighted magnetic resonance imaging for tumour response assessment: why, when and how? Cancer Imaging 2010;10(Spec no A):S179–88.
68. Reischauer C, Froehlich JM, Koh DM, et al. Bone metastases from prostate cancer: assessing treatment response by using diffusion-weighted imaging and functional diffusion maps–initial observations. Radiology 2010;257(2):523–31.
69. Messiou C, Collins DJ, Giles S, et al. Assessing response in bone metastases in prostate cancer with diffusion weighted MRI. Eur Radiol 2011; 21(10):2169–77.
70. Horger M, Weisel K, Horger W, et al. Whole-body diffusion-weighted MRI with apparent diffusion coefficient mapping for early response monitoring in

multiple myeloma: preliminary results. AJR Am J Roentgenol 2011;196(6):W790–5.

71. Wu X, Kellokumpu-Lehtinen PL, Pertovaara H, et al. Diffusion-weighted MRI in early chemotherapy response evaluation of patients with diffuse large B-cell lymphoma–a pilot study: comparison with 2-deoxy-2-fluoro-D-glucose-positron emission tomography/computed tomography. NMR Biomed 2011;24(10):1181–90.
72. Koh DM, Scurr E, Collins D, et al. Predicting response of colorectal hepatic metastasis: value of pretreatment apparent diffusion coefficients. AJR Am J Roentgenol 2007;188(4):1001–8.
73. Park SH, Moon WK, Cho N, et al. Diffusion-weighted MR imaging: pretreatment prediction of response to neoadjuvant chemotherapy in patients with breast cancer. Radiology 2010;257(1):56–63.
74. Ohno Y, Koyama H, Yoshikawa T, et al. Diffusion-weighted MRI versus 18F-FDG PET/CT: performance as predictors of tumor treatment response and patient survival in patients with non-small cell lung cancer receiving chemoradiotherapy. AJR Am J Roentgenol 2012;198(1):75–82.
75. Punwani S, Taylor SA, Saad ZZ, et al. Diffusion-weighted MRI of lymphoma: prognostic utility and implications for PET/MRI? Eur J Nucl Med Mol Imaging 2013;40(3):373–85.
76. Buchbender C, Hartung-Knemeyer V, Heusch P, et al. Does positron emission tomography data acquisition impact simultaneous diffusion-weighted imaging in a whole-body PET/MRI system? Eur J Radiol 2013;82(2):380–4.
77. Blackledge MD, Leach MO, Collins DJ, et al. Computed diffusion-weighted MR imaging may improve tumor detection. Radiology 2011;261(2):573–81.
78. Blackledge MD, Koh DM, Collins DJ, et al. The utility of whole-body diffusion-weighted MRI for delineating regions of interest in PET. Nucl Instrum Methods Phys Res A 2013;702(2):148–51.

Diffusion Magnetic Resonance Imaging and Fiber Tractography

The State of the Art and its Potential Impact on Patient Management

Sjoerd B. Vos, MSc*, Chantal M.W. Tax, MSc, Alexander Leemans, PhD

KEYWORDS

• White matter • Diffusion-weighted MRI (DWI) • Diffusion tensor MRI (DTI) • Fiber tractography
• High angular resolution diffusion imaging (HARDI)

KEY POINTS

- Diffusion magnetic resonance (MR) imaging can characterize microstructural properties of brain tissue based on the random motion of water molecules.
- With diffusion tensor imaging (DTI), valuable quantitative measures can be calculated, such as the magnitude and anisotropy of diffusion.
- Fiber tractography allows for the three-dimensional reconstruction of the tissue architecture such as the trajectories of white matter fiber bundles.
- State of the art diffusion MR imaging approaches beyond DTI can provide more reliable information on the microstructural and architectural tissue organization.
- Clinical uses of diffusion MR imaging include the detection of microstructural abnormalities and the virtual reconstruction of fiber pathways for surgical planning.

INTRODUCTION TO DIFFUSION TENSOR MAGNETIC RESONANCE IMAGING

From Diffusion to Diffusion-Weighted Magnetic Resonance Imaging

To introduce diffusion-weighted magnetic resonance imaging (DWI), we must go back to the nineteenth century. In 1827, Robert Brown observed random motion of pollen particles suspended in water.[1] All molecules in a fluid warmer than absolute zero temperature inherently have thermal energies that cause them to show random motions: a phenomenon now known as Brownian motion. Later, Albert Einstein described this physical process theoretically with the well-known diffusion equation as follows[2]: $\langle x^2 \rangle = 2Dt$. Here, $\langle x^2 \rangle$ denotes the mean squared displacement in 1 dimension, D is the diffusion coefficient of the solution, and t is the diffusion time. So, for a certain value for D, the longer a group of molecules is allowed to move, the larger the spread of these molecules is. In this example, the medium in which particles diffuse is assumed to be homogeneous. In such cases, the mean squared displacement $\langle x^2 \rangle$ is independent of the direction in which particles move (hence, isotropic diffusion), as shown in **Fig. 1**A. If the medium is inhomogeneous (ie, structured in some way), diffusion is not equal in all directions (hence, anisotropic diffusion) (see **Fig. 1**B).

None of the authors has a financial conflict of interest.
Image Sciences Institute, University Medical Center Utrecht, Heidelberglaan 100, Utrecht 3584 CX, The Netherlands
* Corresponding author.
E-mail address: sjoerd@isi.uu.nl

PET Clin 8 (2013) 279–293
http://dx.doi.org/10.1016/j.cpet.2013.04.002
1556-8598/13/$ – see front matter

pet.theclinics.com

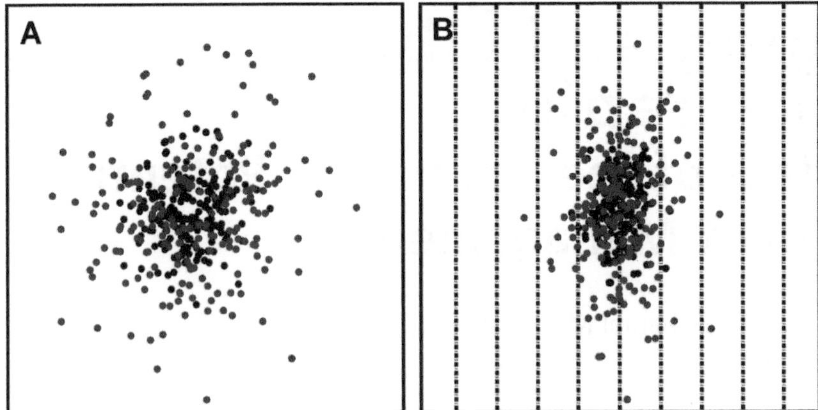

Fig. 1. (*A*) The blue and red dots visualize the displacement of 200 particles over a certain time t (*blue dots*) and 2t (*red dots*). (*B*) Semipermeable barriers, as indicated by the dashed black lines, can hinder diffusion along one direction but not the other. This situation results in diffusion that is not equal in all directions, called anisotropic diffusion.

Diffusion not only takes place in pure fluids; it is also present in tissue that contains fluid particles, such as the brain (more than 75% of the brain consists of water molecules). The brain consists of roughly 100 billion (10^{11}) neurons,[3] and each neuron has a complex cell structure (including cytoskeletal filaments, membranes, a myelin sheath, and so forth) that hinders or restricts diffusion within and between these neurons. As a result, the diffusion medium in the brain is very inhomogeneous, making diffusion highly anisotropic.[4] For a comprehensive overview of the role of each cellular component in diffusion anisotropy, see Beaulieau.[5]

To use diffusion as an image contrast, the conventional magnetic resonance (MR) imaging signal (which originates from the water molecules) must be sensitized to diffusion. During MR imaging acquisition, several magnetic field gradients are applied to generate the images. An example of such an image (T2-weighted image) is shown in **Fig. 2**A. To generate a DW image, additional magnetic field gradients are used, which cause the signal to attenuate as a result of diffusion.[6,7] For a specific orientation of the diffusion gradient (eg, along the z-axis), only diffusion along this axis attenuates the signal. The anisotropic diffusion in the brain can be observed when acquiring DW images with different diffusion gradient directions (see **Fig. 2**B–D).[4]

It can also be appreciated that the diffusion process causes signal attenuation by looking at the

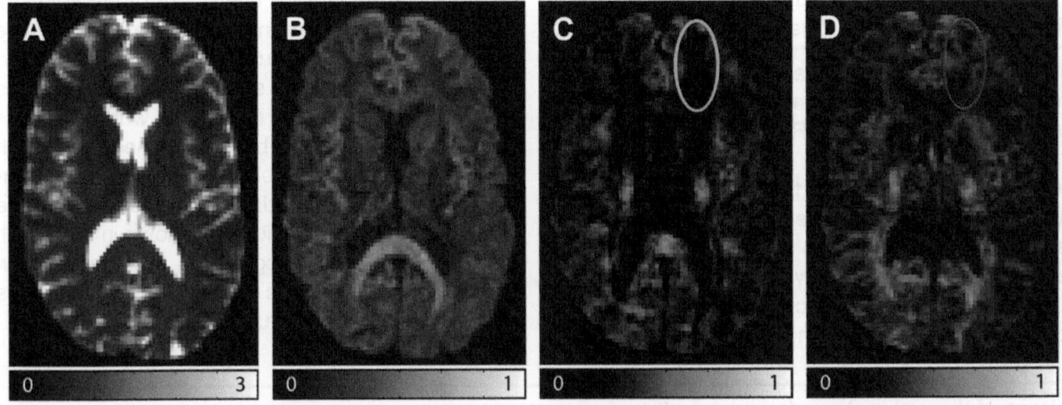

Fig. 2. Non-DW (*A*) and DW images with 3 different diffusion directions: (*B*) inferior-superior, (*C*) anterior-posterior, and (*D*) left-right. Throughout the brain, differences in contrast between the different diffusion directions can be observed, caused by anisotropic diffusion. The green and red ellipses (*C, D*) indicate regions of highly anisotropic diffusion. Diffusion causes signal attenuation, so regions of low intensity (eg, green ellipse in *C*) are caused by a high diffusivity along that direction, whereas hyperintense regions (eg, the red ellipse in *D*) are caused by a low diffusivity along that direction.

diffusion weighting in a more mathematical way. The signal equation for DW (S_{DW}) intensities is[8]

$$S_{DW} = S_0 \times e^{-TE/T2} \times e^{-bD} = S_{b0} \times e^{-bD} \quad [1]$$

where S_0 is the signal after excitation, $T2$ is the tissue-specific transverse relaxation time, TE is the time at which the signal echo is read out, b is the b value (ie, the magnitude of diffusion weighting), and D is the diffusion coefficient. When $b = 0$ s/mm^2, no diffusion weighting is applied, resulting in the T2-weighted image (see **Fig. 2**A), also called the non-DW image or $b = 0$ image.

In DWI, it is common to name the diffusion coefficient the apparent diffusion coefficient (ADC), because it reflects the estimated diffusion from MR measurements, not the true microstructural diffusion. From Eq. [1], the ADC can be quantified based on 1 DW and 1 non-DW measurement. The change in image contrast with b value is shown in **Fig. 3**.

Diffusion Tensor Magnetic Resonance Imaging

Diffusion is largest parallel to the orientation of brain fibers and smallest perpendicular to the fiber orientation.[4,6] Moseley and colleagues[4] suggested using this knowledge to determine fiber orientations from the MR measurements, but a generalized quantification was first described in 1994, when Basser and colleagues[9] proposed Diffusion Tensor magnetic Resonance Imaging (DTI). In DTI, the diffusion profile in each imaging voxel is modeled as a tensor, D:

$$D = \begin{bmatrix} Dxx & Dxy & Dxz \\ Dyx & Dyy & Dyz \\ Dzx & Dzy & Dzz \end{bmatrix} \quad [2]$$

Here, the diagonal components Dxx, Dyy, and Dzz are the ADC values in the x-direction, y-direction, and z-direction, and the off-diagonal components denote the correlations between the diagonal values. For instance, a high Dxy indicates a high correlation between diffusion in the x-direction and y-direction. Conceptually, D can be visualized as an ellipsoid, with its surface representing the probability distribution of the mean squared displacement (**Fig. 4**A). Because diffusion does not occur in a direction (eg, from x to −x) but along an axis (ie, in the orientation of axis x), it is impossible to distinguish between diffusion from −x to x and diffusion from x to −x, which means that Dxy and Dyx are equal (similarly, $Dxz = Dzx$ and $Dyz = Dzy$), and, hence, D is called a symmetric tensor. Because of this symmetry, there are only 6 unknown components in D. To estimate these 6 elements, at least 6 unique diffusion measurements are needed, meaning 6 DW images and 1 non-DW image. In addition, these 6 DW images must be acquired with gradient directions that are noncollinear (ie, orientationally independent of each other).

As seen in Eq. [2], the tensor describes the estimated diffusion profile based on the standard global coordinate system (x, y, z), as used in the MR scanner. This statement means that the values of the tensor elements in each voxel depend on the orientation of the object with respect to these axes. This situation is visualized in **Fig. 4**A, B, where the same tensor is oriented differently. Defining a local coordinate system for each voxel separately enables formulation of the tensor independent of the orientation of the tensor, as shown in **Fig. 4**C, D. With this coordinate transform, the DT can be defined by 3 perpendicular vectors, called eigenvectors, along which diffusion can be measured independently of the other orientations. The magnitudes of diffusion along these 3 eigenvectors (ε_1, ε_2, and ε_3) are called the eigenvalues (λ_1, λ_2, and λ_3). The eigenvectors and eigenvalues

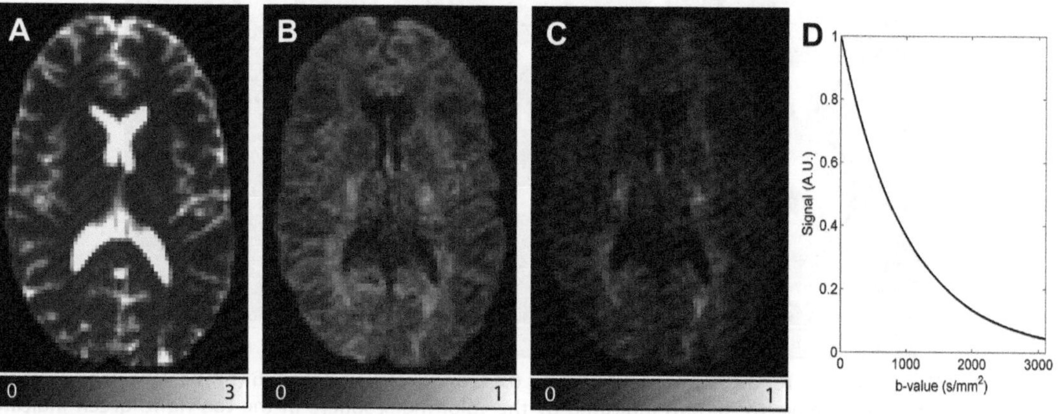

Fig. 3. (*A*) Non-DW image; (*B*) DW image with $b = 1000$ s/mm^2; (*C*) DW image with $b = 2500$ s/mm^2; (*D*) how signal decreases exponentially with the b value.

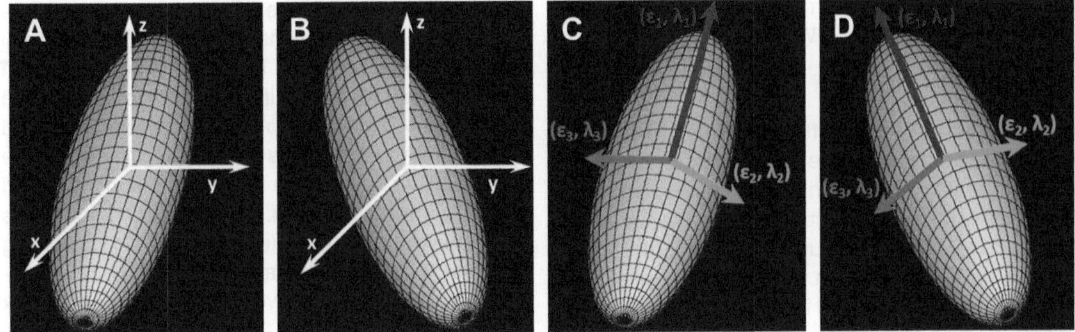

Fig. 4. The DT can be visualized as an ellipsoid, where the surface represents the surface of mean displacement. This situation means that at a given time t, there is equal probability of finding a diffused molecule anywhere on the surface. In a global coordinate system (*A, B*), each tensor component (eg, *Dxx*) is dependent on the orientation of the tensor. In a local coordinate system (*C, D*), the eigenvectors (ε_1–ε_3) and eigenvalues (λ_1–λ_3) describe the principal diffusion directions and their magnitudes, respectively.

are ordered such that the first eigenvector, ε_1, corresponds to the largest eigenvalue, λ_1. The first eigenvector is the orientation along which the diffusion is highest. Assuming that this dominant diffusion oriented is parallel to the fiber pathways, ε_1 reflects the main axis of these fiber trajectories.

DTI and quantitative measures

There are several scalar measures that can be extracted from the DT. In this section, the most popular DTI-based metrics are discussed. The mean diffusivity (MD, equal to the average of the 3 eigenvalues) describes the overall magnitude of the diffusion. In cerebrospinal fluid (CSF) regions, for instance, MD values are in the order of 3×10^{-3} mm^2/s. By contrast, the MD of brain white and gray matter is roughly 0.7×10^{-3} and 0.8×10^{-3} mm^2/s, respectively.[10] Another popular property of the DT is the degree of anisotropy with which diffusion occurs. Although there are several fractional anisotropy,[11] the most common measure is fractional anisotropy (FA), which represents the standard deviation of the eigenvalues, scaled between 0 (isotropic) and 1 (totally anisotropic).[12] Example images of these 2 DTI metrics are shown in **Fig. 5**A, B.

Changes in brain microstructure modulate both the magnitude and anisotropy of diffusion. For instance, Hanyu and colleagues[13] have shown that in Alzheimer disease, these diffusional changes can be observed before any abnormalities can be observed in conventional MR imaging (Alzheimer disease, and other diseases, are discussed in more detail later in this article). Despite being sensitive, it should be clear that changes in FA are not specific. For instance, a decrease in FA could be caused by either a decrease in λ_1, increases in λ_2 or λ_3, or both of these happening simultaneously.

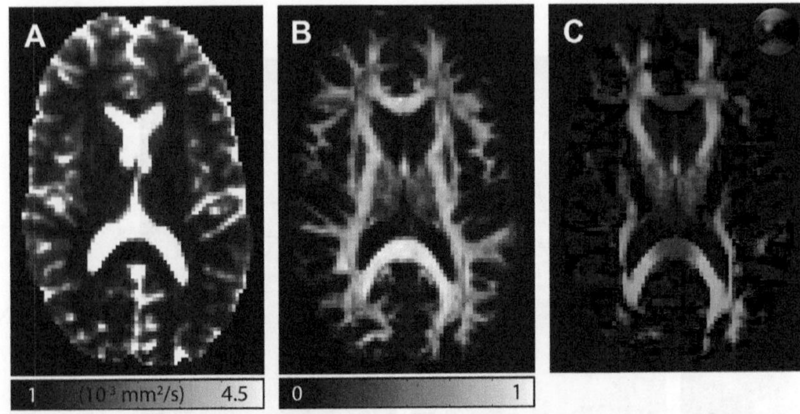

Fig. 5. (*A*) MD; (*B*) FA; and (*C*) diffusion-encoded-color (DEC) map. The DEC map in (*C*) is color encoded by the direction of the first eigenvector (ε_1), as indicated by the color index sphere in the top right: green indicates anterior-posterior; red means left-right; and blue is inferior-superior. The intensity in (*C*) is scaled by the FA, so that regions of low anisotropy, where ε_1 is less informative, have a lower intensity.

To further understand what is driving the diffusion anisotropy, 2 other DTI measures are often used: the axial diffusivity (ie, the diffusion parallel to the fiber orientation [$\lambda_{\|} = \lambda_1$]) and the radial diffusivity (the average of the diffusivities perpendicular to the fiber [$\lambda_{\perp} = (\lambda_2 + \lambda_3)/2$]).[12,14]

The local fiber orientation can be visualized in a diffusion-encoded color (DEC) map (see **Fig. 5**C). In this map, the FA map is color encoded based on the orientation of largest diffusion, ε_1. In this DEC map, green indicates that ε_1 is oriented anterior-posterior, red means left-right, and blue is inferior-superior.

Fiber Tractography

The principal diffusion direction of the DT (ellipsoid) is given by ε_1 and can be calculated for each voxel. Plotting these first eigenvectors therefore yields a discrete representation of the main diffusion directions throughout the brain. This representation is shown in **Fig. 6**A and B, where diffusion ellipsoids (left hemisphere) and first eigenvectors (right hemisphere) are shown. From these voxel-wise glyph objects, or glyphs, the voxel-by-voxel continuity in the diffusion orientations can be appreciated. From the first eigenvectors at each voxel, continuous representations of the principal diffusion orientations can also be created. This virtual reconstruction of fiber tract pathways is called fiber tractography (FT) or fiber tracking.[15,16] Starting from a certain voxel within the brain, a fiber tract pathway can be created in a step-wise way by following ε_1 in each subsequent voxel. This fiber pathway (see **Fig. 6**C) gives a more continuous representation than the eigenvectors, resulting in a more intuitive representation of the data.

Reconstruction of fiber tracts throughout the brain, termed whole-brain tractography, is possible by tract propagation at each location (**Fig. 7**A–C). Although such a set of fiber tracts may seem a big tangle, it can be disentangled with a priori anatomic knowledge of the location of specific fiber bundles. For instance, postmortem anatomic studies have shown that the arcuate fasciculus connects the language areas of Broca and Wernicke.[17,18] Identification of these areas can guide us to select the pathways of the arcuate fasciculus (**Fig. 7**D–F).[19,20]

Analysis of DTI Data

Analysis of DTI data, for instance to compare diffusion measures between healthy controls and individuals with some disease, can be performed in multiple ways, in which each method has its own specific benefits and drawbacks.[21] A short overview is given here of the most widely used approaches; for a more extensive overview, the interested reader is referred to Ref.[22]

Region-of-interest analysis

When interested in a specific white matter (WM) bundle or region, manually delineating a region of interest (ROI) allows for the calculation of diffusion statistics within this ROI. When drawing an ROI on each subject's DTI scan, a comparison between subjects can be made.[23] The need for manual ROI delineation makes this a time-consuming method, especially when one is interested in many different regions or in large-cohort studies. Moreover, it is user subjective and therefore poorly reproducible.

Atlas-based analysis

Instead of manual ROI placement, a predefined atlas with each brain region pre-segmented can also be used, to register each subject to this atlas image. In this way, the brain can be automatically parcellated and average DTI metrics for each

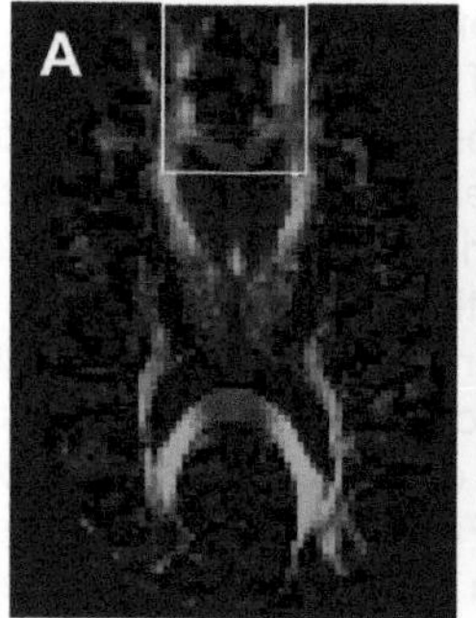

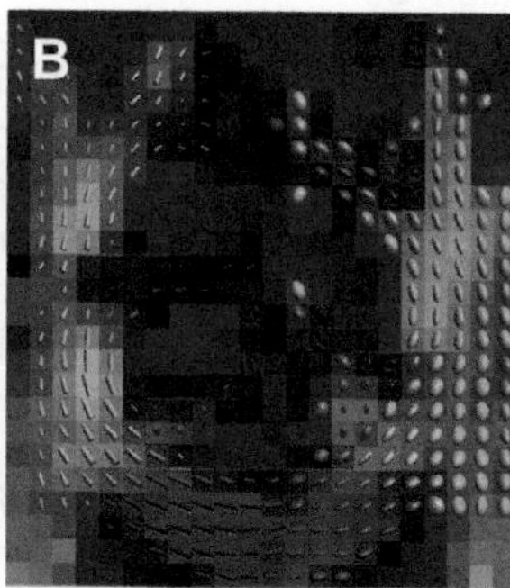

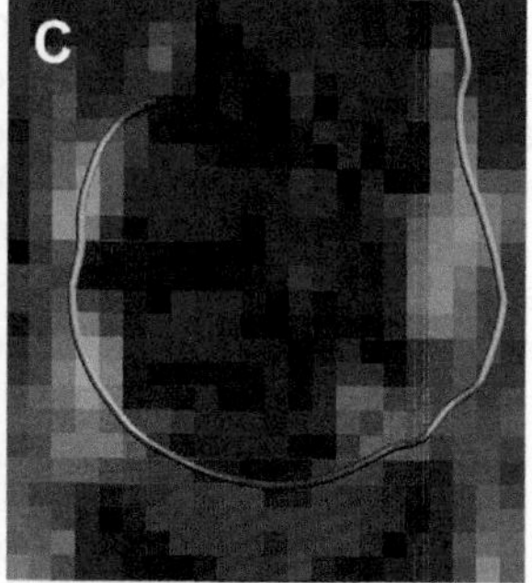

Fig. 6. (*A*) Axial slice of a DEC map. Enlargement of the genu of the corpus callosum outlined in (*A*) is shown in (*B, C*). (*B*) Tensors properties are visualized as voxel-wise glyph objects: the diffusion ellipsoid for the left hemisphere; the first eigenvectors (ε_1), shown as tubes, for the right hemisphere. Like the DEC map, the glyphs are colored by the orientation of ε_1. From these discrete representations, fiber tractography can be used to generate a continuous fiber tract pathway, shown in (*C*).

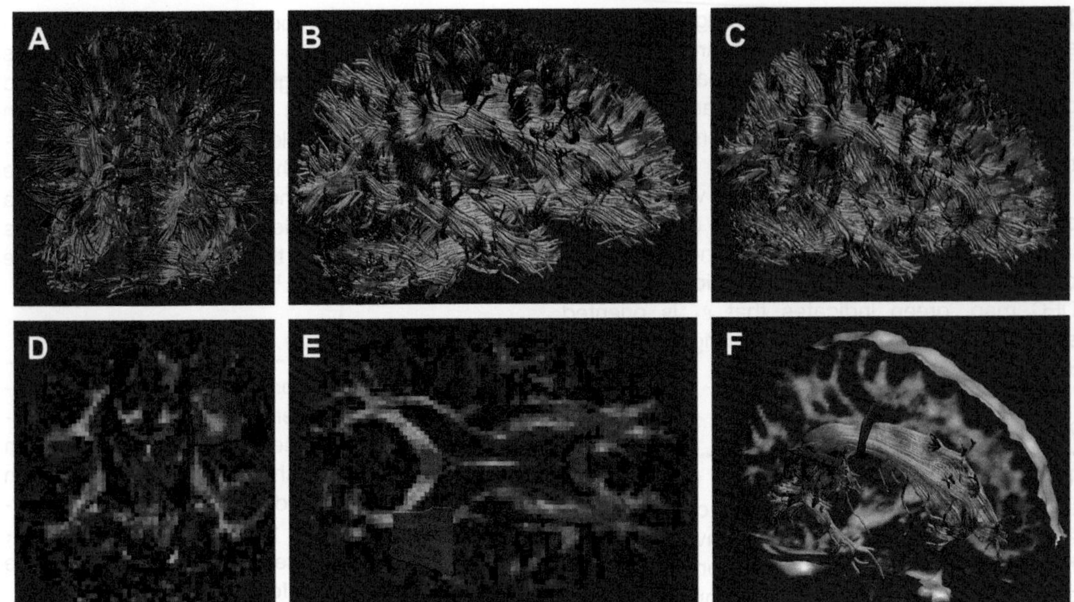

Fig. 7. Whole-brain tractography results shown from a coronal (*A*), sagittal (*B*), and oblique (*C*) angle. By delineating 2 regions of interest (ROIs) around the known locations of a specific white matter fiber bundle, only those reconstructed tract pathways are selected that intersect both these regions. For the left arcuate fasciculus, a coronal (*D*) and axial (*E*) ROI are sufficient to select the whole bundle (*F*), shown in the same orientation as (*C*).

region can be calculated.[24] As an automated and objective method, it does not suffer from many of the limitations of the ROI-based approach. However, large anatomic differences between atlas image and subject population (eg, caused by disease) may limit the reliability and accuracy of the method.[25]

Voxel-based analysis

Voxel-based analysis (VBA) is an automated approach in which scans from all subjects are coregistered for anatomic correspondence between subjects, and then compared on a voxelwise basis.[26] The extent of smoothing, required to compensate for residual misregistration between subjects, has a strong influence on the results, complicating the interpretation of VBA results.[27] Tract-based spatial statistics[28] was proposed as an alternative to ameliorate the drawbacks of VBA and is now one of the most popular methods for voxel-based analyses of DTI data, even although it has shortcomings of its own.[29,30]

FT analysis

Manual delineation of ROIs can also be used to select fiber tracts, as explained in **Fig. 7**. The DTI parameters can be averaged over all voxels within that selected tract, yielding more anatomically specific averages than the ROI-based analysis. Instead of manual ROI delineation to select tracts in each subject individually, it is also possible to do this in a (semi-) automated way,[31] strongly reducing the manual effort required at the possible expense of reduced accuracy/precision.

FROM DTI TO STATE OF THE ART DIFFUSION MR IMAGING

The cellular components that hinder the diffusion, and thus cause the diffusion contrast, include the cell membranes and myelin sheaths around the axons, which have a size in the order of microns.[5] The standard MR imaging voxel in DTI has dimensions in the order of millimeters, a difference in length scale of 10^3 with the diffusion that it aims to estimate. The tensor framework is based on the assumption that the diffusion profile in each imaging voxel can be characterized with a Gaussian distribution (ie, the DT). However, in voxels with multiple fiber populations (eg, fibers crossing within a voxel) or multiple fiber orientations (eg, bending fibers), the diffusion signal can no longer be described accurately by the DT,[32] as shown in **Fig. 8**. This intravoxel heterogeneity causes 2 main problems: (1) with more than 1 fiber population or orientation in a voxel, the principal diffusion direction no longer corresponds to the underlying fiber orientation[33]; and (2) the quantitative metrics derived from DTI do not reflect the measured diffusion profile in an accurate

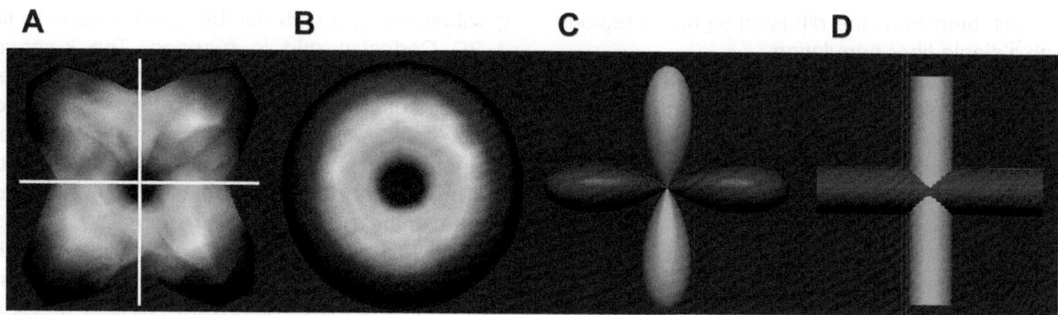

Fig. 8. Simulation of 1 voxel with 2 fiber populations crossing orthogonally in the image plane (orientations indicated by the white lines in *A*). Because of the invalid assumption in DTI, the ADC profile of the tensor (*B*) does not match the true ADC profile calculated directly from the diffusion signals (*A*). In these figures, low ADC is indicated in blue and high ADC in red. The resulting first eigenvector of the tensor is ill defined: depending on the noise, ε_1 is oriented somewhere in the image plane. When calculating the orientation distribution function (ODF) using more advanced models (*C*), the peaks of the ODF ideally represents the fiber orientations (*D*).

way.[34–36] With high percentages of WM voxels estimated to contain 2 or more fiber populations,[37,38] there is a need to go beyond the tensor model to characterize the diffusion profiles in a more reliable manner.

High Angular Resolution Diffusion Imaging

Among the first to propose alternative acquisition and signal estimation methods were Frank[39] and Tuch and colleagues.[40] Commonly known under the term high angular resolution diffusion imaging (HARDI), these techniques used a higher number of DW directions (eg, around 40 or more) to sample the three-dimensional (3D) diffusion attenuation profile at a higher angular resolution. From the measured diffusion signal, a 3D distribution of diffusion directions can be calculated, called the orientation distribution function (ODF). This ODF has its maxima along the orientations of the underlying fiber populations.

In recent years, a multitude of HARDI methods have been proposed to reconstruct the ODF from the diffusion signal. The methods can be divided into 2 main groups: parametric and nonparametric methods. The technique initially proposed by Tuch and colleagues,[40] Q-ball imaging (QBI), is a nonparametric approach, in which a mathematical approximation converts the diffusion signal to the diffusion ODF[41] (dODF). The *q*-value is another feature to describe the diffusion weighting (closely related to the *b*-value), on which the name QBI is based. The parametric methods are originally based on modeling the signal attenuation profile for a single fiber population, and the assumption that the measured signal attenuation profile can then be represented as a sum of these single fiber profiles.[39] One example of this method is spherical deconvolution, in which a single fiber response function can be used to deconvolve the diffusion signal to obtain the fiber ODF[42] (fODF), as shown in **Fig. 9**. This response function can

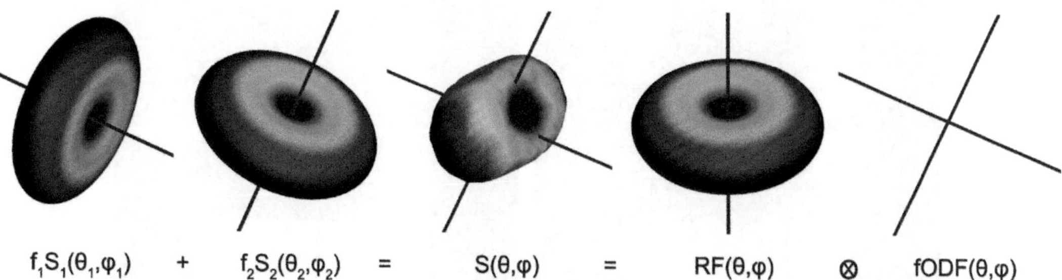

$f_1S_1(\theta_1,\varphi_1)$ + $f_2S_2(\theta_2,\varphi_2)$ = $S(\theta,\varphi)$ = $RF(\theta,\varphi)$ $\otimes$ $fODF(\theta,\varphi)$

Fig. 9. Example of spherical (de-) convolution. Two fiber populations with different orientations are shown as black lines, with the corresponding DW signals, $S_1(\theta_1,\varphi_1)$ and $S_2(\theta_2,\varphi_2)$, and equal volume fractions ($f_1 = f_2 = 0.5$). In the DW profiles, low signal is indicated in blue and high signal in red. The combined diffusion signal is shown in the middle, $S(\theta,\varphi)$. $S(\theta,\varphi)$ can also be expressed as a single fiber response function, with $RF(\theta,\varphi)$ characterizing the diffusion signal of a single fiber, and convoluted (indicated by $\otimes$) with an $fODF(\theta,\varphi)$. In diffusion imaging, the measured signal $S(\theta,\varphi)$ can be deconvoluted with the RF to obtain the fODF.

be estimated from the diffusion signal in regions with a single fiber population.

Using the ODFs from these advanced techniques, multi-fiber tractography uses the peak orientations obtained from the ODFs (**Fig. 8**C, D), as an alternative to the first eigenvector obtained from DTI. Fillard and colleagues[43] and Jeurissen and colleagues[44] have shown that multi-fiber tractography can be used to track through regions of multiple fiber populations, as shown by the simulation in **Fig. 10**.

The ODFs calculated using parametric and nonparametric methods differ. An important difference between parametric and nonparametric methods is that the fODF obtained from spherical deconvolution methods is an absolute measure, in which the size and shape of fODF peaks of different fiber populations within a voxel are independent of each other. This situation has led to the definition of quantitative measures based on the fODF: the apparent fiber density[45] and the hindrance modulated orientational anisotropy.[46] These are scalar values that characterize the diffusion properties for each detected fiber population per voxel. By contrast, the dODF is normalized to have unit probability over the sphere, and the dODF amplitude of 1 peak is therefore dependent on the presence and size of other populations, making it difficult to define similar metrics.

Alternative Diffusion MR Imaging Approaches

Several other approaches have been proposed to describe the measured diffusion signals. Diffusion spectrum imaging[47] (DSI) uses many different *q* values along a high number of directions to fill a 3D Cartesian grid in q-space. The k-space (used in MR image generation) samples the spatial positions of the signal. Similar for the k-space and image space, the Fourier transform is a direct mathematical relation between the q-space and the probability density of diffusion. However, to fill the entire q-space, many more DW images are required and at higher *q* values, putting high demands on scan time for clinical MR systems, resulting in a low use of DSI in (pre-) clinical diffusion MR studies.

Another alternative is diffusion kurtosis imaging[48] (DKI), already extensively used in clinical and preclinical research studies.[49,50] The kurtosis is a measure of how non-Gaussian the diffusion is. Full quantification of the anisotropic kurtosis is achieved by estimating the kurtosis tensor, requiring at least 15 diffusion directions and 2 nonzero *b* values, which can be acquired clinically in acquisition times as low as 5 minutes.

More specific modeling of different tissue components to describe the signal attenuation profile was proposed by Assaf and colleagues[51] and dubbed CHARMED (the composite hindered and restricted model of diffusion). Here, the volume fractions as well as diffusion properties of the hindered (eg, extra-axonal space) and restricted (eg, intra-axonal space) components are estimated, and any observed diffusion changes can therefore be interpreted with a higher specificity. More recently, models have been proposed to estimate axonal diameters and densities in the brain, with initial findings showing strong differences between the genu, midbody, and splenium of the corpus callosum.[52]

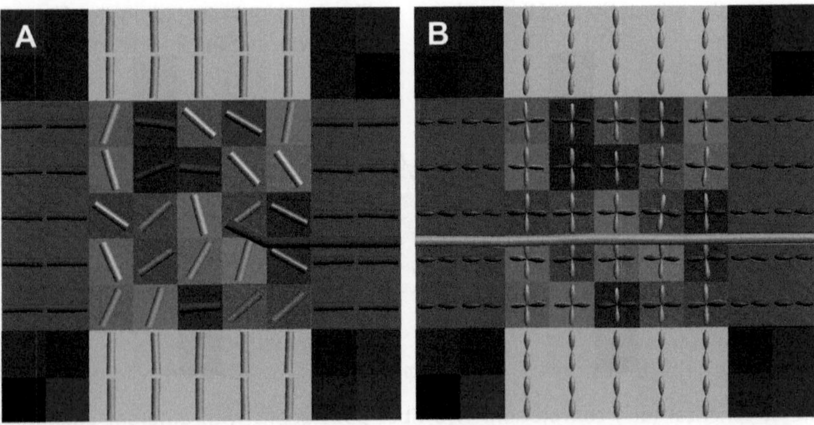

Fig. 10. Simulation of 2 individual fiber populations crossing at a 90° angle. (*A*) The first eigenvectors, ε_1; and (*B*) the ODFs in this region. At such crossings, the ε_1s do not reflect the underlying fiber architecture (*A*). FT through such a region of a crossing is therefore unreliable. The tract terminates at the region of crossing fibers because the angular deviation is too large. The ODFs (*B*) are more robust, and can be used more reliably to perform tractography.

CLINICAL AND PRECLINICAL USE OF DIFFUSION MR IMAGING

The role of DWI is well established in clinical practice, for example in stroke,[53] and radiotherapy treatment evaluation.[54] There are a myriad of brain diseases, with different physiologic underpinnings, which all cause changes in tissue organization and diffusion properties. This diversity means that there is a huge potential for the use of diffusion MR imaging. DTI and more advanced diffusion MR imaging methods are being used extensively in clinical research studies, with most studies comparing DTI parameters like FA and MD between patients and controls, trying to correlate these changes with clinical parameters. However, the use of diffusion MR imaging in clinical practice (ie, on a patient-by-patient basis) is still limited. The next section focuses on a few applications to show its potential for clinical use in more detail.

Alzheimer Disease

In Alzheimer disease, patients initially have deficits in mental functioning like emotional behavior, perception, and memory. Neurons and synapses in the cerebral cortex and subcortical regions degrade, which results in atrophy of the affected structures.[55] Diffusion MR imaging can detect these changes in WM microstructure and can give insight in the type of microstructural damage by looking at changes in MD and FA.[56] Traditional biomarkers such as CSF levels of tau protein and amyloid β_{42} are good diagnostic predictors of conversion from mild cognitive impairment to Alzheimer disease. Recently, FA, MD, and the radial diffusivity have been shown to be even better predictors of disease progression in a small patient population.[57]

Parkinson Disease

Parkinson disease is characterized by tremor and difficulties in coordination and movement. Deep brain stimulation is a therapy that aims at improvement of the patient's motor function by electrical stimulation of the motor part of the subthalamic nucleus. Accurate localization of this part is of crucial importance, because wrong placement of the electrode in the limbic or associative part of the subthalamic nucleus leads to cognitive and emotional side effects in 50% of the patients. Researchers have used DTI and HARDI-based tractography to localize the motor part by looking at its connectivity with other motor areas.[58] This information can then be used by neurosurgeons for better targeting.

Stroke

DWI is very sensitive to early ischemic injury and shows increased signal intensity (and thus decreased signal intensity on ADC maps), and is clinically used for lesion examination. DTI measures might provide more insight in the pathology of stroke, compared with the ADC alone. For instance, FA has been shown to correlate with recovery from stroke, decreasing in correspondence to Wallerian degeneration[33] and sometimes increasing as a result of WM reorganization.[59]

Cancer

Diffusion MR imaging, together with other modalities, can be used in the characterization of tumor tissue. Recently, DKI has been shown to have strong discriminative power to distinguish high-grade from low-grade gliomas in the brain.[50]

Alternatively, DTI is sensitive to microstructural changes after cancer treatment. After chemotherapy treatment of breast cancer, patients experienced cognitive deficits that were correlated with lower FA values in the corpus callosum.[60] In whole-brain VBA studies, changes in FA and MD were detected in patients (compared with controls) throughout the brain, with larger changes in patients with cognitive impairment.[61,62] Concomitant changes in radial diffusivity observed in these studies indicate that myelin degradation is the most likely underlying cause.[14,21] These studies conducted cross-sectional analyses, comparing posttreatment patients with controls. In the first longitudinal study, in which patients who have breast cancer were examined before and 3 to 4 months after treatment, Deprez and colleagues[63] showed that these patients show cognitive decline after treatment, which is strongly correlated with decreased FA in large areas of the WM. Whether these changes remain during years after treatment is still unclear, and strongly depends on the type and dose of the chemotherapeutic agents used in treatment. For an extensive review of chemotherapy-induced changes, the interested reader is referred to Deprez and colleagues.[21]

Traumatic Brain Injury

Whereas conventional MR imaging contrasts (eg, T1-weighted or T2-weighted images) have great use in assessing the acute phase of lesions in patients with traumatic brain injury, DTI has the potential to detect more subtle changes throughout the WM in the subacute or chronic phases, showing axonal injury whereas T1-weighted and T2-weighted images show no change (eg, Arfanakis and colleagues[64]). More detailed investigations have shown that FA is correlated with parameters that indicate clinical severity of the injury.[65] This diffuse brain damage can result in long-term behavioral and cognitive changes, which are associated with changes in DTI parameters.[66] Similar changes can be observed in children and adolescents, with FA and MD in motor pathways correlated with movement control and processing of visual stimuli.[67,68] As a result, DTI measures such as FA may provide an important noninvasive marker of microstructural injury to predict clinical outcome of patients.[69,70]

Epilepsy

Epilepsy is a common neurologic disorder characterized by seizures caused by temporary abnormal brain activity, which can include tonic-clonic phases, loss of consciousness, or change in behavior. Case studies performed between seizures (interictal) show that putative epileptogenic areas and connected brain regions show increased MD and reduced FA values.[71] However, it is not clear whether this finding is cause or effect, and the value of DTI in this evaluation still has to be investigated in more detail.

Tractography in particular can be used to investigate structural abnormalities in patients with epilepsy and has been applied to map epileptogenic networks, revealing structural connections of the epileptic focus with other brain regions. Connections of the medial temporal lobe to the cerebellum and frontal and occipital lobes, for example, may explain seizure characteristics seen in temporal lobe epilepsy, like motor automatisms and auras.[72] Hippocampal sclerosis is the most commonly found cause of temporal lobe epilepsy, and DTI tractography analysis has indicated chronic structural changes (reduction in FA) in the cingulum, fornix, and corpus callosum, suggesting a network of structural changes instead of involvement of only the hippocampus.[73] However, differences in connectivity found in patients with epilepsy have to be interpreted with care, because there is no reference to validate these findings.

Neurosurgery

Since the early development of diffusion MR imaging, the potential of tractography in neurosurgical planning has been evident. Complete removal of the lesion is the primary goal of neurosurgery, but it is important not to cause too much functional damage during surgery, which can worsen the situation of the patient. The position of nearby fiber tract pathways can be visualized relative to the lesion,[74] as shown in **Fig. 11**. The arcuate fasciculus, for instance, is an important WM tract in the language network, and is often subject to investigation in neurosurgical applications. Alternatively, reconstruction of the optic radiation is important in temporal lobe epilepsy surgery, because the anterior extent is often located in the resection area, and damage to that bundle can lead to loss of vision.[75] For these reasons, use of fiber tracking in preoperative planning may improve postsurgical outcome.[76]

In these applications, the reliability and reproducibility of the reconstructed pathways are essential (eg, Kristo and colleagues[77]). The DT model is inaccurate at regions of crossing fibers, and it is therefore important to incorporate more advanced diffusion MR imaging methods. Tractography based on HARDI methods was shown to have improved results, both in the presence of tumors[78] and in treatment target localization.[58] Subsequent integration in neuronavigation systems is promising, but faces challenges like intraoperative brain shift. Diffusion MR imaging can also be combined with functional MR imaging, or other imaging modalities, to map both structure and function before neurosurgery (see Sherman and colleagues[79] for an overview).

FUTURE OUTLOOK OF THE STATE OF THE ART IN DIFFUSION MR IMAGING

DTI is still the most popular approach in diffusion MR imaging. The main reasons are its conceptual simplicity, possibility of extracting intuitive and quantitative scalar diffusion measures, such as FA and MD, and the short acquisition times (in the order of a few minutes). In the following sections, some critical considerations for the use of diffusion MR imaging are discussed, and an outlook over future uses of diffusion MR imaging in clinical settings is presented.

Diffusion MR Imaging Acquisition

Many DW images must be acquired to most accurately measure the DW signal and estimate the diffusion, especially for the advanced methods. Single-shot echo-planar imaging (SS-EPI) is the fastest method for MR image acquisition, and is therefore the method of choice for DWI. However, this acquisition speed comes at the cost of several drawbacks. SS-EPI is prone to susceptibility artifacts, which cause image deformations, which leads to a mismatch between the image and the anatomy it should represent. Second, higher image resolution reduces signal-to-noise ratio and increases these geometric distortions. Even with the use of parallel imaging techniques, which speed

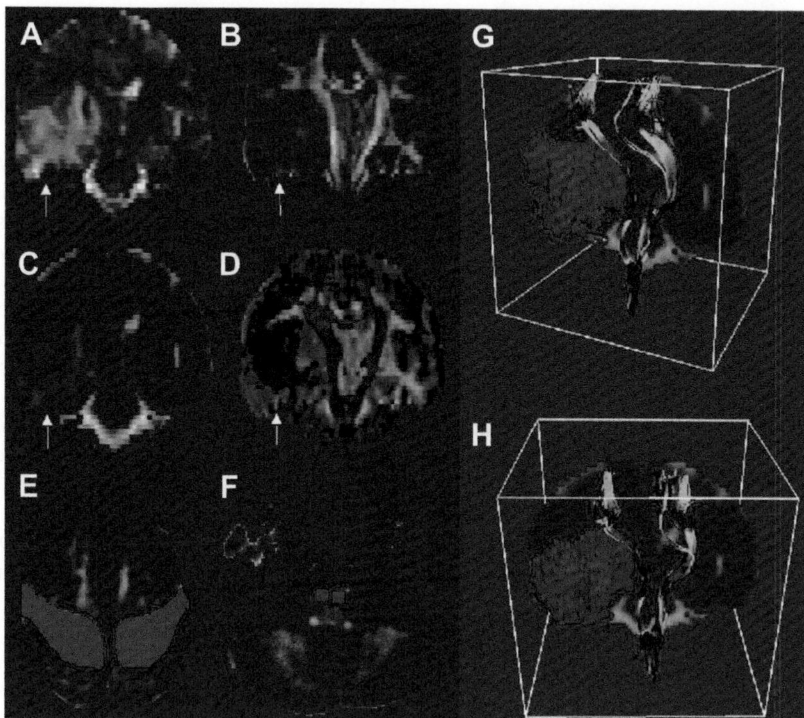

Fig. 11. Coronal images and FT results in a tumor patient. (*A*) T2-weighted image; (*B*) FA image; (*C*) MD image; (*D*) DEC image. In these images, the white arrow indicates the tumor. Tractography was initiated from the motor cortex (*red areas in E*) and the brain stem (*red overlay in F*). The corticospinal tracts connecting these 2 regions are shown in (*G, H*), with the tumor volume shown in red. (*Reproduced from* Clark CA, Barrick TR, Murphy MM, et al. White matter fiber tracking in patients with space-occupying lesions of the brain: a new technique for neurosurgical planning? Neuroimage 2003;20:1603. Fig. 2; with permission.)

up imaging and ameliorate these issues, distortions are still pronounced, with resolutions usually around 2 × 2 × 2 mm or larger. Alternative imaging strategies have been proposed to address these drawbacks, but generally come at the cost of increased scan time, and are not so widely available (eg, Pipe and colleagues[80] and Holdsworth and colleagues[81]). For an extensive overview of these new methods, the interested reader is referred to Bammer and colleagues.[82]

Translating State of the Art Diffusion MR Imaging Approaches to the Clinic

The drawback of most of the advanced diffusion MR imaging methods (eg, DSI or axon diameter estimation) is the requirement for acquisition times that may be excessively long for clinical applications. To reduce acquisition times, these models can be simplified by fixing some of the parameters to be estimated, at the possible cost of less accurate estimates. An example of such a simplification is in the estimation of axonal diameters. Instead of estimating the full distribution of axonal diameters, the average axon diameter only can be estimated based on a shorter acquisition.[52] However, theoretically, disease may cause a broadening in the distribution without changing the average, which might be overlooked in the simplified model. Despite the challenges of translating the state of the art to clinical settings, these methods can provide more specific microstructural tissue properties in vivo, potentially yielding important new insights in microstructural pathologic changes.

Tractography

An important aspect in the use of tractography, especially in a clinical setting, is the accuracy of the reconstructed tracts. Diffusion hardware phantoms allow for an objective evaluation of tractography based on different diffusion MR imaging methods. Comparing tractography results with a ground truth, Fillard and colleagues[43] showed strong improvement in accuracy using multi-fiber versus tensor-based tracking. However, none of the investigated methods performed perfectly. Even although the multi-fiber tractography can track through fiber crossings, it is virtually impossible for tractography algorithms to distinguish between fibers that cross or kiss within a voxel[83] (ie, populations that enter a voxel, but bend instead of crossing). Furthermore, there is no ground truth data set of the wiring of a human brain, which means it is challenging to quantify the accuracy of in vivo tractography. Despite these issues, technical as well as clinical research has already shown benefits of using ODF-based tractography.[43,58,76,78,84]

SUMMARY

Diffusion MR imaging is very sensitive to microstructural changes in tissue, and the DT model is commonly used to describe the orientational preference of diffusion. FA and MD values, which can be derived from the DT, have been shown to change in many neuropathologic conditions. For instance, in preclinical research studies into Alzheimer disease and traumatic brain injury, disease severity is found to correlate with FA. More advanced diffusion models like DKI or CHARMED can describe the diffusion more accurately than DTI, in turn providing more detailed information about the underlying tissue microstructure. In addition to microstructural tissue information, diffusion MR imaging can also provide a 3D architectural representation of the tissue using FT. DT tractography is used extensively in research settings to define WM fiber bundles and then extract FA or MD values from those tracts. Clinically, for instance, it is used in tumor resection, and several studies have shown improved outcome when incorporating it in presurgical planning. Diffusion MR imaging methods that can resolve crossing fibers, such as QBI, constrained spherical deconvolution, or DSI, are used in research studies to provide more accurate tractography results, and provide more feasible reconstructions of fiber tract pathways, especially in pathologic cases.

REFERENCES

1. Brown R. A brief account of microscopical observations made on the particles contained in the pollen of plants. Philosophical Magazine 1828;4:161–73.
2. Einstein A. Über die von der molekularkinetischen Theorie der Wärme geforderte Bewegung von in ruhenden Flüssigkeiten suspendierten Teilchen. Ann Phys 1905;322:549–60 [in German].
3. Lange W. Cell number and cell density in the cerebellar cortex of man and other mammals. Cell Tissue Res 1975;157:115–24.
4. Moseley ME, Cohen Y, Kucharczyk J, et al. Diffusion-weighted MR imaging of anisotropic water diffusion in cat central nervous system. Radiology 1990;176:439–45.
5. Beaulieu C. The basis of anisotropic water diffusion in the nervous system–a technical review. NMR Biomed 2002;15:435–55.
6. Cleveland GG, Chang DC, Hazlewood CF, et al. Nuclear magnetic resonance measurement of skeletal muscle: anisotropy of the diffusion coefficient of the intracellular water. Biophys J 1976;16:1043–53.
7. Le Bihan D, Breton E. Imagerie de diffusion in-vivo par resonance magnetique nucleaire. Compte Rendus de l'Académie des Sciences (Paris) 1985;301:1109–12 [in French].
8. Stejskal EO, Tanner JE. Spin diffusion measurements: spin echoes in the presence of time-dependent field gradient. J Chem Phys 1965;42:288–92.
9. Basser PJ, Mattiello J, Le Bihan D. MR diffusion tensor spectroscopy and imaging. Biophys J 1994;66:259–67.
10. Le Bihan D, Mangin JF, Poupon C, et al. Diffusion tensor imaging; concepts and applications. J Magn Reson Imaging 2001;13:534–46.
11. Pierpaoli C, Basser PJ. Toward a quantitative assessment of diffusion anisotropy. Magn Reson Med 1996;36:893–906.
12. Basser PJ. Inferring microstructural features and the physiological state of tissues from diffusion-weighted images. NMR Biomed 1995;8:333–44.
13. Hanyu H, Shindo H, Kakizaki D, et al. Increased water diffusion in cerebral white matter in Alzheimer's disease. Gerontology 1997;43:343–51.
14. Song SK, Sun SW, Ramsbottom MJ, et al. Dysmyelination revealed through MRI as increased radial (but unchanged axial) diffusion of water. Neuroimage 2002;17:1429–36.
15. Mori S, Brain BJ, Chacko VP, et al. Three-dimensional tracking of axonal projections in the brain by magnetic resonance imaging. Ann Neurol 1999;45:265–9.
16. Basser PJ, Pajevic S, Pierpaoli C, et al. In vivo fiber tractography using DT-MRI data. Magn Reson Med 2000;44:625–32.
17. Dejerine J. Anatomie de centres nerveux, vol. 1. Paris: Rueff et Cie; 1895 [in French].
18. Benson DF, Sheremata WA, Bouchard R, et al. Conduction aphasia: a clinicopathological study. Arch Neurol 1973;28:339–46.
19. Wakana S, Jiang H, Nagae-Poetscher LM, et al. Fiber tract-based atlas of human white matter anatomy. Radiology 2004;230:77–87.
20. Catani M, Jones DK, ffytche DH. Perisylvian language networks of the human brain. Ann Neurol 2005;57:8–16.
21. Deprez S, Billiot T, Sunaert S, et al. Diffusion tensor MIR of chemotherapy-induced cognitive

impairment in non-CNS cancer patients: a review. Brain Imaging Behav 2013. http://dx.doi.org/10.1007/s11682-012-9220-1. [Epub ahead of print].
22. Cercignani M. Strategies for patient-control comparison in diffusion MR data. In: Jones DK, editor. Diffusion MRI: theory, methods, and applications. Oxford, UK: Oxford University Press; 2011. p. 485–99.
23. Snook L, Paulson LA, Roy D, et al. Diffusion tensor imaging in neurodevelopment in children and young adults. Neuroimage 2005;26:1164–73.
24. Mori S, Oishi K, Jiang H, et al. Stereotaxic white matter atlas based on diffusion tensor imaging in an ICBM template. Neuroimage 2008;40:570–82.
25. Oishi K, Faria A, Jiang H, et al. Atlas-based whole brain white matter analysis using large deformation diffeomorphic metric mapping: application to normal elderly and Alzheimer's disease participants. Neuroimage 2009;46:486–99.
26. Ashburner J, Friston K. Voxel-based morphometry–the methods. Neuroimage 2000;11:805–21.
27. Jones DK, Symms MR, Cercignani M, et al. The effect of filter size on VBM analyses of DT-MRI data. Neuroimage 2005;26:546–54.
28. Smith SM, Jenkinson M, Johansen-Berg H, et al. Tract-based spatial statistics: voxelwise analysis of multi-subject diffusion data. Neuroimage 2006;31:1487–505.
29. Van Hecke W, Leemans A, de Backer S, et al. Comparing isotropic and anisotropic smoothing for voxel-based DTI analyses: a simulation study. Hum Brain Mapp 2010;31:98–114.
30. Edden RA, Jones DK. Spatial and orientation heterogeneity in the statistical sensitivity of skeleton-based analyses of diffusion tensor MR imaging data. J Neurosci Methods 2011;201:213–9.
31. Lebel C, Walker L, Leemans A, et al. Microstructural maturation of the human brain from childhood to adulthood. Neuroimage 2008;40:1044–55.
32. Frank LR. Anisotropy in high angular resolution diffusion-weighted MRI. Magn Reson Med 2001;45:935–9.
33. Pierpaoli C, Barnett A, Pajevic S, et al. Water diffusion changes in Wallerian degeneration and their dependence on white matter architecture. Neuroimage 2001;13:1174–85.
34. Alexander AL, Hasan KM, Lazar M, et al. Analysis of partial volume effects in diffusion-tensor MRI. Magn Reson Med 2001;45:770–80.
35. Vos SB, Jones DK, Viergever MA, et al. Partial volume effect as a hidden covariate in DTI analyses. Neuroimage 2011;55:1566–76.
36. Vos SB, Jones DK, Jeurissen B, et al. The influence of complex white matter architecture on the mean diffusivity in diffusion tensor MRI of the human brain. Neuroimage 2012;59:2208–16.
37. Behrens TE, Johansen-Berg H, Jbabdi S, et al. Probabilistic diffusion tractography with multiple fiber orientations: what can we gain? Neuroimage 2007;34:144–55.
38. Jeurissen B, Leemans A, Tournier JD, et al. Investigating the prevalence of complex fiber configurations in white matter tissues with diffusion magnetic resonance imaging. Hum Brain Mapp 2012. http://dx.doi.org/10.1002/hbm.22099. [Epub ahead of print].
39. Frank LR. Characterization of anisotropy in high angular resolution diffusion-weighted MRI. Magn Reson Med 2002;47:1083–99.
40. Tuch DS, Reese TG, Wiegell MR, et al. Diffusion MRI of complex neural architecture. Neuron 2003;40:885–95.
41. Tuch DS. Q-ball imaging. Magn Reson Med 2004;52:1358–72.
42. Tournier JD, Calamante F, Gadian DG, et al. Direct estimation of the fiber orientation distribution from diffusion-weighted MRI data using spherical deconvolution. Neuroimage 2004;23:1176–85.
43. Fillard P, Descoteaux M, Goh A, et al. Quantitative evaluation of 10 tractography algorithms on a realistic diffusion MR phantom. Neuroimage 2011;56:220–34.
44. Jeurissen B, Leemans A, Jones DK, et al. Probabilistic fiber tracking using the residual bootstrap with constrained spherical deconvolution. Hum Brain Mapp 2011;32:461–79.
45. Raffelt D, Tournier JD, Rose S, et al. Apparent fibre density: a novel measure for the analysis of diffusion-weighted magnetic resonance images. Neuroimage 2012;59:3976–94.
46. Dell'Acqua F, Simmons A, Williams SC, et al. Can spherical deconvolution provide more information than fiber orientation? Hindrance modulated orientational anisotropy, a true-tract specific index to characterize white matter diffusion. Hum Brain Mapp 2012. http://dx.doi.org/10.1002/hbm.22080. [Epub ahead of print].
47. Wedeen VJ, Hagmann P, Tseng WY, et al. Mapping complex tissue architecture with diffusion spectrum magnetic resonance imaging. Magn Reson Med 2005;54:1377–86.
48. Jensen JH, Helpern JA, Ramani A, et al. Diffusional Kurtosis imaging: the quantification of non-gaussian water diffusion by means of magnetic resonance imaging. Magn Reson Med 2005;53:1432–40.
49. Fieremans E, Jensen JH, Helpern JA. White matter characterization with diffusional kurtosis imaging. Neuroimage 2011;58:177–88.
50. van Cauter S, Veraart J, Sijbers J, et al. Gliomas: diffusion kurtosis MR imaging in grading. Radiology 2012;263:492–501.
51. Assaf Y, Freidlin RZ, Rohde GK, et al. New modeling and experimental framework to characterize hindered and restricted water diffusion in the brain white matter. Magn Reson Med 2004;52:965–78.

52. Alexander DC, Hubbard PL, Hall MG, et al. Orientationally invariant indices of axon diameter and density from diffusion MRI. Neuroimage 2010;52:1374–89.
53. Albers GW, Thijs VN, Wechsler L, et al. Magnetic resonance imaging profiles predict clinical response to early reperfusion; the DEFUSE study. Ann Neurol 2006;60:508–17.
54. Hermans R. Diffusion-weighted MRI in head and neck cancer. Curr Opin Otolaryngol Head Neck Surg 2010;18:72–8.
55. Fox NC, Scahill RI, Crum WR, et al. Correlations between rates of brain atrophy and cognitive decline in AD. Neurology 1999;52:1687–9.
56. Bozzali M, Falini A, Francheschi M, et al. White matter damage in Alzheimer's disease assessed in vivo using diffusion tensor magnetic resonance imaging. J Neurol Neurosurg Psychiatry 2002;72:742–6.
57. Selnes P, Aarsland D, Bjornerud A, et al. Diffusion tensor imaging surpasses cerebrospinal fluid as predictor of cognitive decline and medial temporal lobe atrophy in subjective cognitive impairment and mild cognitive impairment. J Alzheimers Dis 2013;33:723–36.
58. Brunenberg EJ, Moeskops P, Backes WH, et al. Structural and resting state functional connectivity of the subthalamic nucleus: identification of motor STN parts and the hyperdirect pathway. PLoS One 2012;7:e39061.
59. van der Zijden JP, van der Toorn A, van der Marel K, et al. Longitudinal in vivo MRI of alterations in perilesional tissue after transcient ischemic stroke in rats. Exp Neurol 2008;212:207–12.
60. Abraham J, Haut MW, Moran MT, et al. Adjuvant chemotherapy for breast cancer: effects on cerebral white matter seen in diffusion tensor imaging. Clin Breast cancer 2008;8:88–91.
61. Deprez S, Amant F, Yigit R, et al. Chemotherapy-induced structural changes in cerebral white matter and its correlation with impaired cognitive functioning in breast cancer patients. Hum Brain Mapp 2011;30:480–93.
62. de Ruiter MB, Beneman L, Boogerd W, et al. Late effects of high-dose adjuvant chemotherapy on white and gray matter in breast cancer survivors: converging results from multimodal magnetic resonance imaging. Hum Brain Mapp 2011;33:2971–83.
63. Deprez S, Amant F, Smeets A, et al. Longitudinal assessment of chemotherapy-induced structural changes in cerebral white matter and its correlation with impaired cognitive functioning. J Clin Oncol 2012;30:274–81.
64. Arfanakis K, Haughton VM, Carew JD, et al. Diffusion tensor MR imaging in diffuse axonal injury. AJNR Am J Neuroradiol 2002;23:794–802.
65. Benson R, Meda SA, Vasudevan S, et al. Global white matter analysis of diffusion tensor images is predictive of injury severity in traumatic brain injury. J Neurotrauma 2007;24:446–59.
66. Kraus MF, Susmaras T, Caughlin BP, et al. White matter integrity and cognition in chronic traumatic brain injury: a diffusion tensor imaging study. Brain 2007;130:2508–19.
67. Caeyenberghs K, Leemans A, Geurts M, et al. Brain-behavior relationships in young traumatic brain injury patients: DTI metrics are highly correlated with postural control. Hum Brain Mapp 2010;31:991–1002.
68. Caeyenberghs K, Leemans A, Geurts M, et al. Brain-behavior relationships in young traumatic brain injury patients: fractional anisotropy measures are highly correlated with dynamic visuomotor tracking performance. Neuropsychologia 2010;48:1472–82.
69. Huisman TA, Schwamm LH, Schaefer PW, et al. Diffusion tensor imaging as potential biomarker of white matter injury in diffuse axonal injury. AJNR Am J Neuroradiol 2004;25:370–6.
70. Niogi SN, Mukherjee P. Diffusion tensor imaging of mild traumatic brain injury. J Head Trauma Rehabil 2010;25:241–55.
71. Focke NK, Yogarajah M, Bonelli SB, et al. Voxel-based diffusion tensor imaging in patients with mesial temporal lobe epilepsy and hippocampal sclerosis. Neuroimage 2008;40:728–37.
72. Powell HW, Guye M, Parker GJ, et al. Noninvasive in vivo demonstration of the connections of the human parahippocampal gyrus. Neuroimage 2004;22:740–7.
73. Concha L, Beaulieu C, Gross DW. Bilateral limbic diffusion abnormalities in unilateral temporal lobe epilepsy. Ann Neurol 2005;57:188–96.
74. Clark CA, Barrick TR, Murphy MM, et al. White matter fiber tracking in patients with space-occupying lesions of the brain: a new technique for neurosurgical planning? Neuroimage 2003;20:1601–8.
75. Powell HW, Parker GJ, Alexander DC, et al. MR tractography predicts visual field defects following temporal lobe resection. Neurology 2005;23:596–9.
76. Witwer BP, Moftakhar R, Hasan KM, et al. Diffusion tensor imaging of white matter tracts in patients with cerebral neoplasm. J Neurosurg 2002;97:568–75.
77. Kristo G, Leemans A, Raemaekers M, et al. Reliability of two clinically relevant fiber pathways reconstructed with constrained spherical deconvolution. Magn Reson Med 2013. http://dx.doi.org/10.1002/mrm.24602. [Epub ahead of print].
78. Kuhnt D, Bauer MH, Egger J, et al. Fiber tractography based on diffusion tensor imaging compared with high-angular resolution diffusion imaging with

compressed sensing: Initial experience. Neurosurgery 2013;72(Suppl 1):A165–75.
79. Sherman JH, Hoes K, Marcus J, et al. Neurosurgery for brain tumors: update on recent technical advances. Curr Neurol Neurosci Rep 2011;11:313–9.
80. Pipe JG, Farthing VG, Forbes KP. Multishot diffusion-weighted FSE using PROPELLOR MRI. Magn Reson Med 2002;47:42–52.
81. Holdsworth SJ, Skare S, Newbould RD, et al. Readout-segmented EPI for rapid high resolution diffusion imaging at 3T. Eur J Radiol 2008;65:36–46.
82. Bammer R, Holdsworth SJ, Veldhuis WB, et al. New methods in diffusion-weighted and diffusion tensor imaging. Magn Reson Imaging Clin North Am 2009;17:175–204.
83. Tournier JD, Mori S, Leemans A. Diffusion tensor imaging and beyond. Magn Reson Med 2011;65:1532–56.
84. Reijmer YD, Leemans A, Heringa SM, et al. Improved sensitivity to cerebral white matter abnormalities in Alzheimer's disease with spherical deconvolution based tractography. PLoS One 2012;7:e44074.

Arterial Spin Labeling Magnetic Resonance Imaging

Intracranial and Emerging Extracranial Applications

Jill B. De Vis, MD*, Esben T. Petersen, PhD,
Jeroen Hendrikse, MD, PhD

KEYWORDS

• Arterial Spin Labeling • MR imaging • Perfusion imaging

KEY POINTS

- Arterial Spin Labeling magnetic resonance (MR) imaging offers a noninvasive approach to studying perfusion.
- Arterial Spin Labeling MR imaging can be used to evaluate cerebral blood flow, cerebrovascular reactivity, oxygen extraction fraction, and cerebral metabolic rate of oxygen.
- Territorial-selective Arterial Spin Labeling MR imaging can replace invasive digital subtraction angiography in the evaluation of perfusion territories.
- Arterial Spin Labeling MR imaging is repeatable and can monitor treatment effects.

INTRODUCTION

To date, PET has been the method of choice for obtaining in vivo measurements of organ metabolism, defined by means of cerebral metabolic rate of oxygen ($CMRo_2$), oxygen extraction fraction (OEF), and cerebral metabolic rate of glucose. Disadvantages of PET are the use of radioactive isotopes, and the requirement of a nearby cyclotron. Because organ metabolism is driven by perfusion, which allocates the delivery of oxygen and nutrients toward the tissue, perfusion techniques have been used as a surrogate to evaluate metabolism. However, xenon-enhanced Computed Tomography (CT), contrast-enhanced CT, and dynamic susceptibility contrast (DSC) magnetic resonance (MR) imaging still require the administration of a radioactive tracer, the exposure to radiation, or the injection of a contrast agent, which potentially can lead to the development of nephrogenic systemic fibrosis (NSF).[1] In the 1990s, Arterial Spin Labeling (ASL) MR imaging emerged as a noninvasive tool to evaluate perfusion in the brain. With this technique, water molecules in the neck are inverted and imaging is performed after a certain delay time that allows the inverted arterial water molecules to travel to the brain and exchange with water molecules in the brain tissue. The main asset of ASL is its noninvasiveness, which allows repeated measurements and enables evaluation of perfusion during the disease course. In addition, the ability to assess perfusion territories of individual arteries with territorial-selective ASL (TASL)[2] is a benefit that no other perfusion technique possesses, with the exception of digital subtraction angiography (DSA). A good agreement between noninvasive TASL and DSA has recently been shown,[3] which makes TASL the method of choice for (follow-up) assessment of collaterals, given its noninvasiveness. Since

Department of Radiology, University Medical Center Utrecht, Postbus 85500, Hp. E01.132, 3508 GA Utrecht, The Netherlands
* Corresponding author.
E-mail address: j.devis-2@umcutrecht.nl

PET Clin 8 (2013) 295–309
http://dx.doi.org/10.1016/j.cpet.2013.03.003
1556-8598/13/$ – see front matter

the development of the technique, ASL MR imaging has been implemented in a wide variety of diseases and recent adaptations to the technique make evaluation of $CMRO_2$ and OEF possible. For instance, T_2-Relaxation-Under-Spin-Tagging (TRUST) MR imaging[4] enables measurement of venular oxygen saturation in the sagittal sinus. When arterial partial oxygen pressure is measured, global OEF can be estimated. A combined approach of TRUST-MR imaging and ASL MR imaging allows a global estimation of $CMRO_2$. Another recent advance in ASL MR imaging, velocity-selective spin labeling (VSSL),[5] can direct perfusion signal toward the venular compartment and, as such, makes localized $CMRO_2$ measurements possible when a T_2-based approach is used (QUantitative Imaging of eXtraction of Oxygen and TIssue Consumption [QUIXOTIC]).[6] In addition, a comprehensive neurofunctional workup, providing OEF, arterial O_2 content, $CMRO_2$, cerebral blood flow (CBF), and cerebrovascular reactivity (CVR), can be achieved with quantitative O_2 imaging (QUO_2), in which a dual-echo ASL sequence is acquired during a hyperoxic and hypercapnic gas manipulation.[7] ASL MR imaging recently became part of the standard software package of most of the vendors, which makes assessment of perfusion with ASL MR imaging in daily clinical practice feasible. Further research is necessary to bring OEF and $CMRo_2$ measurements based on new ASL approaches into the clinics. In the following paragraphs the ASL technique will be discussed, and a descriptive overview of the clinical applications is given.

IMAGING TECHNIQUE

ASL MR imaging is a noninvasive tool that magnetizes arterial water molecules in the neck region by applying radiofrequency (RF) pulses. These inverted or saturated water molecules are imaged after a certain delay time that allows the labeled water molecules to reach the capillary vasculature in the brain and exchange with water molecules in the brain tissue. Two phases in ASL MR imaging can be distinguished: the preparation phase, in which inflowing blood is labeled (**Fig. 1**), and the acquisition phase, in which perfusion-weighted images are acquired. By alternating between the acquisition of labeled images and control images, which only differ in the magnetized state of arterial blood, paired label-control images are obtained. A subtraction image, control image minus label image, reflects the perfusion signal. The signal difference between both images is only a small fraction (1%–2%) of the tissue signal. To obtain sufficient signal/noise ratio (SNR), the acquisition of the paired label-control images is repeated multiple times and ASL is preferably performed at higher field strengths. A summation of all the images provides the perfusion-weighted ΔM image. The relation between the ΔM signal and perfusion depends on the longitudinal relaxation rate of tissue (T_{1t}) and blood (T_{1b}), the proton density, and on transit time of the labeled blood toward the brain tissue. Taking all these factors in account, perfusion can be quantified using either a single compartment[8,9] or a multicompartment model,[10] based on the tracer clearance theory.[11]

Based on differences in preparation phase, 4 main ASL MR imaging techniques can be distinguished: pulsed ASL (PASL), continuous ASL (CASL), pseudocontinuous ASL (pCASL), and VSSL (**Fig. 2**, **Table 1**).

PASL

In PASL a thick slab (10–15 cm) of arterial water molecules is inverted proximal to the imaging slice (see **Fig. 2**A) at a single time point using short RF pulses (5–20 ms).[12] Because of the imperfect inversion profile, a gap (of 1–2 cm) is left between the labeling and imaging planes. Labeling is performed at one moment in time, after which the magnetically labeled water molecules perfuse the brain tissue. Within the labeling slab, the arterial water closest to the brain has a shorter travel distance to the brain tissue compared with the arterial water in the arteries at the most caudal part of the labeling slab. The travel distance and travel time of the labeled water consequently differ within the labeling slab. Furthermore, compared with CASL and pCASL, the amount of labeled water is smaller because of the fixed width of the labeling slab leading to lower SNR. In contrast, the inversion efficiency of PASL (95%)[13] is higher and lower levels of RF are deposited into the tissue, which is advantageous in pediatric or neonatal imaging (see **Fig. 2**A, see **Table 1**).

CASL

Contrary to PASL, CASL uses a flow-driven adiabatic inversion in a confined plane in close proximity to the imaging plane (see **Fig. 2**B),[9,14] which minimizes loss of perfusion signal caused by T_1 relaxation, which leads to higher SNR. In addition, the typical duration of the labeling pulses results in a larger labeled bolus of arterial water protons compared with PASL. Disadvantages are the lower inversion efficiency (80%–90%)[13] and the application of continuous RF transmit hardware, which is not available on most scanners. Furthermore, specific absorption rate (SAR) can exceed US Food and Drug Administration (FDA)

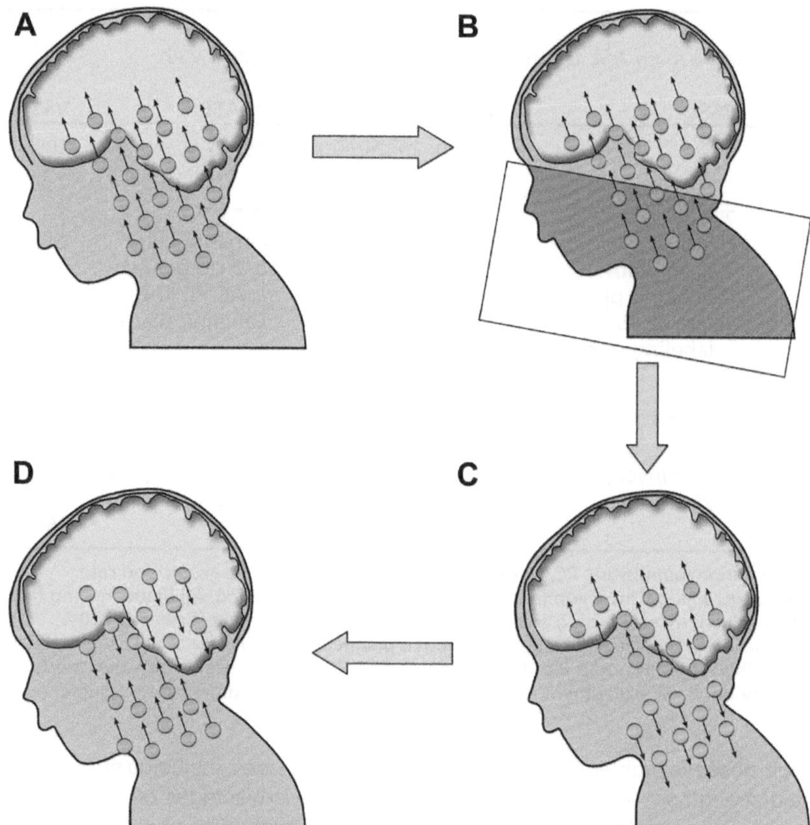

Fig. 1. ASL technique; the preparation phase. (*A*) All water molecules (*green*) align according to the magnetic field after the subject has been positioned in the scanner. (*B*) A pulsed ASL experiment in which a labeling slab of 10 to 15 cm is positioned in the neck region. By applying a single inversion pulse within this plane, the water molecules are inverted. (*C*) All water molecules in the neck region are inverted with the ASL labeling pulse (*blue*). (*D*) The arterial inverted water molecules travel via the blood toward the brain tissue and exchange there with water molecules in the tissue. At this moment, the acquisition phase is started.

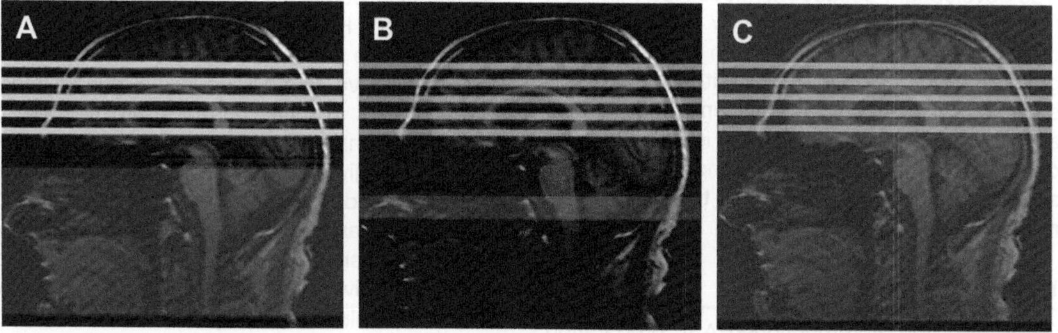

Fig. 2. The labeling plane (*full green plane*) and imaging plane (*green stripes*) in an ASL experiment. (*A*) Pulsed ASL; the labeling plane (10–15 cm) is positioned proximal to the imaging plane, in the neck. (*B*) The labeling and imaging planes for a continuous or a pseudocontinuous ASL experiment. The labeling plane (1–2 cm) is positioned in close proximity to the imaging plane. The continuous ASL technique differs from the pseudocontinuous ASL technique in how the labeling is achieved. The continuous technique inverts hydrogen protons by applying continuous RF pulses; in the pseudocontinuous experiment a train of short RF pulses is applied. (*C*) Positioning of the labeling and imaging planes in a VSSL experiment. Labeling is performed in the same region as imaging. This technique eliminates transit time differences because labeling is performed at the tissue level, which ensures a uniform arrival of labeled signal.

Table 1
The properties of the 4 main ASL techniques: PASL, CASL, pCASL, and VSSL

	PASL	CASL	pCASL	VSSL
Labeling efficiency (%)	95	80–90	85–95	50[a]
SNR	++	+++	++++	+
Labeling area	Fixed 1–2 cm below imaging plane 10-cm to 15-cm labeling slab	Perpendicular[b] 8–9 cm below AC-PC line Labeling plane	Perpendicular[b] 8–9 cm below AC-PC line Labeling plane	Global[a]
SAR	+	+++[c]	++	+
Sensitivity to transit delays	+++++	+++	+++	+
Labeling method	Single inversion pulse 5–20 ms	Continuous RF pulse 1–2 s	Train of RF pulses 1–2 s	Velocity-encoding module[a] 15–30 ms

Abbreviations: AC, anterior commissure; PC, posterior commissure; SAR, specific absorption rate.

[a] In a VSSL experiment, a global inversion (entire-body coil coverage) is applied. All blood moving faster than a predefined velocity cutoff value is inverted using a velocity-encoding module with an efficiency of 50%.

[b] The labeling plane in a (pseudo)continuous experiment is planned perpendicular to both internal carotid arteries and to the basilar artery. This is usually about 8 to 9 cm below the AC-PC line (line drawn between the AC and PC).

[c] The SAR in a continuous ASL experiment may exceed US Food and Drug Administration guidelines at 3 T.

guidelines, which poses a problem when moving on to higher field strengths[15] or when implementing CASL in pediatric or neonatal MR imaging protocols (see **Fig. 2**B, see **Table 1**).

pCASL

To overcome the disadvantages of CASL, such as lower inversion efficiency and high RF power deposition, but still maintain the advantages of higher SNR and uniform travel distance, pCASL[16] was developed. Pseudocontinuous ASL mimics a flow-driven adiabatic inversion by using a train of discrete RF pulses combined with a simultaneous gradient field (see **Fig. 2**C). With this labeling scheme, a higher inversion efficiency (85%–95%) and lower RF power deposition is achieved. To date, pCASL is the most commonly used ASL sequence and is thought to have the best performance (see **Fig. 2**B, see **Table 1**).

VSSL

Contrary to the aforementioned ASL preparation schemes, VSSL[5] saturates arterial water molecules based on velocity rather than spatial location. Blood traveling within the imaging plane is saturated when traveling at a higher speed than the preset cutoff value. With this approach, a uniform transit time is ensured.[17] This property makes VSSL beneficial when slow or collateral flow is encountered, which is the case in several clinical circumstances, including stroke or moyamoya disease. Disadvantages of VSSL are the lower SNR caused by the use of saturation pulses instead of inversion pulses, as applied in PASL, CASL, and pCASL. In general, VSSL is less widely available compared with the other labeling schemes (see **Fig. 2**C, see **Table 1**).

IMAGING FINDINGS

Using the previously described techniques, high signal/noise perfusion-weighted MR images can be obtained. However, ASL MR imaging is still susceptible to a few commonly encountered artifacts that have to be recognized during image interpretation. For this purpose, an overview of the most common artifacts and their respective solutions is given in **Table 2**. ASL MR imaging has been used in a wide variety of diseases with a spectrum ranging from ischemic brain lesions to cystic fibrosis (CF), and an overview of most applications is given in **Box 1**. A descriptive overview of these applications is given, subdivided into adult ASL MR imaging, pediatric ASL MR imaging, and neonatal ASL MR imaging.

ASL MR Imaging in Adult Subjects

Brain perfusion imaging

When evaluating ASL brain perfusion images it is important to be aware of the influence of physiologic properties. For instance, a reduced CBF

Table 2
Causes, representation, and solutions of commonly encountered artifacts on ASL MR imaging

Artifact	Cause	Representation	Solution
Motion and other physiologic noise	Motion, respiration, and so forth	Increase or decrease in signal intensity on a focal or global basis	Prior saturation of imaging plane Background suppression Realignment of images Filter that detects and discards bad subtraction pairs[81]
Transit time artifact			
Healthy volunteers	Late arrival in border zones	Invalid absolute and relative quantification	QUIPSS II[92] Q2-TIPS[93]
Atherosclerosis	Transit time >2.0 s Low perfusion velocity Extensive collateral perfusion	Invalid absolute and relative quantification	Imaging at multiple inversion delays Look-Locker[34] Quasar[33]
Vascular artifact	Labeled arterial blood in vasculature	Error in CBF quantification (overestimation)	Bipolar crusher gradients[94] Longer inversion time
Susceptibility artifact	Echo planar imaging readout	Signal intensity void in case of metallic hardware, blood products, calcification, air	Spiral sequences Multishot 3D sequences
Gadolinium artifact	Gadolinium shortens T_1 in all tissues	Maps with almost no usable signal intensity	ASL imaging before gadolinium administration

Abbreviations: 3D, three-dimensional; QUIPSS, Quantitative Imaging of Perfusion Using a Single Subtraction; Q2-TIPS, QUIPSS II with thin-slice periodic saturation.

and prolonged bolus arrival time and arterial-arteriole transit time with advancing age has been shown with ASL,[18] similar to PET imaging findings,[19] and has to be taken into account when interpreting ASL MR images. In the wide range of diseases that have been studied with ASL, cerebrovascular diseases are the commonest. ASL MR imaging is able to show hypoperfusion,[20] luxury perfusion, and delayed transit time[21] after an ischemic event. These findings were proved to be similar to DSC MR imaging findings.[22] ASL offers some additional opportunities compared with DSC MR imaging. By combining ASL MR imaging with a vasodilatory stimulus, such as acetazolamide or a CO_2 challenge, CVR can be assessed, which provides an insight in the brain's capacity to manage decreased perfusion pressure. Previous ASL studies have shown a decreased CVR in patients with cerebrovascular disease.[23] Examples of ASL perfusion images before and after the administration of acetazolamide, and the resulting reactivity map of a patient with carotid artery occlusion, are shown in **Fig. 3**. Until recently, evaluation of other hemodynamic parameters (such as OEF and $CMRo_2$) that may also be affected when perfusion pressure is decreased[24,25] was only possible with PET. However, recent advances in ASL MR imaging enable full assessment of the hemodynamic cascade. Global OEF can be measured using TRUST-MR imaging[4] and regional OEF values can be obtained with QUIXOTIC.[6] Cerebral metabolic rate of oxygen can be estimated based on regional or global OEF techniques in combination with CBF measurements, or regional $CMRo_2$ can be assessed using QUO_2.[7] In addition to assessment of all hemodynamic parameters, TASL allows perfusion territory assessment, which is especially important because the perfusion territory responsible for infarction is misclassified in 10% of patients when evaluated based on conventional MR imaging alone.[26] Furthermore, TASL can be used to evaluate collateral perfusion pathways after an ischemic event[27] and to assess changes in perfusion territories after extracranial-intracranial bypass surgery.[28] **Fig. 4** shows how labeling is performed in a TASL experiment. In addition, ASL perfusion territory images are shown.

Box 1
Clinical applications of ASL MR imaging

Clinical applications

- Adults
  - Brain perfusion imaging
    - Cerebrovascular diseases
      - Ischemic events
        - Stroke
        - Transient ischemic event
      - Steno-occlusive disease
      - Moyamoya disease
      - Vascular malformations
    - Brain tumors
    - Epilepsy
    - Alzheimer disease
  - Renal perfusion imaging
  - Leg perfusion imaging
  - Cardiac perfusion imaging
- Pediatric imaging
  - Brain perfusion imaging
    - Cerebrovascular disease
      - Ischemic events
        - Stroke
    - Sickle cell disease
  - Lung perfusion imaging
    - CF
- Neonatal imaging
  - Brain perfusion imaging
    - Ischemic events
      - Cerebrovascular disease
        - Stroke
      - Asphyxia
    - Congenital heart defects

Although all these advantages of ASL MR imaging favor its use in daily clinical work-up of patients with stroke or transient ischemic attach (TIA), its use in clinics is still hampered because of the low spatial resolution and low SNR, especially in white matter,[29,30] which means that the perfusion-diffusion mismatch, used to guide treatment in patients with stroke, is still hard to define with ASL. Studies comparing ASL with gold standard DSC MR imaging have shown a low positive predictive value (0.42)[31] and a low interrater agreement (0.51).[29] Arterial transit delays are commonly misinterpreted as penumbra. The implementation of transit time–insensitive approaches, such as acquisition at multiple inversion delays[32–34] or VSSL,[5] could be a breakthrough. In contrast, the transit time sensitivity of ASL is beneficial when evaluating collateral perfusion pathways in patients with moyamoya disease, a progressive occlusive disease of the cerebral vasculature. In these patients, collateral vessels can be identified as bright intravascular signal. Evaluation of collateral pathways is of interest in these patients because they protect against ischemia and, as such, can be used to identify patients at risk. To support the use of ASL in the evaluation of collateral arteries, collateral scoring performed on ASL images was compared with DSA collateral scoring. A sensitivity of 0.83 and specificity of 0.82[35] was shown. In addition, interrater agreement for collateral scoring was higher on ASL images. TASL may further increase identification of collateral pathways[3] in patients with moyamoya. An MR angiography image, a T_2 fluid-attenuated inversion recovery (FLAIR) image, and ASL perfusion images of a patient with moyamoya are shown in **Fig. 5**. ASL MR imaging can also be used in patients with moyamoya to evaluate hyperperfusion[36] after surgical revascularization, which is a marker for the development of transient neurologic deterioration and intracerebral hemorrhage.[37,38] ASL MR imaging can be used to identify vascular malformations such as dural arteriovenous fistula and arteriovenous malformations, both characterized by a shunt between the arterial and venous circulation. Because of this unique anatomic connection, labeled hydrogen protons do not travel through the capillary bed and as such are not extracted. Furthermore, transit time toward the venous circulation is enhanced. A combination of these two properties means that intravascular labeled signal is present in the venous circulation and can be used to identify these vascular malformations.[39,40] A comparison between ASL and gold standard DSA has shown a sensitivity of 78% and a specificity of 85% to detect these lesions with ASL.[41] Furthermore, the added value of ASL MR imaging in addition to other MR imaging sequences has been shown[41,42] and ASL has been used to evaluate treatment efficacy during follow-up.[43] ASL MR imaging is advantageous compared with DSC MR imaging in perfusion evaluation of brain tumors because contrast agent leakage can distort perfusion findings in DSC MR imaging because of T_2* and T_1 effects. Perfusion,

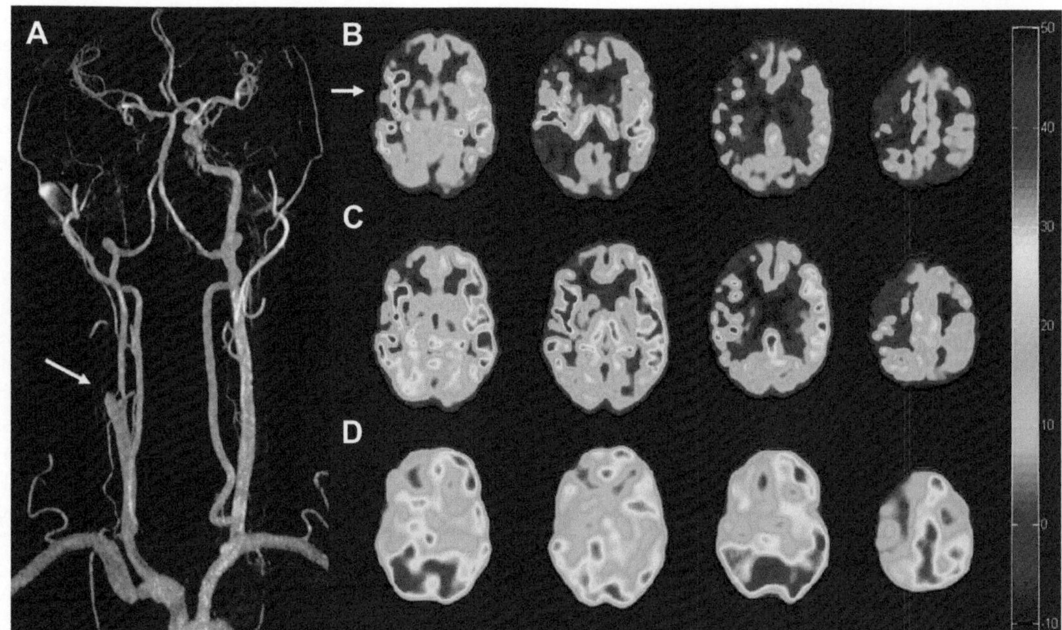

Fig. 3. MR angiography image and ASL perfusion images of a patient with occlusion of the right internal carotid artery. (*A*) MR angiography image shows an occlusion of the right internal carotid artery (*arrow*). (*B*) ASL perfusion images show lower perfusion in the right hemisphere. The color bar denotes perfusion (in mL/100 g/min). In addition, delayed arrival via collateral arteries can be appreciated because labeled signal is still present in the vasculature (*arrow*). (*C*) ASL perfusion images after intravenous administration of acetazolamide. Perfusion is increased compared with the images acquired before the administration of acetazolamide, as shown in *B*. (*D*) Resulting reactivity images; reactivity is lower in the right hemisphere.

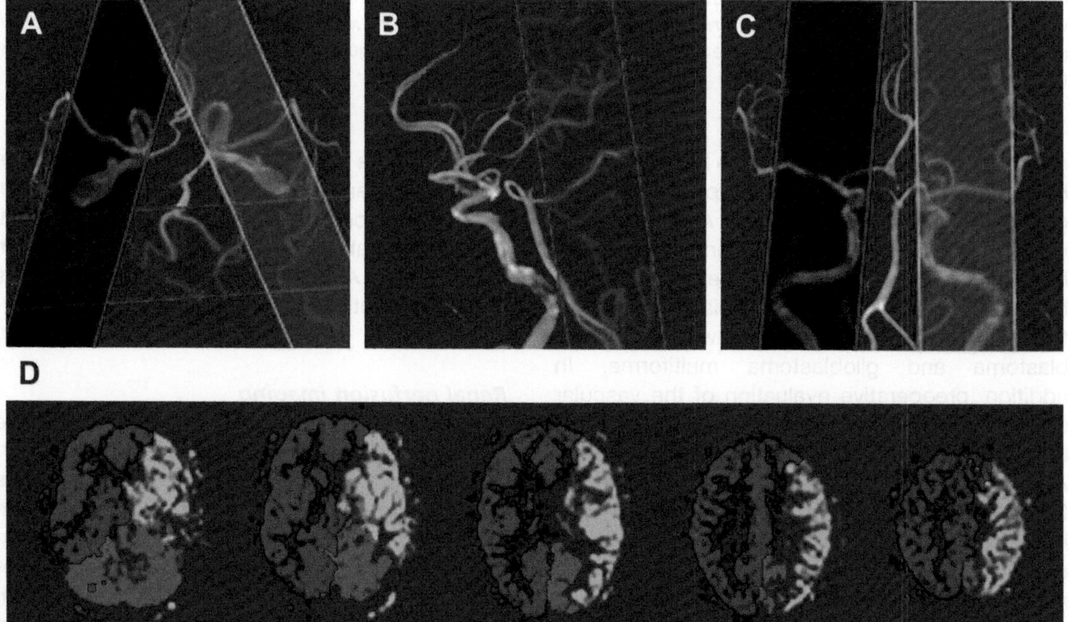

Fig. 4. A TASL experiment. Positioning of the labeling planes shown on transverse (*A*), sagittal (*B*), and coronal (*C*) maximum intensity projections of a time-of-flight image. The labeling plane covering the right internal carotid artery (ICA) is shown in red, the labeling plane covering the left ICA in green, and the labeling plane covering the vertebrobasilar arteries in blue. (*D*) TASL images from caudal to cranial, the perfusion territories of right ICA is shown in red, of the left ICA in green, and of the vertebrobasilar arteries in blue.

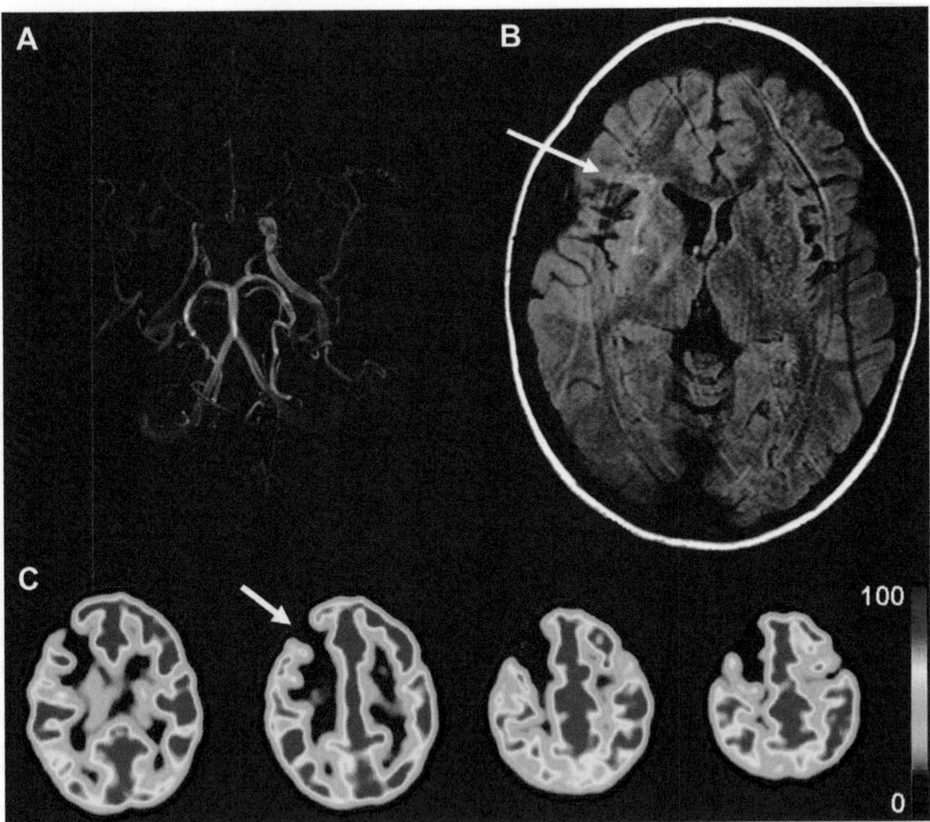

Fig. 5. MR angiography image, T_2-FLAIR image, and ASL perfusion images of a moyamoya patient. (*A*) MR angiography image shows extensive collateral perfusion pathways in this patient. (*B*) A small region of infarction is visualized on the T_2-FLAIR image (*arrow*). (*C*) ASL perfusion images show an area of lower perfusion (*arrow*) corresponding with the infarcted area as visualized on the T_2-FLAIR image. Perfusion is denoted by a color bar (in mL/100 g/min).

evaluated with ASL, was shown to be significantly higher in high-grade gliomas compared with low-grade gliomas.[44] Furthermore, ASL perfusion imaging can be used to differentiate between hemangioblastoma and brain metastasis[45] and between lymphoma and glioblastoma multiforme[46] based on higher blood flow in hemangioblastoma and glioblastoma multiforme. In addition, preoperative evaluation of the vascular supply of brain tumors can be performed using selective ASL MR imaging.[47] In epileptic patients, ASL MR imaging provides similar information as PET; interictal hypoperfusion[48–50] and (peri-)ictal hyperperfusion.[51–53] As such, ASL MR imaging can be used to localize the epileptogenic focus noninvasively. Brain perfusion in patients with Alzheimer disease, evaluated with ASL MR imaging, showed lower perfusion in the temporal, parietal, frontal, and cingulate cortices compared with healthy controls.[54–56] A relationship was shown between regional or global hypoperfusion and severity of the disease, evaluated using the Mini-Mental State Examination.[54,55] Furthermore, results of recent studies show a high correlation between hypoperfused areas shown with ASL and hypometabolic areas with FDG-PET both in patients with Alzheimer disease and in patients with more subtle cognitive impairment.[57–59]

Renal perfusion imaging

Renal ASL MR imaging possesses some unique qualities compared with dynamic contrast-enhanced (DCE) MR imaging; contrast agent is not needed and it is restricted to perfusion signal, which is in contrast with DCE-MR imaging, in which the relative contributions of permeability and blood flow are unclear. Perfusion values have been shown to be in agreement with perfusion scintigraphy measurements,[60,61] and the influence of antiangiogenic therapy on renal blood flow in patients with renal cell carcinoma and with NSF has been evaluated with ASL.[62,63]

Muscle perfusion imaging

At present, the invasive microsphere experiment[64] is the gold standard to measure skeletal muscle perfusion. ASL MR imaging offers a noninvasive approach with better spatial and temporal resolution. Experiments in rats have shown agreement between the microsphere and ASL technique,[65] and ASL MR imaging has been used to measure muscle perfusion in humans.[66–68] In subjects with peripheral artery disease (PAD), calf muscle peak hyperemic flow (PHF) has been shown to decrease and time to peak to increase with increasing disease severity. Time to peak seemed to be an early marker of PAD disease; PHF was only affected in later stages.[69]

Cardiac perfusion

Heart motion in combination with multiple label-control experiments make assessment of cardiac perfusion with ASL MR imaging challenging. Some proof-of-principle studies have been performed[70,71] and more developments are expected in ASL cardiac perfusion MR imaging.

ASL MR Imaging in Pediatric Subjects

ASL MR imaging in the pediatric population possesses some unique properties compared with ASL MR imaging in the adult population. First, increased CBF, peaking around the age of 4 to 11 years[72] and estimated to be 30% higher compared with adults,[72,73] contributes to higher SNR in this population. In addition, the higher water content of the brain increases the equilibrium MR signal (M_0), and the spin-lattice (T_1) and the spin-spin relaxation times (T_2),[73–75] also contributing to higher SNR. Furthermore, the greater the blood water signal (blood M_o) leading to higher tracer quantity, the longer T_1 of blood[76] which impels a longer tracer lifetime and the faster mean transit time also accord to the higher SNR. Overall, SNR increases by 70% in the pediatric population compared with the adult population.[73] Another advantage of pediatric ASL perfusion imaging is the smaller susceptibility artifact in the orbitofrontal region as a result of the sinuses not being fully developed.[77] Both aspects contribute to a better image quality in the pediatric population, which means that ASL MR imaging is increasingly being implemented in pediatric clinical examination or clinical studies.

Brain perfusion imaging

ASL MR imaging can be used to monitor the brain development of infants by evaluating regional perfusion changes with age.[78] It has also been used to evaluate brain perfusion in the (sub)acute stage and at follow-up in pediatric patients with stroke. Hypoperfusion in stroke lesions was shown to be associated with larger infarct volumes at initial examination and at follow-up compared with hyperperfused and normal perfused lesions. Furthermore, it was shown that regions in which delayed arterial transit were visualized did not evolve into infarcted tissue.[79] Another clinical application is the evaluation of brain perfusion in children with sickle cell disease. Sickle cell disease is a chronic disease characterized by a sickle-shaped appearance of deoxygenated red blood cells leading to hemolytic anemia and vascular occlusions. Chronic anemia leads to hyperemia, which presents as increased brain perfusion.[80,81] Detection of sickle cell patients with increased brain perfusion is important because an inverse correlation with normal intelligence quotient has been documented.[82] Hydroxyurea treatment has been shown to decrease gray matter perfusion in these patients, which means that ASL MR imaging can also be used to study therapy effectiveness.[83]

Lung perfusion imaging

ASL MR imaging has recently been used to investigate regional lung function in infants with CF. CF is a chronic lung disease that requires lifelong monitoring. Imaging techniques that are commonly used, such as lung perfusion scintigraphy and ventilation scintigraphy, require ionizing radiation, which poses a problem in this young population with increasing life-span. ASL MR imaging offers a noninvasive alternative that can visualize regional hypoperfusion provoked by regional ventilatory obstruction. One study was able to show lower perfusion in the upper lobes of patients with CF, which corresponds with the pathologic distribution in CF. Furthermore, a correlation between perfusion values and pulmonary function was shown.[84] Although results seem promising, research is still preliminary with only single-slice experiments. In addition, results depend on the patient's compliance with breath-holding experiments, which makes this approach less suited for young patients with CF.

ASL MR Imaging in Neonatal Subjects

In contrast with the advantages experienced in the pediatric population, ASL MR imaging in the neonatal population is challenging. Lower perfusion values[85] result in lower SNR, and a longer longitudinal relaxation rate of blood[86] causes a longer tracer lifetime, resulting in negative perfusion.[87] These technical difficulties have delayed the implementation of ASL MR imaging in the neonatal population.

Brain perfusion imaging

Implementation of ASL MR imaging in the neonatal population has been limited to brain perfusion imaging. ASL MR imaging can be used to evaluate brain development[85]; an increase in whole-brain perfusion with advancing postconceptional age has been shown and regional changes in relative brain perfusion are correlated with brain maturation. **Fig. 6** shows ASL brain perfusion images of neonates scanned at preterm age, at term-equivalent age, and at 3 months–equivalent age; an increase in brain perfusion with increasing postmenstrual age can be appreciated. ASL has also been used to evaluate brain perfusion in neonates with congenital heart defects (CHDs)[88] and in neonates who had an ischemic event such as asphyxia or stroke.[89–91] Promising results were achieved; in infants with CHD-related periventricular leukomalacia, brain perfusion and CVR were shown to be decreased and ASL MR imaging was able to show regions of hypoperfusion and hyperperfusion in infants with perinatal arterial ischemic stroke.[90] In addition, a recent study showed an association between the apparent diffusion coefficient, measured on diffusion-weighted imaging, and perfusion in infants with cerebral ischemic injury, either asphyxia or stroke.[89] **Fig. 7** shows diffusion-weighted images and

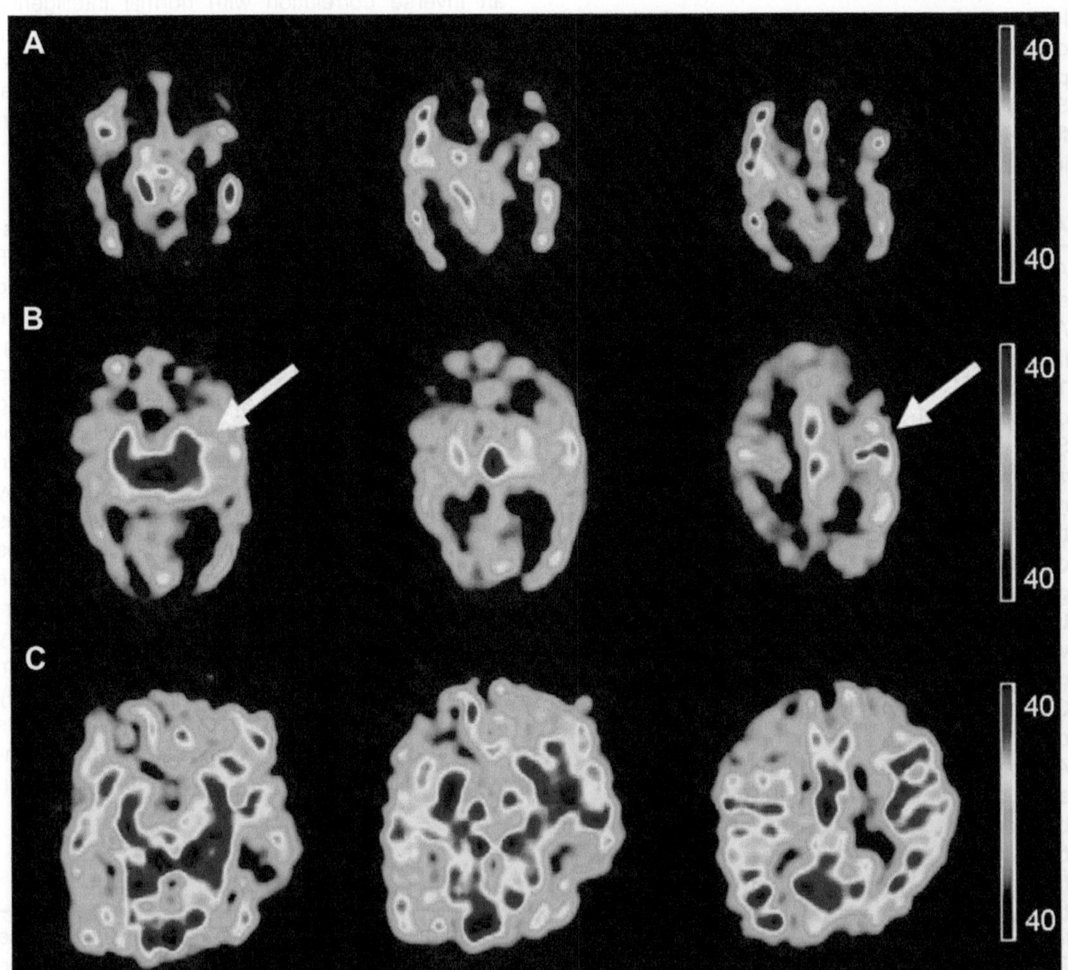

Fig. 6. Transverse ASL MR images of 3 neonates. The color bars denote perfusion given in mL/100 g/min. (*A*) Infant born prematurely at 29 weeks' postconceptional age. ASL MR imaging was performed at a postconceptional age of 31 weeks. (*B*) Preterm infant, born at 28 weeks' postconceptional age, ASL MR imaging was performed at 41 weeks' postconceptional age. (*C*) Infant born at 36 weeks' postconceptional age, scan performed at 49 weeks' postconceptional age. Note the increase in brain perfusion with increasing postconceptional age at the time of scan. Also note the higher perfusion visualized in the area corresponding with the basal ganglia and the sensorimotor cortex in the second neonate (*arrows*).

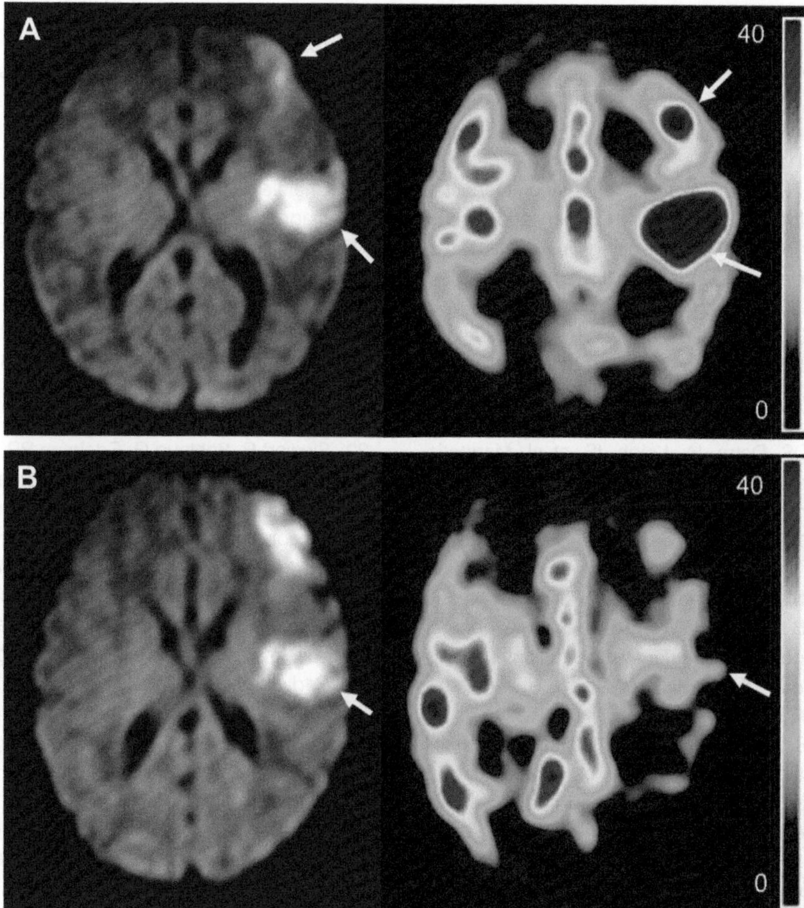

Fig. 7. Infant with perinatal arterial ischemic stroke at day 2 after birth. Stroke in the territory of the left middle cerebral artery (MCA) was confirmed with MR imaging performed on day 3. (*A*) Diffusion-weighted imaging shows diffusion restriction in 2 areas within the territory of the left MCA (*arrows*). Corresponding ASL image shows luxury perfusion in these 2 areas (*arrows*). (*B*) Follow-up MR imaging performed on day 6. Diffusion restriction is still visible in the two areas. Corresponding ASL perfusion MR images show no more luxury perfusion. A hypoperfused area is visible within the territory of the left MCA compared with the contralateral hemisphere (*arrow*).

corresponding ASL perfusion images of a neonate with perinatal stroke.

SUMMARY

ASL MR imaging offers a noninvasive approach to assessing perfusion. This perfusion technique has been successfully implemented in a wide variety of diseases, of which cerebrovascular diseases have been investigated most commonly. ASL software recently became part of the standard software package on clinical MR scanners, which has led to the increasing implementation of ASL in daily clinical practice. Furthermore, recent developments in ASL techniques enable full hemodynamic assessment, offering a window for future opportunities.

ACKNOWLEDGMENTS

We thank Dr Nolan S. Hartkamp and Dr Reinoud P.H. Bokkers for providing images.

REFERENCES

1. Grobner T. Gadolinium–a specific trigger for the development of nephrogenic fibrosing dermopathy and nephrogenic systemic fibrosis? Nephrol Dial Transplant 2006;21:1104–8.
2. Hendrikse J, van der GJ, Lu H, et al. Flow territory mapping of the cerebral arteries with regional perfusion MRI. Stroke 2004;35:882–7.
3. Chng SM, Petersen ET, Zimine I, et al. Territorial arterial spin labeling in the assessment of collateral circulation: comparison with digital subtraction angiography. Stroke 2008;39:3248–54.

4. Lu H, Ge Y. Quantitative evaluation of oxygenation in venous vessels using T2-relaxation-under-spin-tagging MRI. Magn Reson Med 2008;60:357–63.
5. Wong EC, Cronin M, Wu WC, et al. Velocity-selective arterial spin labeling. Magn Reson Med 2006; 55:1334–41.
6. Bolar DS, Rosen BR, Sorensen AG, et al. Quantitative Imaging of Extraction of Oxygen and Tissue Consumption (QUIXOTIC) using venular-targeted velocity-selective spin labeling. Magn Reson Med 2011;66:1550–62.
7. Gauthier CJ, Hoge RD. Magnetic resonance imaging of resting OEF and CMRO(2) using a generalized calibration model for hypercapnia and hyperoxia. Neuroimage 2012;60:1212–25.
8. Williams DS, Detre JA, Leigh JS, et al. Magnetic resonance imaging of perfusion using spin inversion of arterial water. Proc Natl Acad Sci U S A 1992;89:212–6.
9. Detre JA, Leigh JS, Williams DS, et al. Perfusion imaging. Magn Reson Med 1992;23:37–45.
10. Buxton RB, Frank LR, Wong EC, et al. A general kinetic model for quantitative perfusion imaging with arterial spin labeling. Magn Reson Med 1998;40:383–96.
11. Kety SS, Schmidt CF. The nitrous oxide method for the quantitative determination of cerebral blood flow in man: theory, procedure and normal values. J Clin Invest 1948;27:476–83.
12. Edelman RR, Siewert B, Darby DG, et al. Qualitative mapping of cerebral blood flow and functional localization with echo-planar MR imaging and signal targeting with alternating radio frequency. Radiology 1994;192:513–20.
13. Petersen ET, Zimine I, Ho YC, et al. Non-invasive measurement of perfusion: a critical review of arterial spin labelling techniques. Br J Radiol 2006;79: 688–701.
14. Williams DS, Grandis DJ, Zhang W, et al. Magnetic resonance imaging of perfusion in the isolated rat heart using spin inversion of arterial water. Magn Reson Med 1993;30:361–5.
15. Wang J, Zhang Y, Wolf RL, et al. Amplitude-modulated continuous arterial spin-labeling 3.0-T perfusion MR imaging with a single coil: feasibility study. Radiology 2005;235:218–28.
16. Dai W, Garcia D, de Bazelaire C, et al. Continuous flow-driven inversion for arterial spin labeling using pulsed radio frequency and gradient fields. Magn Reson Med 2008;60:1488–97.
17. Qiu D, Straka M, Zun Z, et al. CBF measurements using multidelay pseudocontinuous and velocity-selective arterial spin labeling in patients with long arterial transit delays: comparison with xenon CT CBF. J Magn Reson Imaging 2012;36:110–9.
18. Liu Y, Zhu X, Feinberg D, et al. Arterial spin labeling MRI study of age and gender effects on brain perfusion hemodynamics. Magn Reson Med 2012;68:912–22.
19. Leenders KL, Perani D, Lammertsma AA, et al. Cerebral blood flow, blood volume and oxygen utilization. Normal values and effect of age. Brain 1990;113:27–47.
20. Chalela JA, Alsop DC, Gonzalez-Atavales JB, et al. Magnetic resonance perfusion imaging in acute ischemic stroke using continuous arterial spin labeling. Stroke 2000;31:680–7.
21. MacIntosh BJ, Lindsay AC, Kylintireas I, et al. Multiple inflow pulsed arterial spin-labeling reveals delays in the arterial arrival time in minor stroke and transient ischemic attack. AJNR Am J Neuroradiol 2010;31:1892–4.
22. Siewert B, Schlaug G, Edelman RR, et al. Comparison of EPISTAR and T2*-weighted gadolinium-enhanced perfusion imaging in patients with acute cerebral ischemia. Neurology 1997;48:673–9.
23. Bokkers RP, van Osch MJ, van der Worp HB, et al. Symptomatic carotid artery stenosis: impairment of cerebral autoregulation measured at the brain tissue level with arterial spin-labeling MR imaging. Radiology 2010;256:201–8.
24. Derdeyn CP, Videen TO, Yundt KD, et al. Variability of cerebral blood volume and oxygen extraction: stages of cerebral haemodynamic impairment revisited. Brain 2002;125:595–607.
25. Powers WJ. Cerebral hemodynamics in ischemic cerebrovascular disease. Ann Neurol 1991;29: 231–40.
26. Hendrikse J, Petersen ET, Cheze A, et al. Relation between cerebral perfusion territories and location of cerebral infarcts. Stroke 2009;40:1617–22.
27. van Laar PJ, Hendrikse J, Klijn CJ, et al. Symptomatic carotid artery occlusion: flow territories of major brain-feeding arteries. Radiology 2007;242: 526–34.
28. Golay X, Hendrikse J, van der GJ. Application of regional perfusion imaging to extra-intracranial bypass surgery and severe stenoses. J Neuroradiol 2005;32:321–4.
29. Bokkers RP, Hernandez DA, Merino JG, et al. Whole-brain arterial spin labeling perfusion MRI in patients with acute stroke. Stroke 2012;43:1290–4.
30. Viallon M, Altrichter S, Pereira VM, et al. Combined use of pulsed arterial spin-labeling and susceptibility-weighted imaging in stroke at 3T. Eur Neurol 2010;64:286–96.
31. Zaharchuk G, El Mogy IS, Fischbein NJ, et al. Comparison of arterial spin labeling and bolus perfusion-weighted imaging for detecting mismatch in acute stroke. Stroke 2012;43:1843–8.
32. Hendrikse J, van Osch MJ, Rutgers DR, et al. Internal carotid artery occlusion assessed at pulsed arterial spin-labeling perfusion MR imaging at multiple delay times. Radiology 2004;233:899–904.

33. Petersen ET, Lim T, Golay X. Model-free arterial spin labeling quantification approach for perfusion MRI. Magn Reson Med 2006;55:219–32.
34. Gunther M, Bock M, Schad LR. Arterial spin labeling in combination with a look-locker sampling strategy: inflow turbo-sampling EPI-FAIR (ITS-FAIR). Magn Reson Med 2001;46:974–84.
35. Zaharchuk G, Do HM, Marks MP, et al. Arterial spin-labeling MRI can identify the presence and intensity of collateral perfusion in patients with moyamoya disease. Stroke 2011;42:2485–91.
36. Sugino T, Mikami T, Miyata K, et al. Arterial spin-labeling magnetic resonance imaging after revascularization of moyamoya disease. J Stroke Cerebrovasc Dis 2012. [Epub ahead of print].
37. Fujimura M, Shimizu H, Mugikura S, et al. Delayed intracerebral hemorrhage after superficial temporal artery-middle cerebral artery anastomosis in a patient with moyamoya disease: possible involvement of cerebral hyperperfusion and increased vascular permeability. Surg Neurol 2009;71:223–7.
38. Fujimura M, Shimizu H, Inoue T, et al. Significance of focal cerebral hyperperfusion as a cause of transient neurologic deterioration after extracranial-intracranial bypass for moyamoya disease: comparative study with non-moyamoya patients using *N*-isopropyl-p-[(123)I]iodoamphetamine single-photon emission computed tomography. Neurosurgery 2011;68:957–64.
39. Wolf RL, Wang J, Detre JA, et al. Arteriovenous shunt visualization in arteriovenous malformations with arterial spin-labeling MR imaging. AJNR Am J Neuroradiol 2008;29:681–7.
40. Noguchi K, Kuwayama N, Kubo M, et al. Flow-sensitive alternating inversion recovery (fair) imaging for retrograde cortical venous drainage related to intracranial dural arteriovenous fistula. Neuroradiology 2011;53:153–8.
41. Le TT, Fischbein NJ, Andre JB, et al. Identification of venous signal on arterial spin labeling improves diagnosis of dural arteriovenous fistulas and small arteriovenous malformations. AJNR Am J Neuroradiol 2012;33:61–8.
42. Kukuk GM, Hadizadeh DR, Bostrom A, et al. Cerebral arteriovenous malformations at 3.0 T: intraindividual comparative study of 4D-MRA in combination with selective arterial spin labeling and digital subtraction angiography. Invest Radiol 2010;45:126–32.
43. Pollock JM, Whitlow CT, Simonds J, et al. Response of arteriovenous malformations to gamma knife therapy evaluated with pulsed arterial spin-labeling MRI perfusion. AJR Am J Roentgenol 2011;196:15–22.
44. Warmuth C, Gunther M, Zimmer C. Quantification of blood flow in brain tumors: comparison of arterial spin labeling and dynamic susceptibility-weighted contrast-enhanced MR imaging. Radiology 2003; 228:523–32.
45. Yamashita K, Yoshiura T, Hiwatashi A, et al. Arterial spin labeling of hemangioblastoma: differentiation from metastatic brain tumors based on quantitative blood flow measurement. Neuroradiology 2012;54: 809–13.
46. Yamashita K, Yoshiura T, Hiwatashi A, et al. Differentiating primary CNS lymphoma from glioblastoma multiforme: assessment using arterial spin labeling, diffusion-weighted imaging, and (18)F-fluorodeoxyglucose positron emission tomography. Neuroradiology 2012;55(2):135–43.
47. Helle M, Janssen O. Presurgical assessment of the feeding vasculature in extra-axial tumors with superselective arterial spin labeling. Proceedings of the 19th annual meeting ISMRM. Montreal (Québec): 2011.
48. Lim YM, Cho YW, Shamim S, et al. Usefulness of pulsed arterial spin labeling MR imaging in mesial temporal lobe epilepsy. Epilepsy Res 2008;82: 183–9.
49. Wolf RL, Alsop DC, Levy-Reis I, et al. Detection of mesial temporal lobe hypoperfusion in patients with temporal lobe epilepsy by use of arterial spin labeled perfusion MR imaging. AJNR Am J Neuroradiol 2001;22:1334–41.
50. Pendse N, Wissmeyer M, Altrichter S, et al. Interictal arterial spin-labeling MRI perfusion in intractable epilepsy. J Neuroradiol 2010;37:60–3.
51. Oishi M, Ishida G, Morii K, et al. Ictal focal hyperperfusion demonstrated by arterial spin-labeling perfusion MRI in partial epilepsy status. Neuroradiology 2012;54:653–6.
52. Pizzini F, Farace P, Zanoni T, et al. Pulsed-arterial-spin-labeling perfusion 3T MRI following single seizure: a first case report study. Epilepsy Res 2008;81:225–7.
53. Toledo M, Munuera J, Salas-Puig X, et al. Localisation value of ictal arterial spin-labelled sequences in partial seizures. Epileptic Disord 2011;13:336–9.
54. Alsop DC, Detre JA, Grossman M. Assessment of cerebral blood flow in Alzheimer's disease by spin-labeled magnetic resonance imaging. Ann Neurol 2000;47:93–100.
55. Mak HK, Chan Q, Zhang Z, et al. Quantitative assessment of cerebral hemodynamic parameters by QUASAR arterial spin labeling in Alzheimer's disease and cognitively normal elderly adults at 3-Tesla. J Alzheimers Dis 2012;31:33–44.
56. Yoshiura T, Hiwatashi A, Yamashita K, et al. Simultaneous measurement of arterial transit time, arterial blood volume, and cerebral blood flow using arterial spin-labeling in patients with Alzheimer disease. AJNR Am J Neuroradiol 2009;30:1388–93.
57. Chen Y, Wolk DA, Reddin JS, et al. Voxel-level comparison of arterial spin-labeled perfusion MRI and

FDG-PET in Alzheimer disease. Neurology 2011; 77:1977–85.
58. Musiek ES, Chen Y, Korczykowski M, et al. Direct comparison of fluorodeoxyglucose positron emission tomography and arterial spin labeling magnetic resonance imaging in Alzheimer's disease. Alzheimers Dement 2012;8:51–9.
59. Xu G, Rowley HA, Wu G, et al. Reliability and precision of pseudo-continuous arterial spin labeling perfusion MRI on 3.0 T and comparison with 15O-water PET in elderly subjects at risk for Alzheimer's disease. NMR Biomed 2010;23:286–93.
60. Michaely HJ, Schoenberg SO, Ittrich C, et al. Renal disease: value of functional magnetic resonance imaging with flow and perfusion measurements. Invest Radiol 2004;39:698–705.
61. Cutajar M, Thomas DL, Banks T, et al. Repeatability of renal arterial spin labelling MRI in healthy subjects. MAGMA 2012;25:145–53.
62. de BC, Rofsky NM, Duhamel G, et al. Arterial spin labeling blood flow magnetic resonance imaging for the characterization of metastatic renal cell carcinoma. Acad Radiol 2005;12:347–57.
63. de BC, Alsop DC, George D, et al. Magnetic resonance imaging-measured blood flow change after antiangiogenic therapy with PTK787/ZK 222584 correlates with clinical outcome in metastatic renal cell carcinoma. Clin Cancer Res 2008;14:5548–54.
64. Laughlin MH, Korthuis RJ, Sexton WL, et al. Regional muscle blood flow capacity and exercise hyperemia in high-intensity trained rats. J Appl Phys 1988;64:2420–7.
65. Pohmann R, Kunnecke B, Fingerle J, et al. Fast perfusion measurements in rat skeletal muscle at rest and during exercise with single-voxel FAIR (flow-sensitive alternating inversion recovery). Magn Reson Med 2006;55:108–15.
66. Lebon V, Carlier PG, Brillault-Salvat C, et al. Simultaneous measurement of perfusion and oxygenation changes using a multiple gradient-echo sequence: application to human muscle study. Magn Reson Imaging 1998;16:721–9.
67. Frank LR, Wong EC, Haseler LJ, et al. Dynamic imaging of perfusion in human skeletal muscle during exercise with arterial spin labeling. Magn Reson Med 1999;42:258–67.
68. Wu WC, Wang J, Detre JA, et al. Transit delay and flow quantification in muscle with continuous arterial spin labeling perfusion-MRI. J Magn Reson Imaging 2008;28:445–52.
69. Wu WC, Mohler E 3rd, Ratcliffe SJ, et al. Skeletal muscle microvascular flow in progressive peripheral artery disease: assessment with continuous arterial spin-labeling perfusion magnetic resonance imaging. J Am Coll Cardiol 2009;53:2372–7.
70. Iltis I, Kober F, Desrois M, et al. Defective myocardial blood flow and altered function of the left ventricle in type 2 diabetic rats: a noninvasive in vivo study using perfusion and cine magnetic resonance imaging. Invest Radiol 2005;40:19–26.
71. Waller C, Engelhorn T, Hiller KH, et al. Impaired resting perfusion in viable myocardium distal to chronic coronary stenosis in rats. Am J Physiol Heart Circ Physiol 2005;288:H2588–93.
72. Pollock JM, Tan H, Kraft RA, et al. Arterial spin-labeled MR perfusion imaging: clinical applications. Magn Reson Imaging Clin N Am 2009;17: 315–38.
73. Wang J, Licht DJ, Jahng G-H, et al. Pediatric perfusion imaging using pulsed arterial spin labeling. J Magn Reson Imaging 2003;18:404–13.
74. Dobbing J, Sands J. Quantitative growth and development of human brain. Arch Dis Child 1973;48:757–67.
75. Holland BA, Haas DK, Norman D, et al. MRI of normal brain maturation. AJNR Am J Neuroradiol 1986;7:201–8.
76. Herscovitch P, Raichle ME. What is the correct value for the brain–blood partition coefficient for water? J Cereb Blood Flow Metab 1985;5:65–9.
77. Gaillard WD, Grandin CB, Xu B. Developmental aspects of pediatric fMRI: considerations for image acquisition, analysis, and interpretation. Neuroimage 2001;13:239–49.
78. Wang Z, Fernandez-Seara M, Alsop DC, et al. Assessment of functional development in normal infant brain using arterial spin labeled perfusion MRI. Neuroimage 2008;39:973–8.
79. Chen J, Licht DJ, Smith SE, et al. Arterial spin labeling perfusion MRI in pediatric arterial ischemic stroke: initial experiences. J Magn Reson Imaging 2009;29:282–90.
80. Gevers S, Nederveen AJ, Fijnvandraat K, et al. Arterial spin labeling measurement of cerebral perfusion in children with sickle cell disease. J Magn Reson Imaging 2012;35:779–87.
81. Oguz KK, Golay X, Pizzini FB, et al. Sickle cell disease: continuous arterial spin-labeling perfusion MR imaging in children. Radiology 2003;227: 567–74.
82. Strouse JJ, Cox CS, Melhem ER, et al. Inverse correlation between cerebral blood flow measured by continuous arterial spin-labeling (CASL) MRI and neurocognitive function in children with sickle cell anemia (SCA). Blood 2006;108:379–81.
83. Helton KJ, Paydar A, Glass J, et al. Arterial spin-labeled perfusion combined with segmentation techniques to evaluate cerebral blood flow in white and gray matter of children with sickle cell anemia. Pediatr Blood Cancer 2009;52:85–91.
84. Schraml C, Schwenzer NF, Martirosian P, et al. Non-invasive pulmonary perfusion assessment in young patients with cystic fibrosis using an arterial spin

labeling MR technique at 1.5 T. MAGMA 2012;25: 155–62.
85. Miranda MJ, Olofsson K, Sidaros K. Noninvasive measurements of regional cerebral perfusion in preterm and term neonates by magnetic resonance arterial spin labeling. Pediatr Res 2006;60: 359–63.
86. Varela M, Hajnal JV, Petersen ET, et al. A method for rapid in vivo measurement of blood T1. NMR Biomed 2011;24:80–8.
87. Wang J, Licht DJ, Silvestre DW, et al. Why perfusion in neonates with congenital heart defects is negative–technical issues related to pulsed arterial spin labeling. Magn Reson Imaging 2006;24: 249–54.
88. Licht DJ, Wang J, Silvestre DW, et al. Preoperative cerebral blood flow is diminished in neonates with severe congenital heart defects. J Thorac Cardiovasc Surg 2004;128:841–9.
89. Pienaar R, Paldino MJ, Madan N, et al. A quantitative method for correlating observations of decreased apparent diffusion coefficient with elevated cerebral blood perfusion in newborns presenting cerebral ischemic insults. Neuroimage 2012;63(3):1510–8.
90. Wintermark P, Warfield S. New insights in perinatal arterial ischemic stroke by assessing brain perfusion. Transl Stroke Res 2012;2:255–62.
91. Wintermark P, Hansen A, Gregas MC, et al. Brain perfusion in asphyxiated newborns treated with therapeutic hypothermia. AJNR Am J Neuroradiol 2011;32:2023–9.
92. Wong EC, Buxton RB, Frank LR. Quantitative imaging of perfusion using a single subtraction (QUIPSS and QUIPSS II). Magn Reson Med 1998;39:702–8.
93. Luh WM, Wong EC, Bandettini PA, et al. QUIPSS II with thin-slice TI1 periodic saturation: a method for improving accuracy of quantitative perfusion imaging using pulsed arterial spin labeling. Magn Reson Med 1999;41:1246–54.
94. Ye FQ, Mattay VS, Jezzard P, et al. Correction for vascular artifacts in cerebral blood flow values measured by using arterial spin tagging techniques. Magn Reson Med 1997;37:226–35.

Ultra-High-Field MR Imaging
Research Tool or Clinical Need?

Jaco J.M. Zwanenburg, PhD*, Anja G. van der Kolk, MD,
Peter R. Luijten, PhD

KEYWORDS

• Ultra-high-field MRI • Hyperthermia • Neuroimaging • Postmortem MRI • Breast • Prostate • Heart • Extremities

KEY POINTS

- Most of the current ultra-high-field imaging has been performed in neuroimaging, for which a comprehensive imaging protocol, including spin-echo-based sequences, has become available.
- The applications of ultra-high-field neuroimaging in patients show a trend toward bridging the gap between anatomy and function, between imaging and histology, and between imaging and (surgical) intervention.
- Additional development is needed before ultra-high-field brain magnetic resonance imaging will be integrated into clinical practice, which includes improved image homogeneity for routine imaging of the whole brain, including the temporal lobes and the cerebellum, and testing the safety of metallic implants to reduce the number of contraindications.
- Imaging beyond the brain, is, thus far, predominantly at the stage of technical development and explorative studies on volunteers, except for certain areas like the breast and joints.
- For some applications, like the breast and the extremities, dedicated coils emerge that could become sufficiently robust to eventually allow widespread clinical use.

INTRODUCTION

Since the first human magnetic resonance (MR) image was made, about 35 years ago, MR imaging has been developing continuously. Image quality has improved dramatically from low-resolution (several millimeters), low signal-to-noise (SNR) images, to high-resolution (submillimeter) images with high SNR and a high contrast-to-noise ratio (CNR) (**Fig. 1**). Most of the improvements have come gradually, by the accumulation of many incremental technical and methodological improvements. The current drive toward ultra-high magnetic field strengths (7 T and higher) is a logical next development in the history of MR imaging.[1]

Although the first MR imaging scanners operated at low field strengths (up to 0.5 T), the commonly used field strength of 1.5 T entered the hospitals around 1985, quite early in the history of MR imaging. It took about 15 years before the next step, to 3 T, was made in the clinic. During these years, technical developments focused mainly on the improvement of the gradient system, aiming for faster and stronger gradients, continuing until the gradient strengths and slew-rates were no longer restricted by technical limitations, but by the physiology of the human body. Faster switching of the gradients would lead to peripheral nerve stimulation, and involuntary muscle contraction. A next major development was the use of multiple surface coils for parallel imaging.[2] Until that time, multiple (typically less than 8) surface coils had been used for optimal signal reception

Disclosures: Nothing to disclose.
Department of Radiology, University Medical Center Utrecht, HP E 01.132, PO Box 85500, Utrecht 3508 GA, The Netherlands
* Corresponding author.
E-mail address: j.j.m.zwanenburg@umcutrecht.nl

PET Clin 8 (2013) 311–328
http://dx.doi.org/10.1016/j.cpet.2013.03.004
1556-8598/13/$ – see front matter

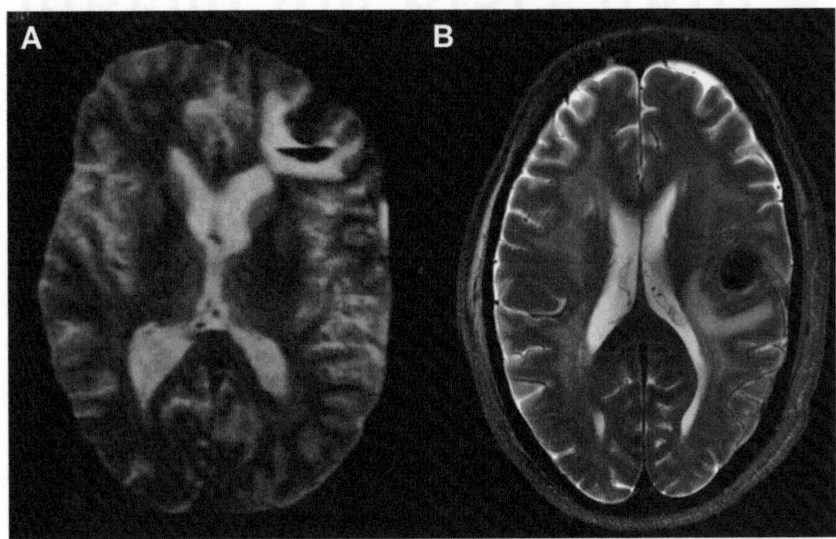

Fig. 1. Practical illustration of the development in image quality over the years. (*A*) T_2-weighted image of a 47-year-old man with head trauma, obtained at a 1.5 T MR imaging scanner in 1985. (*B*) T_2-weighted image of a 42-year-old man with a history of hypertension, with a cerebral hemorrhage and widespread white matter hyperintensities, obtained at a 7 T MR imaging scanner with volume transmit coil and 16-channel receive coil, in 2008. ([*A*] *Adapted from* Gomori JM, Grossman RI, Goldberg HI, et al. Intracranial hematomas: imaging by high-field MR. Radiology 1985;157(1):87–93; with permission; [*B*] *Courtesy of* GJ Biessels, MD, PhD, University Medical Center, Utrecht.)

only. In parallel imaging, the local sensitivity of the coil is used to perform part of the spatial encoding of the MR imaging signal, which allows for reduced scanning time. This new application for surface coils lead to an ongoing increase in the number of receive coils (32 elements are no exception for current receive coil arrays).

Fast scanning, enabled by both imaging with high bandwidths (strong gradients) and parallel imaging with high acceleration factors, comes at the cost of a reduced SNR. Moreover, fast imaging would allow the acquisition of high spatial resolution datasets within reasonable scan times, but a high spatial resolution reduces the SNR of the images even further. As the intrinsic SNR of MR imaging increases approximately linearly with increasing field strength, the development of ultra-high-field ($\geq$7 T) MR imaging is a natural step in the ongoing evolution of MR imaging, to provide high-resolution images with sufficient SNR.[1] However, ultra-high-field MR imaging comes with a new technical challenge, which concerns mainly the radiofrequency (RF) fields.

The aim of this article is to describe the opportunities and challenges of ultra-high-field MR imaging for patient-related research. In principle, all MR imaging–based imaging techniques would benefit from the increase in SNR as a result of an increased field strength and the technical challenges must be addressed for successful implementation. Because other articles in this issue of *PET Clinics* address advanced MR imaging techniques, like spectroscopy, functional MR imaging, chemical exchange saturation transfer, diffusion-weighted imaging, and perfusion measurements, the current article focuses mainly on conventional imaging, including anatomic (structural) imaging with different contrast weightings.

OPPORTUNITIES AND TECHNICAL CHALLENGES OF ULTRA-HIGH-FIELD MR IMAGING

Increased SNR

When a (human) subject is placed in a strong magnetic field, the magnetic moments (or "spins") of the hydrogen nuclei (mainly present in water molecules and fat) will align in either a parallel or an anti-parallel orientation to the external magnetic field. Even at 3 T, the difference between the number of parallel and anti-parallel spins is as small as 10 in one million, meaning that only a small fraction of 1×10^{-5} of the available spins contribute to the observed MR imaging signal at 3 T.[1] This explains the relatively low sensitivity of MR imaging compared with nuclear imaging techniques like PET and single-photon emission computed tomography.

Increasing the field strength will increase the fraction of spins that contribute to the MR imaging signal and, thus, the SNR. As illustrated in **Fig. 2**, SNR in MR imaging can be used in the central tradeoff between SNR, spatial resolution, and scan time. Although the increase in SNR or, alternatively, spatial resolution, is substantial, the field-strength-related changes in tissue properties are just as important as the gain in SNR. In general, the T_1 relaxation time constants become longer, whereas the T_2 and particularly the T_2* relaxation time constants become shorter. The frequency differences induced by differences in magnetic susceptibility increase. Finally, the ability to distinguish different metabolites using spectroscopy improves, as the separation between different spectral peaks improves.

Prolongation of T_1 Relaxation Time Constants

Initially, it was feared that T_1 relaxation times would converge for tissues in the brain, leading to reduced contrast at 7 T.[3] However, this appeared not to be the case.[4,5] An increased T_1 can be regarded as a disadvantage, as longer T_1 values require longer repetition times for full signal recovery, and, thus, reduce the SNR efficiency (attainable SNR per unit of scan time). However, in applications in which magnetization is labeled before imaging, longer T_1 values mean less decay of the label, and hence improved sensitivity for the labeled spins. Examples are arterial spin labeling,[6] in which blood is labeled to obtain perfusion-weighted images, and myocardial tagging,[7] in which lines of saturated magnetization enable the visualization of the muscular contraction over the cardiac cycle. Another application for which prolonged T_1 values are beneficial is time-of-flight angiography. With time-of-flight angiography, static background tissue is suppressed by repetitive excitation with relatively high flip angle and repetition times that are much shorter than T_1 to prevent signal recovery. Fresh blood entering the tissue has not experienced the train of RF pulses and will give full signal with good contrast to the suppressed static tissue. With increased T_1 relaxation times, the background suppression will improve, on top of the intrinsically increased signal from the blood as a result of the increased field strength.[8–10]

Shorter T_2* Relaxation Time Constants

The reduced T_2* values make ultra-high-field MR imaging more sensitive for the detection of small deposits of material with deviating magnetic susceptibility, like calcifications, and iron in microbleeds and hemorrhages, leading, for example, to increased detection rates of microbleeds in patients,[11,12] improved depiction of small venules,[13,14] and better

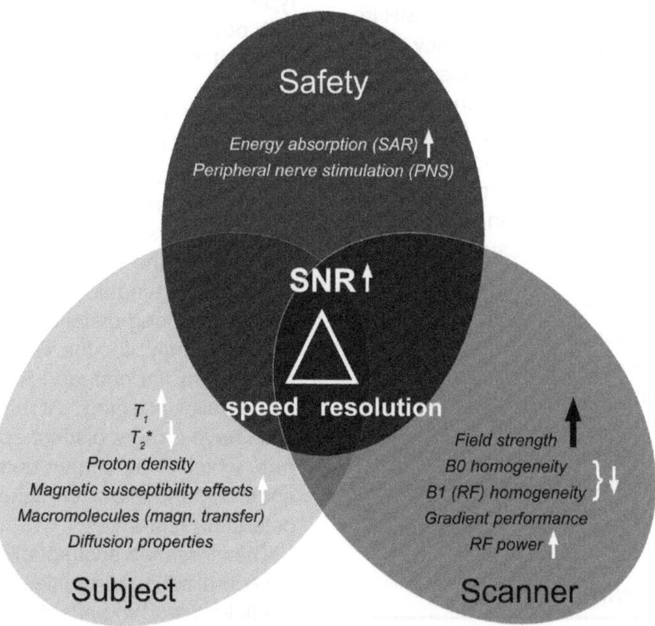

Fig. 2. Schematic visualization of the central tradeoff between SNR, speed and resolution of MR imaging, and the boundary conditions that constrain the room for image protocol optimization, which are imposed by the technology of the scanner, the properties of the imaged subject, and safety. *White arrows*: the effect of an increase in the static field of the MR imaging scanner (*black arrow*). (*Modified from* van der Kolk AG, Hendrikse J, Zwanenburg JJ et al. Clinical applications of 7T MRI in the brain. Eur J Radiol 2013;82:708–18; with permission.)

visualization of deep brain nuclei.[15,16] Also, the increase in T_1 relaxation times, together with a reduction in the T_2* relaxation times, allows for simultaneous acquisition of a time-of-flight angiogram (in which the static background is suppressed relative to freshly inflowing blood, by repetitive RF pulses and a long T_1) with a venogram (in which the veins are dark due to the short T_2*).[17] Furthermore, the sensitivity of blood-oxygen-level-dependent (BOLD) functional MR imaging (fMRI) is higher at ultra-high-field. The localization of the functional areas with fMRI is also improved, because of both a reduced contribution from the intravascular signal of large draining veins (due to the short T_2* of venous blood), and an increased contribution from the extravascular signal of the capillary bed (due to the increased BOLD sensitivity).[18,19]

Increased Magnetic Susceptibility Effects

The magnetic susceptibility is a tissue (or material) property describing how much an applied external magnetic field is changed inside this tissue or material. Different tissues have subtle differences in magnetic susceptibility, and hence, slightly different MR frequencies. Even at 7 T these frequency differences are generally small: the frequency difference between gray matter and white matter at 7 T is approximately only 5 Hz, relative to the resonance frequency of approximately 300 MHz.[20] Nonetheless, the phase of the MR imaging signal is sensitive to small frequency differences, and the SNR of the phase images increases quadratically with field strength, which can lead to an order of magnitude higher CNR for phase images than for magnitude images in the brain.[20] This increase allows, for example, for acquiring high-resolution (200 μm in-plane resolution) images of the layers in the visual cortex with high contrast.[20]

It is possible to obtain quantitative estimations of the local magnetic susceptibility by measuring the subtle phase differences induced by the local magnetic susceptibility.[21] Quantitative susceptibility mapping benefits from the quadratic increase in CNR of the phase images with increasing field strength, and can, for example, be used to distinguish iron-containing blood products from calcifications.[22]

Increased Chemical Shift

The MR frequency of hydrogen nuclei (protons) depends on their chemical bond. Different chemical compounds, therefore, have slightly shifted resonance frequencies ("chemical shift"). This aspect is used in MR spectroscopy to study the presence of different metabolites in different tissues, such as tumors or brain tissue. The frequency difference between different spectral peaks increases with increasing field strength, which is beneficial for separating peaks that are close or overlapping at lower field strengths. Protons in fat tissue have a considerable chemical shift with respect to water, which makes it possible to suppress the often unwanted bright fat signal in anatomic images. Increased chemical shifts at higher field strength make it, in principle, easier to perform fat suppression at high field.[23]

Technical Challenges

The main challenge of ultra-high-field is the management of the RF transmit fields. The wavelength of the RF waves becomes shorter at higher field (due to the higher resonance frequency), while dielectric properties of the tissue increasingly effect the RF penetration.[24] This results in spatially inhomogeneous flip angles, SNR, and contrast, particularly in the abdomen. Moreover, the specific absorption rate (SAR) increases quadratically with field strength, limiting the amount of RF pulses that can be applied in a certain sequence before the SAR limits are reached. The inhomogeneity in the transmit fields can also lead to hot spots in SAR, which requires careful modeling of the transmit antenna performance and the effect of various tissue types and geometries.

A potential solution to the inhomogeneous RF transmit fields is parallel transmission with multiple channels. The additional channels provide extra degrees of freedom to homogenize the RF transmit field and can simultaneously be used to reduce the inhomogeneity in SAR as well.[25] A completely different approach to RF excitation is the use of traveling waves, which makes use of the fact that the bore of the MR imaging scanner at 7 T can serve as a waveguide, which allows the use of antennas at a long distance for transmission.[26,27]

Interestingly, for the RF reception, it has been shown that the changed RF behavior is favorable for parallel imaging. At ultra-high-field, surface coils have a more distinct spatial sensitivity structure, which makes them better suitable for spatial encoding and allow for higher parallel imaging acceleration factors.[28]

The increased susceptibility effects that provide new contrast opportunities have the drawback that the field-disturbing effects of air-tissue boundaries and bone-tissue boundaries are much more pronounced as well, which leads to larger inhomogeneity of the B_0 field, which can lead to image distortion and signal dropouts, particularly in T_2*-weighted images.

Finally, safety of implants in patients needs to be reconsidered at 7 T. Implants that are safe at 1.5 T or 3 T are not necessarily safe at 7 T. Due to the shorter wavelength of the RF fields, coupling with implants like stents, leads of stimulators, and dental wires are expected to occur more easily. Therefore, not only are a large number of (mainly) older patients excluded from 7 T imaging, due to a history of surgery or metallic implants, but also many younger healthy volunteers due to the presence of a dental wire, reducing the number of subjects to be scanned in patient studies considerably.[29] Although it will take time before all implants and materials are tested for their safety, several recent studies on RF heating of dental wires and peripheral stents showed promising results.[30–32]

Return of Hyperthermia?

It is interesting to observe that the challenges of managing RF fields in ultra-high-field MR imaging, and hyperthermia for cancer treatment, are very similar.[33] Hyperthermia uses RF fields with frequencies ranging from 100 to 400 MHz, to increase the temperature in the target area of radiation. 7 T MR imaging works at a resonance frequency of approximately 300 MHz, which is in the same range of the RF frequencies used in hyperthermia. As mentioned above, SAR hot spots can occur due to the inhomogeneity in the transmit field. Current multi-transmit technology at 7 T MR imaging aims at homogenizing both the SAR and the flip angle and can benefit from the knowledge of hyperthermia techniques. Both multi-transmit MR imaging and hyperthermia require careful steering of the individual antennas to obtain the desired field distribution, which requires managing the mutual coupling between antennas, and between antennas and cables. Hyperthermia treatment needs a feedback system to verify the location and extent of the heated tissue volume, for which MR imaging temperature mapping methods could be valuable. Although not yet on the near horizon, it is not unthinkable that hyperthermia and ultra-high-field MR imaging can be merged into a single system that both applies hyperthermia and monitors the treatment.[33–35]

BRAIN IMAGING

Most of the ultra-high-field imaging has been performed in neuroimaging, mainly because the potential benefit of ultra-high-field is most obvious for this area, and because the head is relatively small, which allows the use of local transmit coils with conventional RF technology.

Initial results were entirely based on gradient echo imaging, because the benefit of increased sensitivity to the magnetic susceptibility difference between different tissues is only seen in gradient echo images with susceptibility or T_2*-weighting. Spin-echo-based imaging is much more challenging to implement at ultra-high-field, because of both the sensitivity to inhomogeneities in the RF transmit field and the generally higher SAR demands of spin-echo-based sequences. Nonetheless, a comprehensive neuroimaging protocol requires spin-echo-based sequences like the fluid-attenuated-inversion-recovery (FLAIR) sequence, which is the working horse for neuroimaging at clinical field strengths. Successful implementation of spin-echo-based sequences[36] has shown that also T_2-weighted spin-echo imaging has a strong potential for neuroimaging at ultra-high-field: it has a high sensitivity for small cortical lesions in multiple sclerosis patients[37,38] and shows multiple layers in the normal cerebral cortex.[39] A spin-echo-based sequence with T_1-weighting allows imaging of intracranial vessel wall lesions with lesion enhancement in patients with stroke.[29] An overview of the currently available spin-echo-based sequences is given in **Fig. 3**, and an illustration of the increased sensitivity to cortical lesions in multiple sclerosis is given in **Fig. 4**.

Several recent reviews are available that provide detailed discussions of neuroimaging at 7 T, and the clinical implications for different diseases, including neurodegenerative disease, stroke, and multiple sclerosis.[40–43] This section, therefore, aims to identify more general trends, which are illustrated with elected examples.

Bridging the Gap Between Tissue Anatomy and Function

With the increase in SNR, contrast and resolution at ultra-high-field MR imaging, the gap between structure (anatomy) and function becomes smaller. An early publication on the potential of phase imaging at 7 T clearly showed layering within the visual cortex,[20] which can be used to distinguish different functional areas, not only in the visual cortex but also in principle throughout the entire brain.[44] While Brodmann, over a century ago, studied postmortem tissues with staining to identify the several functional areas,[45] ultra-high-field MR imaging now makes it feasible to identify at least some functional areas individually in a living human, without the use of invasive techniques or contrast agents. Besides susceptibility effects (signal phase and/or T_2*), also T_1-weighting,[46,47] T_2-weighting,[39] and combined

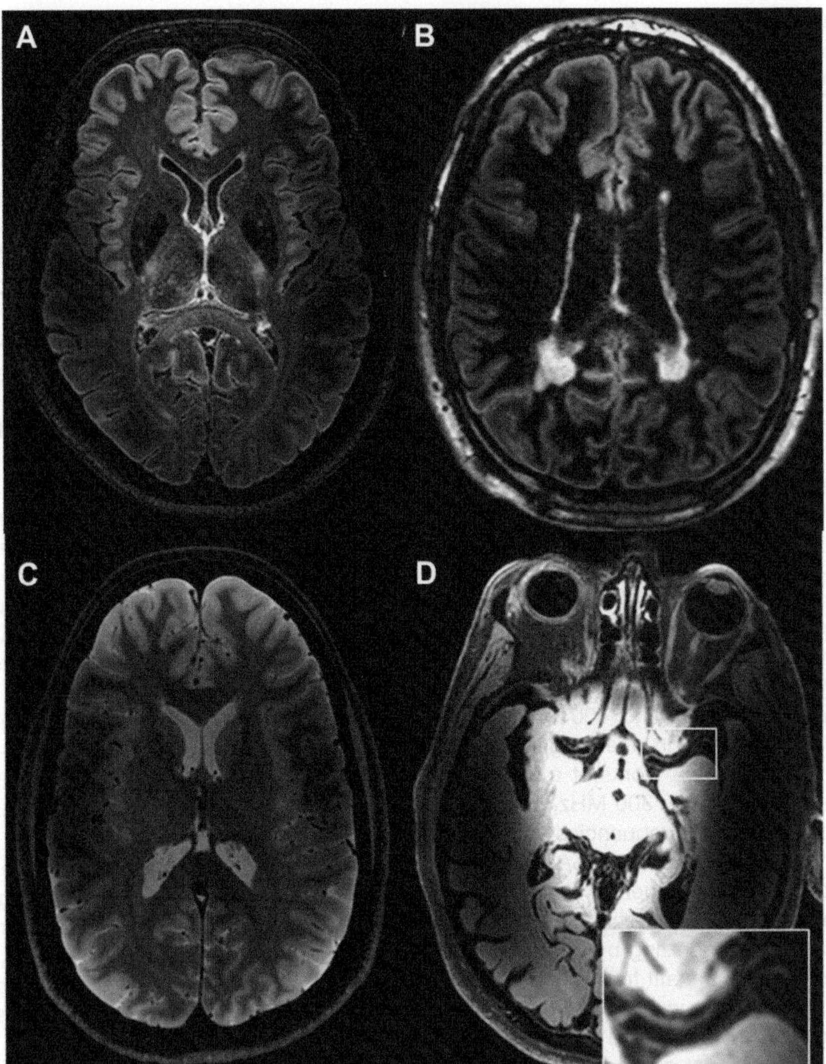

Fig. 3. Overview of turbo-spin-echo-based sequences at ultra-high-field (7 T) MR imaging in the University Medical Center Utrecht. (*A*) Fluid-attenuated inversion recovery sequence (FLAIR, 0.8 mm isotropic resolution[36]) in a healthy volunteer. (*B*) Dual inversion recovery sequence ($1.0 \times 1.0 \times 1.1$ mm^3 resolution[90]) with suppression of both cerebrospinal fluid and white matter in a patient with multiple sclerosis. (*C*) Turbo-spin-echo sequence (TSE, 0.7 mm isotropic resolution[91]) in a healthy volunteer. (*D*) Magnetization prepared inversion recovery TSE (0.8 mm isotropic resolution[42]) for visualization of the intracranial vessel wall in a healthy elderly volunteer. The inset shows the vessel walls of the left middle cerebral artery, which appear as a "rail track." (*A–C*) Transverse reformats of volumetric (3D) datasets with full brain coverage.

T_1- and T_2-weighting[48] are explored for their potential of mapping of different cortical areas based on differences in myelin content or cell density, for example.

BOLD fMRI also allows for identifying different functional areas. At ultra-high-field MR imaging, the sensitivity to BOLD contrast increases, whereas it is more constrained to the tissue as the blood in large draining veins contributes much less to the signal due to its short T_2* relaxation time constant,[18] bringing ultra-high-field to the unique position of both developing the high-resolution anatomic imaging methods that might differentiate different functional areas, and validating these techniques with high-resolution fMRI.[49]

An intriguing example of the close link between anatomy and (dys)function is given in a recent publication that showed that Parkinson disease could be directly visualized from the anatomy of the substantia nigra on T_2*-weighted images at 7 T (**Fig. 5**).[50] It is tempting to speculate that also

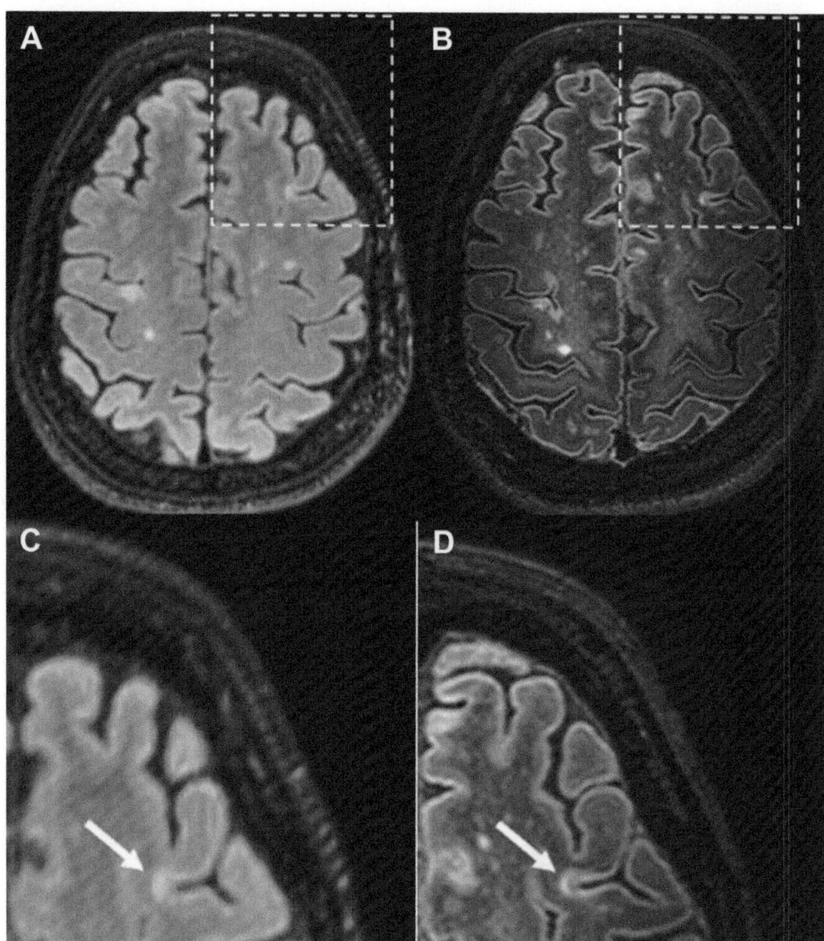

Fig. 4. (*A*) 3 T transverse FLAIR image with 1.1 × 1.1 × 1.2 mm^3 resolution and (*B*) corresponding 7-T FLAIR image with 0.8 mm isotropic resolution in a 37-year-old woman with secondary progressive multiple sclerosis. (*C, D*) Corresponding magnifications of the regions indicated in (*A* and *B*). The cortical lesion clearly visible on the 7-T FLAIR was only seen in retrospect on the 3 T FLAIR image as a very subtle change in intensity (*white arrows*). In a study with 38 multiple sclerosis patients, 238% (230 vs 68) more gray matter lesions were detected on 7 T as compared with 3 T. (*Data from* de Graaf WL, Kilsdonk ID, Lopez-Soriano A, et al. Clinical application of multi-contrast 7-T MR imaging in multiple sclerosis: increased lesion detection compared to 3 T confined to grey matter. Eur Radiol 2013;23(2):528–40; and *Courtesy:* ID Kilsdonk, MD and WL de Graaf, PhD, VU Medical Center, Amsterdam.)

other diseases like schizophrenia might show distinct changes in the cortical layers, for example, which might eventually be visualized on an individual basis.

Bridging the Gap Between in Vivo Imaging and Histology

Ultra-high-field MR imaging not only starts to bridge the gap between anatomy and function, it is also increasingly used for postmortem imaging in a way that is complementary to both in vivo imaging and histology. Ultra-high-field postmortem imaging allows for acquiring high-resolution (approximately 100–200 μm isotropic voxels) images, which cannot be acquired in vivo, because of subject motion and long scan durations of up to several hours. Relative to histology, this resolution is limited, but the MR imaging scan covers a complete volume (typical volume ranging from 15 × 10 × 3 cm^3 for high-resolution scans to full brain coverage for somewhat lower resolutions), whereas histopathological examinations sample only a limited number of very thin (approximately 4 μm) slices.

There are different applications for which postmortem MR imaging is valuable. First, it can be used to validate the interpretation of in vivo MR imaging findings, by comparing similar findings on postmortem MR imaging with histology. A

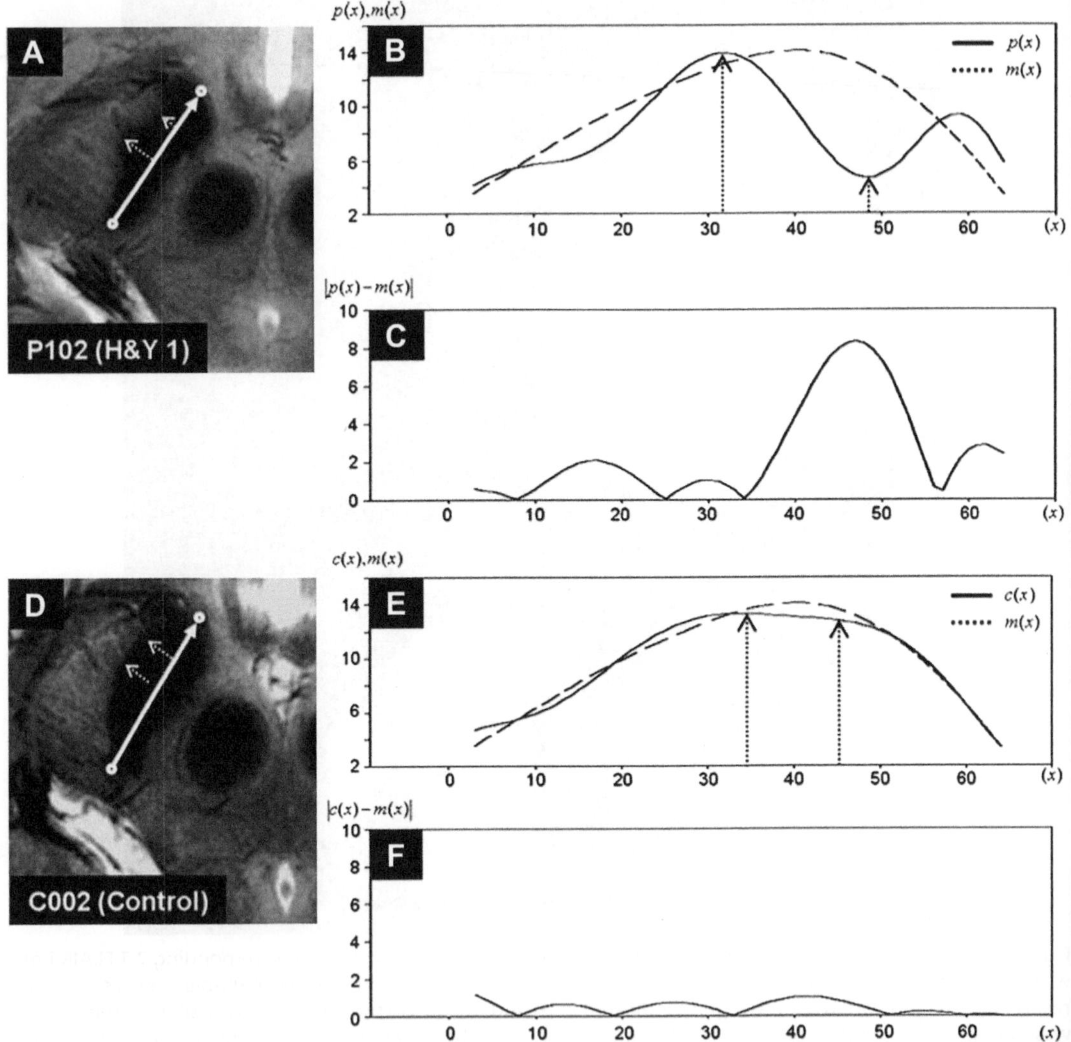

Fig. 5. Illustration of detailed anatomic imaging of the substantia nigra at ultra-high-field, and how anatomy might reflect (dys)function, for a patient with Parkinson disease (PD). (*A, D*) High-resolution T_2*-weighted images of the substantia nigra (SN) at 7 T, for a patient with PD and a healthy control, respectively. For the quantification of PD, Cho and colleagues[50] measured distance profiles of the individual PD patients [p(x)] and normal controls [c(x)] along the white arrow. (*B, E*) The profiles are measured along the white arrows as indicated in (*A, D*). The solid line shows the individual data, while the dotted line is the reference data [m(x)] obtained by averaging of the 9 normal healthy controls. (*C, F*) Distance profiles of absolute differences measured between the individual (both PD and normal control) and reference data. (*Adapted from* Cho ZH, Oh SH, Kim JM, et al. Direct visualization of Parkinson's disease by in vivo human brain imaging using 7.0T magnetic resonance imaging. Mov Disord 2011;26(4):713–8; with permission.)

clinical example of this is the in vivo detection of microinfarcts in the aging human brain. 7 T MR imaging of postmortem brain slices containing histologically validated microinfarcts has provided strong evidence that small cortical lesions observed in vivo in the brain images of elderly individuals are indeed microinfarcts, as can be seen in **Figs. 6** and **7**.[51] Examples in the field of neuroscience are studies that combined postmortem MR imaging with histology to understand the contrast mechanisms that lead to contrast between gray and white matter,[52] and between the cerebral cortical layers[53] as observed with ultra-high-field MR imaging. A second application of postmortem MR imaging is to study complex anatomy,[54] and 3D (microscopic) tissue structure.[55] Finally, postmortem MR imaging is also useful to search for potential endogenous MR imaging contrasts for detecting certain pathologies, like detecting metastatic lymph nodes in breast

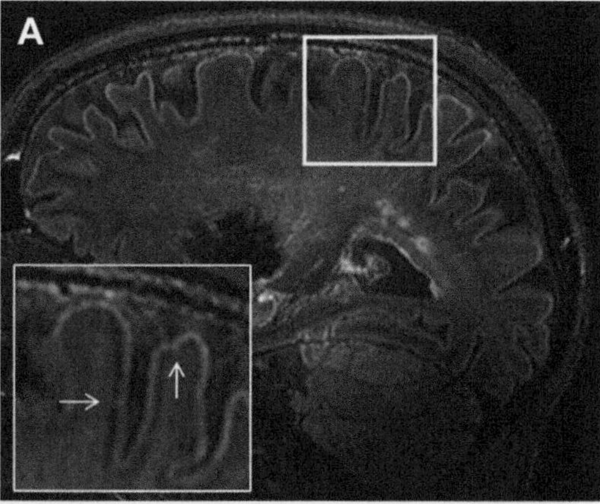

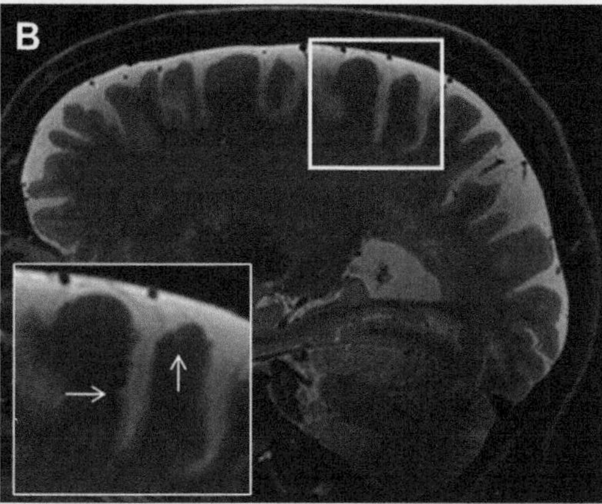

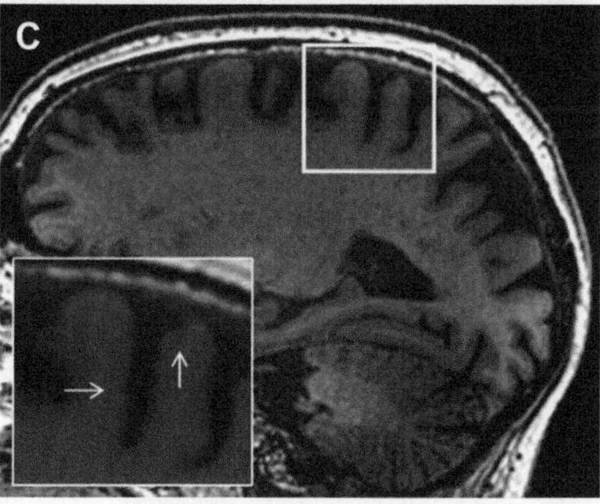

Fig. 6. Example of cortical lesions in a 76-year-old man, suggestive of a microinfarct. (*A*) Sagittal T_2-weighted FLAIR image (0.8 mm isotropic resolution), clearly showing 2 small hyperintense lesions in the cortical gray matter (*arrows* in the enlarged insets). The lesions were also visible on (*B*) the sagittal T_2-weighted turbo-spin-echo image (0.7 mm isotropic resolution), and, with much less contrast, on (*C*) the T_1-weighted image (1 mm isotropic resolution). (*Courtesy of* SJ van Veluw, MSc, and GJ Biessels, MD, PhD, University Medical Center, Utrecht.)

cancer patients[56] or scar tissue in cardiovascular disease.[57]

Bridging the Gap Between Imaging and (Surgical) Intervention

A third trend visible with the advance of ultra-high-field MR imaging is the reduction of the gap between imaging and (surgical) intervention. Although neurosurgeons and neurointerventionalists are very skilled in anticipating the actual anatomy during the procedure, advanced imaging can provide important details, like small blood vessels or the location of vital brain functions, which can improve treatment planning and, thus, reduce the risk of complications.

In treatment of intracranial aneurysms, it is important to know whether or not small perforating arteries arise from the (neck of the) aneurysm. Occluding such a vessel while coiling or clipping the aneurysm might lead to an ischemic stroke with significant functional loss for the patient. **Fig. 8** gives an example of how small perforating arteries can be visualized in relation to the aneurysm.

Other examples are surgery for tumor resection in tumor patients and seizure focus resection in patients with epilepsy. In both cases, it is important to know the location of vital functions like language and motor control with respect to the area that is to be resected. On the one hand, as much tissue as possible should be removed to minimize the risk of recurrence of the tumor or epileptic seizures, whereas on the other hand, vital function should be spared. fMRI is capable of locating specific functional brain areas and has both increased sensitivity and localization accuracy at ultra-high-field, which can make an fMRI-based assessment of patients who are eligible for brain surgery a valuable application of ultra-high-field MR imaging. For tumor resection, detailed visualization of the blood vessels surrounding the tumor is of additional value as well. An example of fMRI in a tumor patient with low-grade glioma near the language area is shown in **Fig. 9**.

IMAGING BEYOND THE BRAIN

Although brain imaging at ultra-high-field MR imaging has been applied in a considerable number of patient studies for different diseases, imaging beyond the brain is, thus far, predominantly at the stage of technical development and explorative studies on volunteers. Because of the shorter wavelength of the RF transmit fields, it is not possible to use a large volume coil for body imaging, such as used in clinical MR imaging scanners at 1.5 T and 3 T. Instead, local transmit coils are

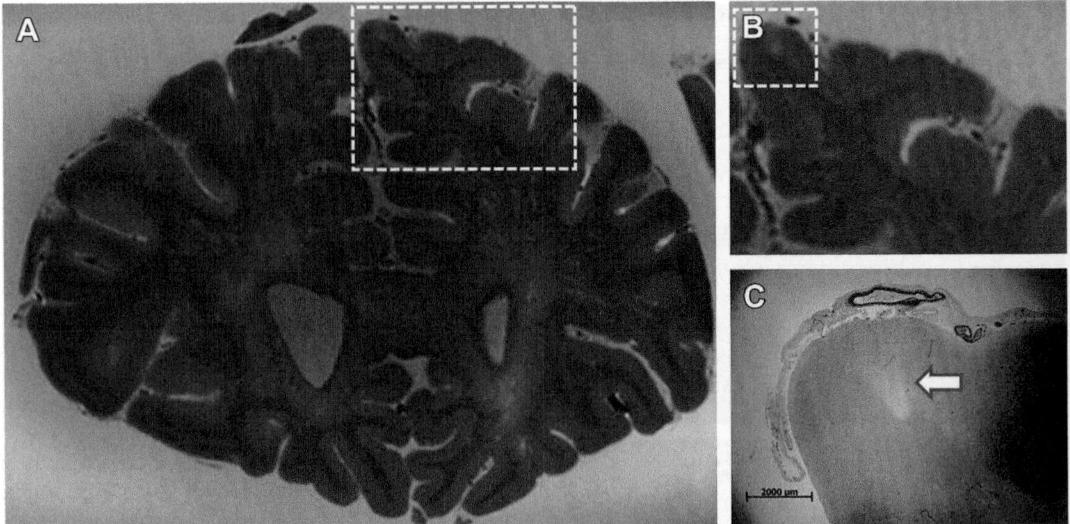

Fig. 7. Postmortem tissue of a 71-year-old man with extensive ischemic damage due to hypertension, showing a similar cortical lesion as observed in vivo in **Fig. 6**. (*A*) T_2-weighted turbo-spin-echo image (0.4 mm isotropic resolution). (*B*) Zoomed detail as indicated by dashed box in (*A*). (*C*) Histologic slice corresponding to dashed box in (*B*), confirming that this lesion (*arrow*) is a microinfarct (L&P stain, scale bar as indicated). (*Courtesy of* SJ van Veluw, MSc, and GJ Biessels, MD, PhD, University Medical Center, Utrecht.)

being developed that are tailored to specific anatomic areas. Using multiple local transmit coils, the result of the combined RF transmit fields can be homogenized by tailoring the waveforms sent to the individual coils.[58,59] A concomitant advantage of using local transmit coils is that the overall SAR levels are lower for a given RF amplitude. This section provides an impression of the progress of imaging beyond the brain at ultra-high-field, by showing examples from different selected anatomic areas.

Head and Neck

Because of the complex anatomy in the head and neck region, imaging can be a valuable tool for planning surgery or radiation treatment. The parotid glands are situated relatively close to the surface, which allows the use of a plain transmit/receive loop surface coil for imaging at 7 T MR imaging. Using such a coil, the potential of 7 T MR imaging as a future alternative to standard radiographic sialography was demonstrated in a small

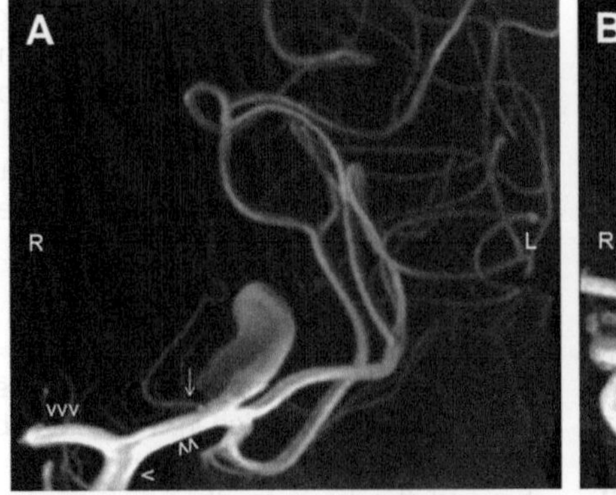

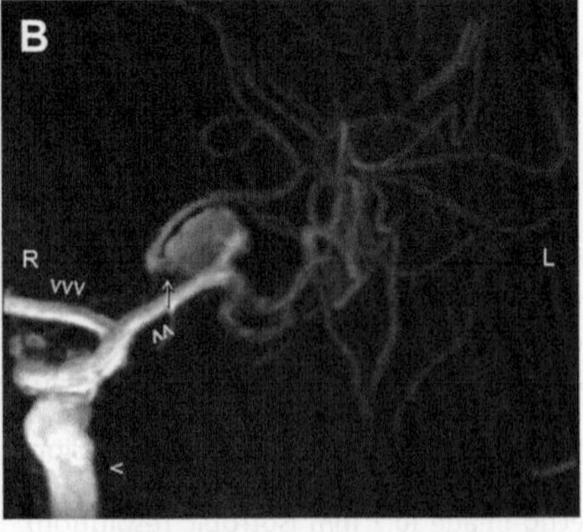

Fig. 8. Coronal maximum intensity projections of 7-T time-of-flight MR angiograms ($0.25 \times 0.3 \times 0.4$ mm^3, 10-minute scan duration) of 2 different patients with a left middle cerebral artery (MCA) aneurysm. (*A*) A case in which the perforating arteries originate from the MCA, separate from the aneurysm (*arrow*). (*B*) A case in which an artery (the M2 frontal branch) originates from the aneurysm (*arrow*), which complicates clipping of the aneurysm at the neck. These configurations were confirmed during surgery. Single open arrowheads: Left internal carotid artery; double open arrowheads: MCA; triple open arrowheads: Anterior cerebral artery. (*Courtesy of* R Kleinloog, MD, and BH Verweij, MD, PhD, University Medical Center, Utrecht.)

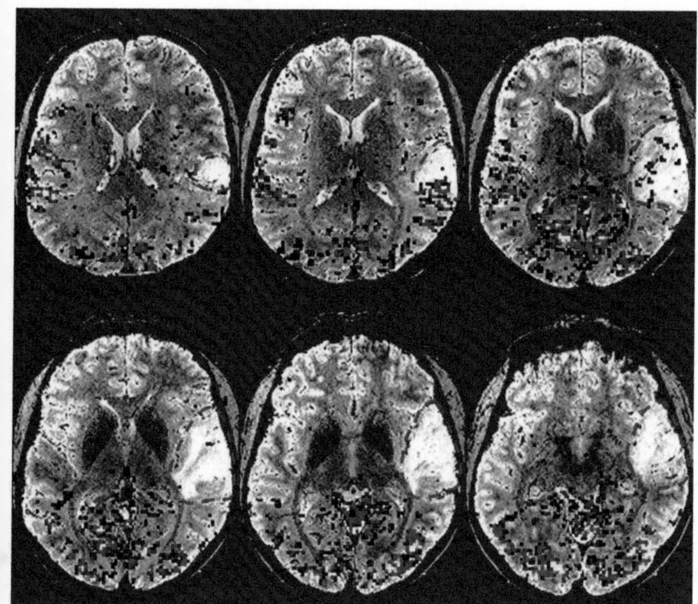

Fig. 9. fMRI results for a 36-year-old man with a low-grade glioma near the language area in the left side of the brain, before surgical tumor removal. Scanning was performed at 7 T using an EPI protocol with volume transmit coil and 16-channel receive coil. The tumor is indicated by the dashed red line. The highlighted areas are the areas activated during a language-related task (verb generation). Some activity is found inside the tumor area ($P<0.001$). (*Courtesy of* AF Rijlaarsdam, MSc, JM Jansma, PhD, and NF Ramsey, PhD, University Medical Center, Utrecht.)

number of patients with various pathologies of the parotid gland and duct.[60]

Imaging the different plaque components in the carotid vessel wall is another important target for which ultra-high-field MR imaging might provide the required improved resolution and contrast. Using a surface loop coil, improved SNR and CNR have been demonstrated at 7 T MR imaging, relative to 3 T MR imaging.[61] A more advanced coil design with multiple transmit/receive coils was recently presented and demonstrated in volunteers and a single patient.[62] Koning and colleagues[63] designed a neck coil with separate dedicated arrays for RF transmission and reception, leading to improved SNR in high-resolution images of the carotid vessel wall, as compared with 3 T, as shown in **Fig. 10**. A patient study in which the potential of this setup for imaging different plaque components is assessed is currently ongoing.

Breast

MR imaging is a valuable tool for diagnosing, staging, and monitoring treatment efficacy of breast cancer. Of all the extracranial imaging at ultra-high-field, breast imaging may be closest to clinical application. Using a dedicated RF transmit coil with separate receive array, the potential of breast imaging in patients has been demonstrated, showing a large gain in SNR, and allowing high-resolution (0.45 mm isotropic voxels) T_1-weighted structural imaging of the breast.[64] The initial results of contrast-enhanced MR imaging suggest that 7 T may be capable of classifying lesions according to the BI-RADS system, provided a suitable coil is used.[65,66] Apart from increased conspicuity of potentially small breast lesions, ultra-high-field MR imaging is also promising in identifying molecular markers with spectroscopy, which might enhance tumor characterization and monitoring of treatment.[67]

Prostate

Prostate tumors occur in a large part of the older male population. Most of these tumors are slow-growing and need no intervention. However, the distinction between indolent tumors and

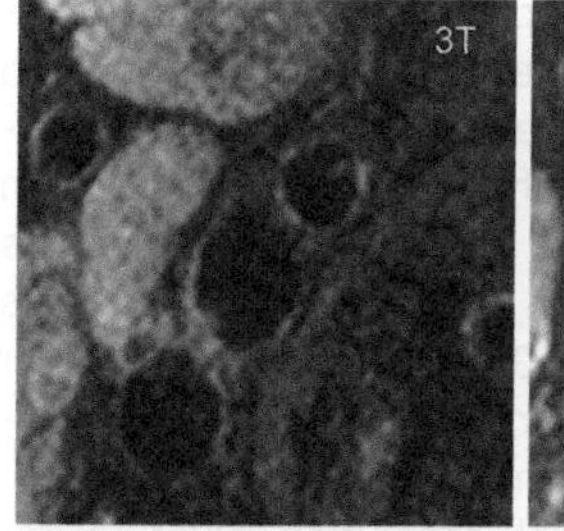

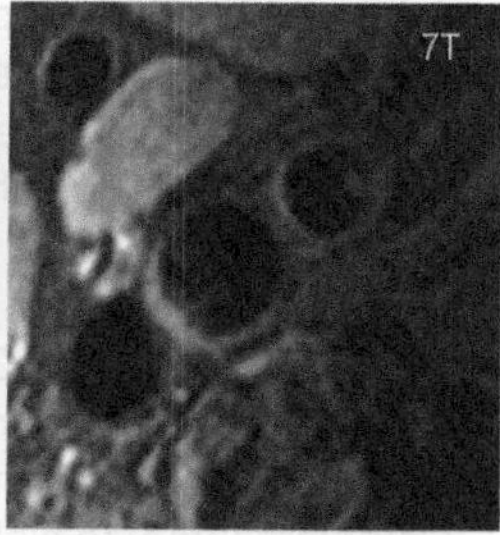

Fig. 10. High-resolution T_1-weighted images ($0.4 \times 0.4 \times 1.5$ mm^3) of the carotid arteries, just beyond the bifurcation. The same volunteer was scanned at 3 T (*left*) and 7 T (*right*). Note the improved signal-to-noise ratio at 7 T, which allows better depiction of the thin-vessel wall of this healthy volunteer. (*Courtesy of* W. Koning, MSc, University Medical Center, Utrecht.)

aggressive tumors is currently not readily made. In the case of suspected aggressive prostate cancer, biopsies are taken, which can easily miss small tumors. Spectroscopic imaging of metabolites like spermine, choline, creatine, and citrate can identify tumor tissue,[68] and benefits from the increased separation of spectral peaks at ultra-high-field strength. Using a dedicated endorectal coil, the feasibility of metabolic prostate imaging at 7 T has been shown in a small number of patients, and a larger study is ongoing to assess the potential value of 7 T MR imaging for staging prostate cancer and treatment monitoring.[69–71]

Extremities

Musculoskeletal MR imaging predominantly targets small structures with complex anatomy, like tendons, ligaments, thin layers of cartilage, and trabecular bone architecture,[72,73] making musculoskeletal MR imaging an interesting potential application at ultra-high-field, which can provide higher resolution and CNR. Compared to other anatomic areas, the extremities have the advantage that the allowed local maximum SAR levels are higher than for other body parts, giving somewhat more freedom for MR imaging sequence design, and a higher tolerance to inhomogeneity of the local SAR of an RF transmit coil. Besides, common areas of interest like the knee, ankle, and wrist have limited dimensions, which make them less prone to the inhomogeneity in RF transmit fields induced by the shorter RF wavelength at ultra-high-field. Therefore, relatively plain RF transmit coil designs already give satisfactory results for these areas.[72,74,75] Still, similar to brain imaging, spin-echo imaging is more difficult to implement successfully than gradient echo imaging.[76] As clinical musculoskeletal imaging heavily relies on turbo spin-echo imaging with various weightings (T_1, T_2, and proton density), this challenge needs to be solved.[77] A potential solution is the use of long spin-echo trains with low refocusing angles, for which an example is given in **Fig. 11**.[78] Nonetheless, for common indications for which the current diagnostic accuracy is already high at 1.5 T or 3 T, it is not clear whether improved resolution and contrast would significantly improve the diagnostic accuracy.[77]

Complementary to high-resolution structural imaging, quantitative imaging techniques, like T_2 mapping, T_2* mapping, and imaging with other nuclei (^{23}Na and ^{31}P), may be of particular interest for musculoskeletal imaging at ultra-high-field, as they allow quantitative assessment of tissue properties. Sodium MR imaging has the potential to measure the glycosaminoglycan content in articulate cartilage, which can be used to assess cartilage degeneration before structural changes become apparent on proton MR imaging.[79] Potential applications are the assessment of osteoarthritis and monitoring of treatment effects. As sodium MR imaging has a very low intrinsic SNR (about 4 thousand-fold smaller than the intrinsic SNR of proton MR imaging[77,79]), it needs long scan durations for signal averaging. Ultra-high-field may provide sufficient SNR at reduced scan times, which is needed to make sodium imaging more suitable for clinical applications. Sodium imaging at ultra-high-field does not suffer from the unfavorable wavelength effects that lead to inhomogeneous image contrast for proton imaging, as sodium has a much lower resonance frequency. More detailed reviews on both advanced imaging techniques[79] and clinical potential[77] for musculoskeletal imaging at ultra-high-field imaging have been published recently.

Another potential application of ultra-high-field MR imaging in the area of the extremities is peripheral angiography. Contrast-enhanced MR imaging angiography is currently a valuable tool in the diagnostic workup of patients with peripheral arterial disease. A challenge of contrast-enhanced MR imaging is the suppression of venous contamination of the arteriogram. Further, the use of contrast agents carries a risk for patients with renal insufficiency or allergy to the contrast agent.[80] Ultra-high-field angiography allows for the separation of arteries and veins on intrinsic contrast, due to the short T_2* of venous blood. Together with the improved contrast in time-of-flight angiography at ultra-high-field, high-quality non-contrast-enhanced angiography may become feasible. An example of the potential quality of non-contrast-enhanced angiography in the legs is shown in **Fig. 12**.

Heart

Cardiac MR imaging can noninvasively assess coronary artery disease, myocarditis, and other cardiomyopathies and the presence of viable tissue, which all are important for disease management. Although the increased SNR and CNR (translatable into imaging speed) at ultra-high-field MR imaging could improve structural and functional cardiac imaging, cardiac imaging proves to be very challenging. Anatomic imaging with balanced steady-state free precession provides excellent contrast at 1.5 T, but has a high SAR level and is, thus, difficult to translate to ultra-high-field strength. Although feasibility of 7T balanced steady state free precession at 7T has been shown,[81] steady-state free precession

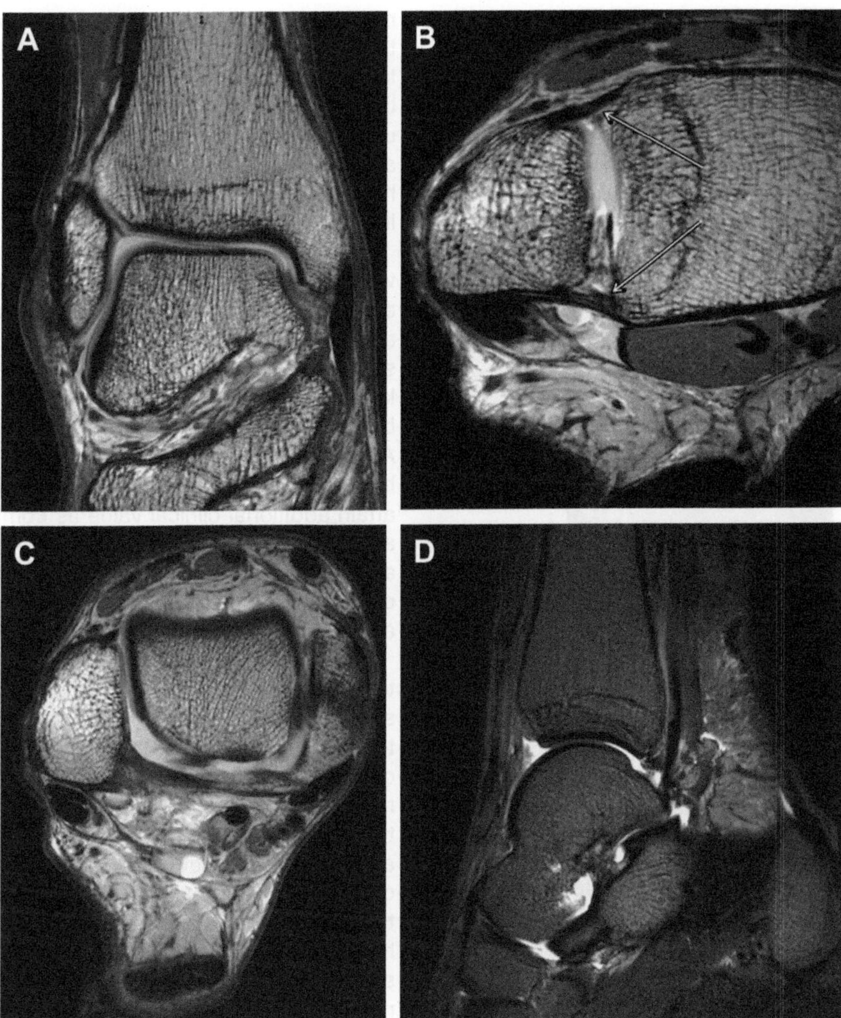

Fig. 11. High-resolution (0.2 × 0.2 × 1.0 mm^3) images of the ankle at 7 T MR imaging with proton density weighted turbo spin-echo sequence, acquired in (*A*) coronal orientation, (*B*) Oblique orientation showing anterior and posterior tibiofibular ligaments (*arrows*), and (*C*) transverse orientation. (*D*) Fat-suppressed (STIR) turbo spin-echo in sagittal orientation (0.4 × 0.4 × 1.0 mm^3). All images were acquired with a local single channel volume coil for transmission and a flexible 32-channel high-density loop array for reception. (*Data from* Visser F, Korteweg MA, Italiaander M, et al. High resolution PDw-TSE of the ankle with the use of a flexible high density receive array at 7 Tesla. Proceedings of ISMRM 20th Scientific Meeting and Exhibition. Melbourne, Australia: 2012. p. 1449; and *Courtesy of* F Visser, University Medical Center, Utrecht.)

remains challenging, even at 3T.[82] Moreover, due to the location of the heart, cardiac imaging at ultra-high-field suffers greatly from the inhomogeneity in the RF transmit fields, and from the large susceptibility difference between cardiac muscle and lung tissue. The challenges due to the inhomogeneity in the RF fields are one of the motivators for the ongoing technical developments regarding RF shimming and parallel transmission with multiple transmit coils.[83]

Although cardiac imaging at ultra-high-field is still in need of major technological developments, several studies show initial results on human subjects. Cardiac function assessment is feasible,[84,85] and coronary artery imaging shows similar or slightly improved quality as compared with 3 T MR imaging, even though using only a plain local quadrature loop coil at 7 T (**Fig. 13**).[86] A new potential application that may be particularly interesting at ultra-high-field is the detection of collagen in the myocardium, based on endogenous contrast. The presence of collagen can be detected with T_2*-weighted imaging,[57,87] and higher field strengths may improve the sensitivity for collagen, although increased B_0

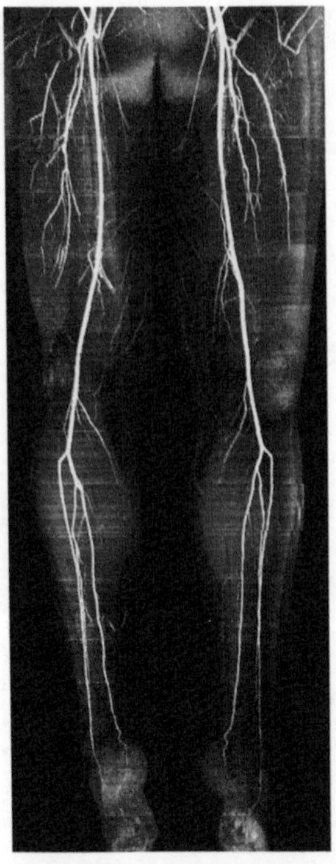

Fig. 12. Non-contrast-enhanced imaging of the lower extremity arteries in a healthy subject at 7 T, using a T_1-weighted gradient echo sequence with phonocardiogram cardiac gating. Images were acquired with a custom-built 16-channel transmit/receive coil and a manually positionable table for multistation imaging. Time-Interleaved Acquisition of Modes[58] was integrated to reduce transmit RF artifacts and to obtain near homogeneous image quality of the arteries. (*Courtesy of* M.E. Ladd, PhD, Erwin L. Hahn Institute for MRI, Essen, Germany.)

inhomogeneity makes T_2*-weighted imaging and T_2*-mapping more challenging at ultra-high-field.[88] A more detailed and elaborate discussion of the potential and the challenges of cardiac imaging of ultra-high-field can be found in a recent review by Niendorf and colleagues.[83]

DISCUSSION—THE FUTURE

When looking forward, one might ask to what extent ultra-high-field will become widely used in the clinic. Regarding brain imaging, the improvement in contrast and spatial resolution at ultra-high-field is evident and will find its way to more and more clinical applications. Nonetheless, even for brain imaging, some additional steps need to be taken before ultra-high-field MR imaging can be integrated into clinical practice. First, the homogeneity of the RF transmit field needs further improvement, to such extent that also the temporal lobes and the cerebellum can be scanned routinely, with a safe and robust setup. Second, the safety of implants has to be tested to reduce the number of contraindications for undergoing ultra-high-field MR imaging. Last, a clinical ultra-high-field MR imaging scanner should be actively shielded and affordable and have similar housing requirements as conventional clinical MR imaging scanners to become generally applicable.

For extracranial applications, the question of whether ultra-high-field MR imaging will become a common clinical tool is less straightforward to answer. The challenges to obtain a robust and safe setup that yields homogeneous images are larger, especially for organs deep inside the body, like the heart and the abdominal organs. Also, for musculoskeletal imaging inside the body (like the spine) it proved to be difficult to attain additional clinical value as compared 1.5 T and 3 T.[89] For other applications like the breast and the extremities, dedicated coils emerge that could become sufficiently robust to eventually allow widespread clinical use.

Obviously, it is difficult to predict to what extent the main magnetic field of human MR imaging scanners will increase in the future. Given the technical limitations of the currently used superconducting material (Niobium–Titanium), the current technical horizon is roughly 12 T.[40] Similar to the maximum gradient performance in MR imaging, it is likely that human physiology will finally determine the maximum field strength, rather than technological limitations. As there are no harmful effects known of static magnetic field strengths to the body at any field strength, the maximum field strength will be rather indirectly determined by human physiology. Most likely, the maximum static field strength will be limited by tissue heating due to the RF transmit fields. The rate of tissue heating increases approximately quadratically with field strength, while increased inhomogeneity of the RF fields increases the risk of local hot spots. Recently, a detailed review addressing the future of ultra-high-field MR imaging for the brain has been published, discussing these effects and its implications in much more detail.[40]

In summary, ultra-high-field MR imaging provides higher SNR and changed tissue contrast, which both have the potential for improved imaging with high-resolution and high-image contrast. In neuroimaging, the technology is sufficiently robust for patient studies, and a comprehensive set of imaging protocols including spin-echo-based sequences has been successfully implemented. Inhomogeneity in image contrast is still present because of inhomogeneity in the RF transmit field, affecting predominantly the temporal lobes and cerebellum. Outside the brain, the

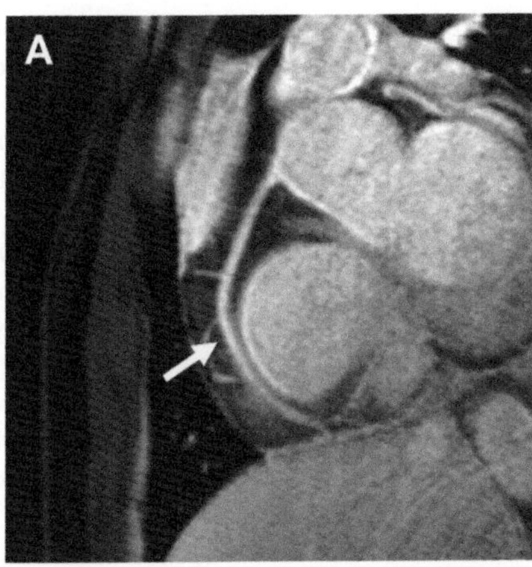

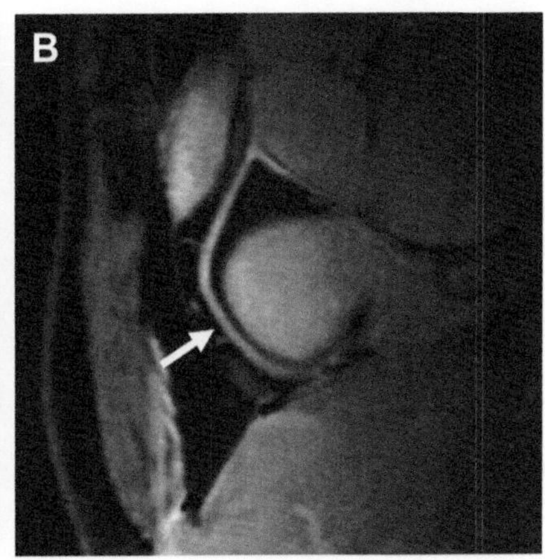

Fig. 13. (*A*) Example of coronary artery (*arrow*) imaging at 3 T MR imaging (0.8 × 0.8 × 2.0 mm^3), using the volume body coil for transmission, and a local 6-element receive coil for reception. (*B*) Corresponding 7 T MR imaging image of the same subject, using a local transmit/receive coil with 2 elements, driven in quadrature. Despite the plain setup at 7 T, the image quality in a group of 10 subjects was at least similar at 7 T compared with 3 T. (*Data from* van Elderen SG, Versluis MJ, Westenberg JJ, et al. Right coronary MR angiography at 7 T: a direct quantitative and qualitative comparison with 3 T in young healthy volunteers. Radiology 2010;257(1):254–9; and *Courtesy of* MJ Versluis, MSc and AG Webb, PhD, Leiden University Medical Center.)

challenges with inhomogeneous RF fields are generally much larger, especially for the heart and abdomen, and require major technical developments in RF transmit technology. Patient studies regarding areas outside the brain are still rare, but begin to emerge for anatomic areas that are accessible with relatively plain surface transmit/receive coils, such as the breast, the neck (carotid arteries), and the joints.

ACKNOWLEDGMENTS

The authors want to thank the contributors to the figures, and F. Visser, C.A.T. van den Berg, PhD, D.W.J. Klomp, PhD, and N. Petridou, PhD, for discussions and comments.

REFERENCES

1. Schick F. Whole-body MRI at high field: technical limits and clinical potential. Eur Radiol 2005;15(5): 946–59.
2. Pruessmann KP, Weiger M, Scheidegger MB, et al. SENSE: sensitivity encoding for fast MRI. Magn Reson Med 1999;42(5):952–62.
3. Fischer HW, Rinck PA, Van HY, et al. Nuclear relaxation of human brain gray and white matter: analysis of field dependence and implications for MRI. Magn Reson Med 1990;16(2):317–34.
4. Ugurbil K, Adriany G, Andersen P, et al. Ultrahigh field magnetic resonance imaging and spectroscopy. Magn Reson Imaging 2003; 21(10):1263–81.
5. Rooney WD, Johnson G, Li X, et al. Magnetic field and tissue dependencies of human brain longitudinal 1H2O relaxation in vivo. Magn Reson Med 2007;57(2):308–18.
6. Golay X, Petersen ET. Arterial spin labeling: benefits and pitfalls of high magnetic field. Neuroimaging Clin N Am 2006;16(2):259–68, x.
7. Ibrahim el-SH. Myocardial tagging by cardiovascular magnetic resonance: evolution of techniques–pulse sequences, analysis algorithms, and applications. J Cardiovasc Magn Reson 2011;13:36.
8. Hendrikse J, Zwanenburg JJ, Visser F, et al. Noninvasive depiction of the Lenticulostriate arteries with time-of-flight MR angiography at 7.0 T. Cerebrovasc Dis 2008;26(6):624–9.
9. Cho ZH, Kang CK, Han JY, et al. Observation of the Lenticulostriate arteries in the human brain in vivo using 7.0T MR angiography. Stroke 2008;39(5):1604–6.
10. Johst S, Wrede KH, Ladd ME, et al. Time-of-flight magnetic resonance angiography at 7 T using venous saturation pulses with reduced flip angles. Invest Radiol 2012;47(8):445–50.
11. Brundel M, Heringa SM, de BJ, et al. High prevalence of cerebral microbleeds at 7Tesla MRI in patients with early Alzheimer's disease. J Alzheimers Dis 2012;31(2):259–63.
12. Conijn MM, Geerlings MI, Biessels GJ, et al. Cerebral microbleeds on MR imaging: comparison between 1.5 and 7T. AJNR Am J Neuroradiol 2011; 32(6):1043–9.
13. Tallantyre EC, Brookes MJ, Dixon JE, et al. Demonstrating the perivascular distribution of MS lesions in vivo with 7-Tesla MRI. Neurology 2008;70(22): 2076–8.

14. Ge Y, Zohrabian VM, Grossman RI. Seven-Tesla magnetic resonance imaging: new vision of microvascular abnormalities in multiple sclerosis. Arch Neurol 2008;65(6):812–6.
15. Cho ZH, Min HK, Oh SH, et al. Direct visualization of deep brain stimulation targets in Parkinson disease with the use of 7-tesla magnetic resonance imaging. J Neurosurg 2010;113(3):639–47.
16. Lenglet C, Abosch A, Yacoub E, et al. Comprehensive in vivo mapping of the human basal ganglia and thalamic connectome in individuals using 7T MRI. PLoS One 2012;7(1):e29153.
17. Bae KT, Park SH, Moon CH, et al. Dual-echo arteriovenography imaging with 7T MRI. J Magn Reson Imaging 2010;31(1):255–61.
18. Donahue MJ, Hoogduin H, van Zijl PC, et al. Blood oxygenation level-dependent (BOLD) total and extravascular signal changes and DeltaR2* in human visual cortex at 1.5, 3.0 and 7.0 T. NMR Biomed 2011;24(1):25–34.
19. Yacoub E, Shmuel A, Pfeuffer J, et al. Imaging brain function in humans at 7 Tesla. Magn Reson Med 2001;45(4):588–94.
20. Duyn JH, van Gelderen P, Li TQ, et al. High-field MRI of brain cortical substructure based on signal phase. Proc Natl Acad Sci U S A 2007;104(28): 11796–801.
21. Wharton S, Schafer A, Bowtell R. Susceptibility mapping in the human brain using threshold-based k-space division. Magn Reson Med 2010; 63(5):1292–304.
22. Schweser F, Deistung A, Lehr BW, et al. Differentiation between diamagnetic and paramagnetic cerebral lesions based on magnetic susceptibility mapping. Med Phys 2010;37(10):5165–78.
23. Ivanov D, Schafer A, Streicher MN, et al. A simple low-SAR technique for chemical-shift selection with high-field spin-echo imaging. Magn Reson Med 2010;64(2):319–26.
24. Ladd ME. High-field-strength magnetic resonance: potential and limits. Top Magn Reson Imaging 2007;18(2):139–52.
25. Van den Berg CA, van den Bergen B, Van de Kamer JB, et al. Simultaneous B1 + homogenization and specific absorption rate hotspot suppression using a magnetic resonance phased array transmit coil. Magn Reson Med 2007; 57(3):577–86.
26. Webb AG, Collins CM, Versluis MJ, et al. MRI and localized proton spectroscopy in human leg muscle at 7 Tesla using longitudinal traveling waves. Magn Reson Med 2010;63(2):297–302.
27. Brunner DO, De ZN, Frohlich J, et al. Travelling-wave nuclear magnetic resonance. Nature 2009; 457(7232):994–8.
28. Wiesinger F, van de Moortele PF, Adriany G, et al. Parallel imaging performance as a function of field strength–an experimental investigation using electrodynamic scaling. Magn Reson Med 2004;52(5): 953–64.
29. van der Kolk AG, Zwanenburg JJ, Brundel M, et al. Intracranial vessel wall imaging at 7.0-T MRI. Stroke 2011;42(9):2478–84.
30. Santoro D, Winter L, Muller A, et al. Detailing radio frequency heating induced by coronary stents: a 7.0 Tesla magnetic resonance study. PLoS One 2012;7(11):e49963.
31. Wezel J, Brink W, Kooij BJ, et al. Simulation study on safety of dental implants at 7T. Proceedings of ISMRM 20th Scientific Meeting and Exhibition. Melbourne, Australia: 2012. p. 2766.
32. Ansems J, van der Kolk AG, Kroeze H, et al. MR imaging of patients with stents is safe at 7.0 Tesla. Proceedings of ISMRM 20th Scientific Meeting and Exhibition. Melbourne, Australia: 2012. p. 2764.
33. Van den Berg CA, Bluemink JJ, van Lier AL, et al. MR and Hyperthermia: exploiting similarities for mutual benefit. Proceedings of European Microwave Week. Amsterdam, The Netherlands: 2012.
34. Jayasundar R, Hall LD, Bleehen NM. RF coils for combined MR and hyperthermia studies: I. Hyperthermia applicator as an MR coil. Magn Reson Imaging 2001;19(1):111–6.
35. Jayasundar R, Hall LD, Bleehen NM. RF coils for combined MR and hyperthermia studies: II. MR coil as an hyperthermic applicator. Magn Reson Imaging 2001;19(1):117–22.
36. Visser F, Zwanenburg JJ, Hoogduin JM, et al. High-resolution magnetization prepared 3D-FLAIR imaging at 7.0 Tesla. Magn Reson Med 2010;64(1): 194–202.
37. Kilsdonk ID, de Graaf WL, Lopez SA, et al. Multi-contrast MR imaging at 7T in multiple sclerosis: highest lesion detection in cortical gray matter with 3D-FLAIR. AJNR Am J Neuroradiol 2013; 34(4):791–6.
38. de Graaf WL, Kilsdonk ID, Lopez-Soriano A, et al. Clinical application of multi-contrast 7-T MR imaging in multiple sclerosis: increased lesion detection compared to 3 T confined to grey matter. Eur Radiol 2013;23(2):528–40.
39. Zwanenburg JJ, Hendrikse J, Luijten PR. Generalized multiple-layer appearance of the cerebral cortex with 3D FLAIR 7.0-T MR imaging. Radiology 2012;262(3):995–1001.
40. Duyn JH. The future of ultra-high field MRI and fMRI for study of the human brain. Neuroimage 2012; 62(2):1241–8.
41. van der Kolk AG, Hendrikse J, Zwanenburg JJ, et al. Clinical applications of 7T MRI in the brain. Eur J Radiol 2013;82(5):708–18.
42. van der Kolk AG, Hendrikse J, Luijten PR. Ultrahigh-field magnetic resonance imaging: the clinical potential for anatomy, pathogenesis, diagnosis, and

treatment planning in brain disease. Neuroimaging Clin N Am 2012;22(2):343–62, xii.
43. Versluis MJ, van der Grond J, van Buchem MA, et al. High-field imaging of neurodegenerative diseases. Neuroimaging Clin N Am 2012;22(2):159–71, ix.
44. Zwanenburg JJ, Versluis MJ, Luijten PR, et al. Fast high resolution whole brain T2* weighted imaging using echo planar imaging at 7T. Neuroimage 2011;56(4):1902–7.
45. Brodmann K. Vergleichende Lokalisationslehre der Großhirnrinde in ihren Prinzipien dargestellt auf Grund des Zellenbaues. Leipzig (Germany): Barth; 1909.
46. Barbier EL, Marrett S, Danek A, et al. Imaging cortical anatomy by high-resolution MR at 3.0T: detection of the stripe of Gennari in visual area 17. Magn Reson Med 2002;48(4):735–8.
47. Bock NA, Hashim E, Janik R, et al. Optimizing T1-weighted imaging of cortical myelin content at 3.0 T. Neuroimage 2013;65:1–12.
48. Glasser MF, Van Essen DC. Mapping human cortical areas in vivo based on myelin content as revealed by T1- and T2-weighted MRI. J Neurosci 2011;31(32):11597–616.
49. Sereno MI, Lutti A, Weiskopf N, et al. Mapping the human cortical surface by combining quantitative T1 with Retinotopy. Cereb Cortex 2012. [Epub ahead of print].
50. Cho ZH, Oh SH, Kim JM, et al. Direct visualization of Parkinson's disease by in vivo human brain imaging using 7.0T magnetic resonance imaging. Mov Disord 2011;26(4):713–8.
51. van Veluw SJ, Zwanenburg JJ, Engelen-Lee J, et al. In vivo detection of cerebral cortical microinfarcts with high-resolution 7T MRI. J Cereb Blood Flow Metab 2013;33(3):322–9.
52. Shmueli K, Dodd SJ, Li TQ, et al. The contribution of chemical exchange to MRI frequency shifts in brain tissue. Magn Reson Med 2011; 65(1):35–43.
53. Fukunaga M, Li TQ, van Gelderen P, et al. Layer-specific variation of iron content in cerebral cortex as a source of MRI contrast. Proc Natl Acad Sci U S A 2010;107(8):3834–9.
54. Oomen KP, Pameijer FA, Zwanenburg JJ, et al. Improved depiction of pterygopalatine fossa anatomy using ultrahigh-resolution magnetic resonance imaging at 7 tesla. ScientificWorldJournal 2012; 2012:691095.
55. Lee J, Shmueli K, Fukunaga M, et al. Sensitivity of MRI resonance frequency to the orientation of brain tissue microstructure. Proc Natl Acad Sci U S A 2010;107(11):5130–5.
56. Korteweg MA, Zwanenburg JJ, Hoogduin JM, et al. Dissected sentinel lymph nodes of breast cancer patients: characterization with high-spatial-resolution 7-T MR imaging. Radiology 2011;261(1):127–35.
57. de Jong S, Zwanenburg JJ, Visser F, et al. Direct detection of myocardial fibrosis by MRI. J Mol Cell Cardiol 2011;51(6):974–9.
58. Orzada S, Maderwald S, Poser BA, et al. RF excitation using time interleaved acquisition of modes (TIAMO) to address B1 inhomogeneity in high-field MRI. Magn Reson Med 2010;64(2):327–33.
59. Katscher U, Bornert P. Parallel RF transmission in MRI. NMR Biomed 2006;19(3):393–400.
60. Kraff O, Theysohn JM, Maderwald S, et al. High-resolution MRI of the human parotid gland and duct at 7 Tesla. Invest Radiol 2009;44(9):518–24.
61. Kroner ES, van Schinkel LD, Versluis MJ, et al. Ultrahigh-field 7-T magnetic resonance carotid vessel wall imaging: initial experience in comparison with 3-T field strength. Invest Radiol 2012; 47(12):697–704.
62. Kraff O, Bitz AK, Breyer T, et al. A transmit/receive radiofrequency array for imaging the carotid arteries at 7 Tesla: coil design and first in vivo results. Invest Radiol 2011;46(4):246–54.
63. Koning W, Bluemink JJ, Langenhuizen EA, et al. High-resolution MRI of the carotid arteries using a leaky waveguide transmitter and a high-density receive array at 7 T. Magn Reson Med 2013; 69(4):1186–93.
64. Korteweg MA, Veldhuis WB, Visser F, et al. Feasibility of 7 Tesla breast magnetic resonance imaging determination of intrinsic sensitivity and high-resolution magnetic resonance imaging, diffusion-weighted imaging, and (1)H-magnetic resonance spectroscopy of breast cancer patients receiving neoadjuvant therapy. Invest Radiol 2011;46(6): 370–6.
65. Stehouwer BL, Klomp DW, Korteweg MA, et al. 7T versus 3T contrast-enhanced breast Magnetic Resonance Imaging of invasive ductulolobular carcinoma: first clinical experience. Magn Reson Imaging 2013;31(4):613–7.
66. Umutlu L, Maderwald S, Kraff O, et al. Dynamic contrast-enhanced breast MRI at 7 Tesla utilizing a single-loop coil: a feasibility trial. Acad Radiol 2010;17(8):1050–6.
67. Klomp DW, van de Bank BL, Raaijmakers A, et al. 31P MRSI and 1H MRS at 7 T: initial results in human breast cancer. NMR Biomed 2011;24(10):1337–42.
68. Wu CL, Jordan KW, Ratai EM, et al. Metabolomic imaging for human prostate cancer detection. Sci Transl Med 2010;2(16):16ra8.
69. Klomp DW, Scheenen TW, Arteaga CS, et al. Detection of fully refocused polyamine spins in prostate cancer at 7 T. NMR Biomed 2011;24(3): 299–306.
70. Arteaga de Castro CS, van den Bergen B, Luijten PR, et al. Improving SNR and B1 transmit field for an endorectal coil in 7 T MRI and MRS of prostate cancer. Magn Reson Med 2012;68(1):311–8.

71. Kobus T, Bitz AK, van Uden MJ, et al. In vivo 31P MR spectroscopic imaging of the human prostate at 7 T: safety and feasibility. Magn Reson Med 2012;68(6):1683–95.
72. Pakin SK, Cavalcanti C, La RR, et al. Ultra-high-field MRI of knee joint at 7.0T: preliminary experience. Acad Radiol 2006;13(9):1135–42.
73. Krug R, Carballido-Gamio J, Banerjee S, et al. In vivo ultra-high-field magnetic resonance imaging of trabecular bone microarchitecture at 7 T. J Magn Reson Imaging 2008;27(4):854–9.
74. Wright AC, Lemdiasov R, Connick TJ, et al. Helmholtz-pair transmit coil with integrated receive array for high-resolution MRI of trabecular bone in the distal tibia at 7T. J Magn Reson 2011; 210(1):113–22.
75. Regatte RR, Schweitzer ME. Ultra-high-field MRI of the musculoskeletal system at 7.0T. J Magn Reson Imaging 2007;25(2):262–9.
76. Stahl R, Krug R, Kelley DA, et al. Assessment of cartilage-dedicated sequences at ultra-high-field MRI: comparison of imaging performance and diagnostic confidence between 3.0 and 7.0 T with respect to osteoarthritis-induced changes at the knee joint. Skeletal Radiol 2009;38(8):771–83.
77. Moser E, Stahlberg F, Ladd ME, et al. 7-T MR–from research to clinical applications? NMR Biomed 2012;25(5):695–716.
78. Visser F, Korteweg MA, Italiaander M, et al. High resolution PDw-TSE of the ankle with the use of a flexible high density receive array at 7 Tesla. Proceedings of ISMRM 20th Scientific Meeting and Exhibition. Melbourne, Australia: 2012. p. 1449.
79. Trattnig S, Zbyn S, Schmitt B, et al. Advanced MR methods at ultra-high field (7 Tesla) for clinical musculoskeletal applications. Eur Radiol 2012; 22(11):2338–46.
80. Agarwal R, Brunelli SM, Williams K, et al. Gadolinium-based contrast agents and nephrogenic systemic fibrosis: a systematic review and meta-analysis. Nephrol Dial Transplant 2009;24(3):856–63.
81. Suttie JJ, Delabarre L, Pitcher A, et al. 7 Tesla (T) human cardiovascular magnetic resonance imaging using FLASH and SSFP to assess cardiac function: validation against 1.5 T and 3 T. NMR Biomed 2012;25(1):27–34.
82. Hays AG, Schar M, Kelle S. Clinical applications for cardiovascular magnetic resonance imaging at 3 tesla. Curr Cardiol Rev 2009;5(3):237–42.
83. Niendorf T, Graessl A, Thalhammer C, et al. Progress and promises of human cardiac magnetic resonance at ultrahigh fields: a physics perspective. J Magn Reson 2013;229:208–22.
84. Brandts A, Westenberg JJ, Versluis MJ, et al. Quantitative assessment of left ventricular function in humans at 7 T. Magn Reson Med 2010;64(5): 1471–7.
85. Winter L, Kellman P, Renz W, et al. Comparison of three multichannel transmit/receive radiofrequency coil configurations for anatomic and functional cardiac MRI at 7.0T: implications for clinical imaging. Eur Radiol 2012;22(10):2211–20.
86. van Elderen SG, Versluis MJ, Westenberg JJ, et al. Right coronary MR angiography at 7 T: a direct quantitative and qualitative comparison with 3 T in young healthy volunteers. Radiology 2010; 257(1):254–9.
87. Kohler S, Hiller KH, Waller C, et al. Visualization of myocardial microstructure using high-resolution T*2 imaging at high magnetic field. Magn Reson Med 2003;49(2):371–5.
88. Hezel F, Thalhammer C, Waiczies S, et al. High spatial resolution and temporally resolved t(2) (*) mapping of normal human myocardium at 7.0 tesla: an ultrahigh field magnetic resonance feasibility study. PLoS One 2012;7(12):e52324.
89. Grams AE, Kraff O, Umutlu L, et al. MRI of the lumbar spine at 7 Tesla in healthy volunteers and a patient with congenital malformations. Skeletal Radiol 2012;41(5):509–14.
90. de Graaf WL, Zwanenburg JJ, Visser F, et al. Lesion detection at seven Tesla in multiple sclerosis using magnetisation prepared 3D-FLAIR and 3D-DIR. Eur Radiol 2012;22(1):221–31.
91. Wisse LE, Gerritsen L, Zwanenburg JJ, et al. Subfields of the hippocampal formation at 7T MRI in vivo volumetric assessment. Neuroimage 2012; 61(4):1043–9.

Blood Oxygenation Level–dependent/Functional Magnetic Resonance Imaging

Underpinnings, Practice, and Perspectives

Jeroen C.W. Siero, PhD[a,*], Alex Bhogal, MSc[a],
J. Martijn Jansma, PhD[b]

KEYWORDS

• Brain function • Blood oxygenation level–dependent contrast • Functional MR imaging
• Neuroimaging • Resting state • Tumor surgery • Epilepsy • Cerebrovascular reactivity

KEY POINTS

- Blood oxygenation level–dependent (BOLD) functional magnetic resonance (fMR) imaging offers a fully noninvasive technique to study brain function and can give measures of cerebrovascular reactivity.
- BOLD fMR imaging is sensitive to the local changes in cerebral blood flow, blood volume, and cerebral metabolic rate of oxygen.
- The BOLD contrast benefits greatly from ultrahigh field strength MR imaging (7 T), pushing the attainable spatiotemporal resolution and vascular specificity toward the submillimeter scale.
- BOLD imaging can aid presurgical planning in patients with brain tumors, identification of brain regions involved in epilepsy, and the diagnosis of certain cerebrovascular diseases.

INTRODUCTION

Technological advancements in the last 2 decades have facilitated increasing understanding of human brain structure and physiology. The development of high-field magnetic resonance (MR) imaging systems and acquisition methodology, in combination with a greater physiologic understanding, has given researchers the tools to examine the processes underlying brain function in more detail. To date, the technique most frequently used to probe brain function has relied on the blood oxygenation level–dependent (BOLD) contrast mechanism. The BOLD contrast is sensitive to changes in cerebral blood flow (CBF), cerebral blood volume (CBV), and the cerebral metabolic rate of oxygen ($CMRO_2$).

The notion of a relationship between neural activation and changes in CBF was first conceptualized by neurophysiologists Roy and Sherrington[1] in 1890. Their description of a local neurovascular coupling mechanism suggested that the energy demand of active neuronal tissue was responsible for a local increase in CBF, thus increasing the supply of O_2 and glucose. The idea of a locally controlled neurovascular unit is fundamental for many functional imaging modalities that are sensitive to changes in CBF, especially in functional mapping experiments having high spatial detail.[2–5] PET[6] was one of the first imaging techniques to

Disclosures: The authors have nothing to disclose.

[a] Department of Radiology, University Medical Center Utrecht, Heidelberglaan 100, 3584 CX Utrecht, HP E 01.132, The Netherlands; [b] Department of Neurology and Neurosurgery, Rudolf Magnus Institute of Neuroscience, University Medical Center Utrecht, Utrecht, The Netherlands
* Corresponding author. Department of Radiology, University Medical Center Utrecht, Heidelberglaan 100, 3584 CX Utrecht, HP E 01.132, The Netherlands.
E-mail address: j.c.w.siero@umcutrecht.nl

PET Clin 8 (2013) 329–344
http://dx.doi.org/10.1016/j.cpet.2013.04.003
1556-8598/13/$ – see front matter

exploit the neurovascular coupling concept for mapping brain function. Fox and colleagues[7–9] used PET imaging for focusing on the visual cortex, to reveal the metabolic and hemodynamic processes apparent during neuronal activation. Their work was a crucial step toward the discovery of the BOLD contrast mechanism. The increases in CBF greatly exceeded the oxygen demand of the neuronal active tissue. It is this mismatch/uncoupling between $CMRo_2$ and CBF (or oxygen supply) during activation that gives rise to the signal changes typical of BOLD functional MR (fMR) imaging (in contrast, glucose metabolism seems to be a better predictor for the induced CBF changes during neuronal activation.[9,10] However, using PET, Powers and colleagues[10] showed that the demand for glucose cannot explain the apparent close coupling to CBF). In 1992, the first 3 papers were published on measuring brain function using BOLD fMR imaging.[11–13] These three key papers showed that changes in brain state could be measured reliably and, in contrast with PET, noninvasively. Since its discovery, BOLD fMR imaging has been the workhorse in neuroscience. It has been used as a tool to delineate active brain regions, but has also been used to identify regional deactivation.[14–17] Furthermore, BOLD fMR imaging has shed light on the interactions between different cerebral networks.[18] With the advent of ultrahigh-field MR systems ($\geq$7 T), BOLD fMR imaging promises to reveal human brain function and hemodynamic processes at the fine level of cortical columns and layers (spatial scale $\leq$1 mm).[19–25]

Besides functional mapping, the BOLD contrast can also be used to investigate neurovascular coupling and venous vessel reactivity, which can be useful for investigating disorders such as vascular stenosis, stroke, and Alzheimer disease, and also for tumor characterization and delineation. Much information can be gained when combining BOLD fMR imaging with the arterial spin labeling (ASL) MR method (discussed elsewhere in this issue by Jill B. De Vis). ASL is primarily sensitive to changes in CBF, and its use in combination with respiratory challenges allows for separation of the relative contributions of CBF, CBV, and $CMRo_2$ to the BOLD signal (calibrated BOLD[26]). Other clinical applications of BOLD fMR imaging are presurgical functional mapping before tumor resection, and in relation to epileptic foci.

This article gives an overview of the mechanisms behind the BOLD contrast, the important factors that determine the specificity and sensitivity of BOLD fMR imaging, and the common scanning methods and image artifacts. The main neuroscientific and clinical applications of BOLD fMR imaging are discussed, as well as future directions and possibilities.

BOLD FMR: IMAGING TECHNIQUE

The BOLD Contrast Mechanism

The BOLD contrast mechanism is based on the endogenous contrast agent deoxyhemoglobin. BOLD imaging techniques are sensitive to the changes in relative blood deoxyhemoglobin concentrations following neuronal activation, and can therefore be used to detect impaired cerebral vascular reactivity (CVR) or altered tissue oxygenation. The BOLD contrast originates from the magnetic susceptibility effects within (intravascular) and around (extravascular) the blood vessels, which are caused by deoxyhemoglobin. Depending on the local vasculature, these effects scale linearly or supralinearly with the main magnetic field strength (B_0) of the MR system.[27,28] The deoxyhemoglobin molecule is paramagnetic, in contrast with the diamagnetic susceptibility of surrounding brain tissue (gray matter). An increase in deoxyhemoglobin leads to an increase in the magnetic susceptibility difference between blood and the surrounding tissue, thus producing local field distortions that change the resonance frequencies of affected protons. As a result, the net magnetization of protons within a given imaging voxel diphase, causing a dropout of the MR signal. In BOLD fMR imaging, the typical local CBF increase on neuronal activation significantly exceeds the $CMRo_2$, causing a net washout of the local deoxyhemoglobin content[29–31] and, thus, an increase of the MR signal because of less intravoxel dephasing. In contrast, oxyhemoglobin is diamagnetic, and so fully oxygenated blood (eg, arterial blood) has a similar magnetic susceptibility to that of the surrounding tissue, resulting in a negligible BOLD signal (a low BOLD contrast). The degree of BOLD-dependent signal changes observed depends on the local deoxyhemoglobin content, and is related to the B_0 field-dependent T_2 and T_2* relaxation parameters of blood and extravascular tissue.

There are multiple models and simulations that can describe the expected BOLD signal evolution for certain conditions of the vascular system (baseline and changes in CBF, CBV, $CMRo_2$, and hematocrit but also vascular architecture such as vessel size and orientation).[26,32–35] For instance, two well-known models are the balloon model and the windkessel model.[29–31] Both models describe the dynamics of CBF and deoxyhemoglobin and how they are transformed into a BOLD signal. The underlying principles are similar: the venous compartment is modeled as an expandable (compliant) balloon receiving blood from the capillary bed. The compliancy of the venous compartment gives rise to viscoelastic effects, observable as a delayed CBV return to baseline that mismatches the CBF return to baseline (ie, a poststimulus undershoot; discussed later). In the cortical vasculature, deoxyhemoglobin changes are largest at the venous side of the vascular bed, and hence standard BOLD fMR imaging predominantly measures changes in blood oxygenation of capillaries, intracortical venules and veins, as well as the draining veins on the pial surface.[3]

The BOLD Response

When a subject performs a mental task or receives a functional stimulus during a BOLD fMR imaging experiment (eg, a flashing checkerboard), neuronal activity in the brain exhibits regional increases and decreases. Within each region, the associated BOLD response manifests as a relative signal change from baseline with the dynamic interplay of CBF, CBV, and $CMRo_2$ determining the amplitude of the signal changes. The generally accepted model on local blood flow regulation states that synaptic activity in these brain regions causes the release of vasoactive agents that dilate the arterioles supplying the neuronal tissue.[36,37] Dilation has the effect of decreasing vascular resistance, resulting in an increase in CBF and the BOLD signal.

A typical positive BOLD response (**Fig. 1**) consists of 3 parts: (1) a small, short-lived negative deflection of the BOLD signal during the first 1 to 2 seconds called the initial dip. The initial dip is thought to indicate an increase in $CMRo_2$ before the CBF response (controversy still exists regarding the origin and mechanisms behind the initial dip of the BOLD response because it is not robustly detected and because of disagreement between MR data and data obtained from optical imaging studies).[38–40] (2) A larger signal increase caused by a large CBF increase that peaks around 3 to 6 seconds, followed by a signal decrease. (3) A subsequent poststimulus undershoot before returning to baseline after 12 to 30 seconds (see **Fig. 1**). There is ongoing debate on the exact physiologic origin of the poststimulus undershoot. At present, MR and optical data suggest that the undershoot is dominated by a sustained increase in $CMRo_2$; however, prolonged CBV increase (vascular compliance) or a CBF decrease may also contribute.[32,41,42] The temporal profile of the BOLD response depends on the stimulus conditions and brain region under examination but also on the biology (including the disorder) of the local vasculature and underlying neurovascular coupling mechanisms.[21,22,24,43,44]

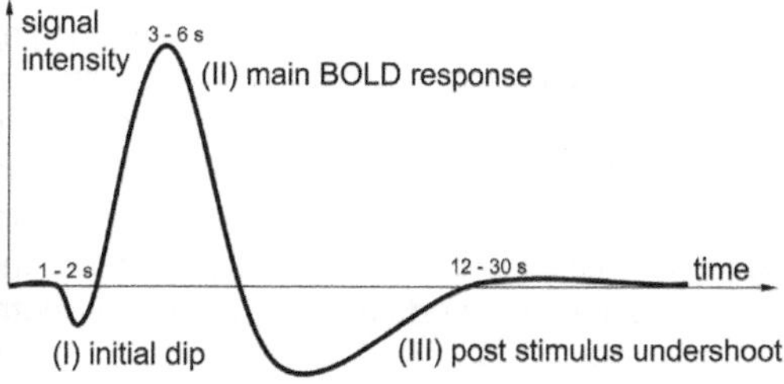

Fig. 1. Depiction of a typical BOLD hemodynamic response function. The shape can vary depending on the stimulus conditions, cortical area, and the biology of the local vasculature.

BOLD Sensitivity and Specificity

Sufficient sensitivity is crucial to performing fMR imaging with high spatial and temporal accuracy. Sensitivity of the BOLD contrast is amplified when increasing the B_0 field strength. Higher B_0 field strength increases the image signal/noise ratio (SNR) but also magnifies the aforementioned magnetic susceptibility differences in the body. As an alternative, sensitivity can be boosted by using dedicated surface receive coils.[45] In the ideal scenario, BOLD fMR imaging is specific to only the BOLD changes in the capillary bed that is closest to the neuronally active tissue (downstream from the capillary bed are, in order of decreasing specificity and increasing vessel size, the venules, intracortical veins oriented perpendicular to the cortical surface, followed by the pial veins and larger draining veins located on the cortical surface).[3] As indicated previously, the vasculature that feeds neuronal tissue consists of several vessel types having different vessel sizes that contribute to the measured signal in their own ways. Vascular properties can affect BOLD fMR imaging specificity, which also depends on both the B_0 field strength and the fMR imaging scan parameters. To clarify the effect of these factors, the BOLD effect must be evaluated in more detail.

The source of the BOLD signal can be separated into internal and external blood vessel components: intravascular and extravascular BOLD signal components. As previously mentioned, a blood vessel containing deoxyhemoglobin has a different magnetic susceptibility from the surrounding tissue. This difference results in a resonance frequency shift between intravascular and extravascular water protons. Increasing the B_0 field strength increases the frequency offsets induced by deoxyhemoglobin and hence allows greater BOLD contrast. Only the extravascular effects have a spatial dependency that scales with the vessel radius.[28] The BOLD signal from a given imaging voxel depends, in a complex manner, on the structural organization of the capillaries and draining veins that give increase to the intravascular and extravascular signal effects, as well as the scan parameters, pulse sequences used, and B_0 field strength. Numerous studies have investigated the combined effects on the BOLD contrast sensitivity and specificity using simulations or analytical approaches.[27,28,34,46–48]

As the strength of the B_0 field increases, especially at 7 T, the BOLD behavior changes as signal contributions shift from predominantly intravascular to extravascular.[27] Compared with lower field strengths, BOLD fMR imaging at 7 T shows an increased weighting toward microvascular signals (capillary and small venules) because of the strong B_0 field dependence of intravascular contributions. The increased specificity comes from the almost complete removal of intravascular contributions from the nonspecific macrovasculature (ie, the pial and larger draining veins).[27] At 7 T, the T_2 and T_2* of venous blood (intravascular) are shorter than the T_2 and T_2* of the extravascular gray matter tissue (**Table 1**). The echo time (TE) is the time at which the MR signal is acquired and acts as a filter for certain T_2 or T_2* values. Setting the TE of the BOLD fMR imaging scan equal to the gray matter T_2 or T_2* results in maximal sensitivity for BOLD signal changes in gray matter and essentially no contribution from intravascular signals (<1%).[27,52] At 7 T, BOLD fMR imaging is thus dominated by extravascular contributions. However, at 1.5 T, the opposite is true: venous blood has a longer T_2 and T_2* than gray matter (see **Table 1**), and hence the BOLD signal is dominated by the enhanced intravascular contributions coming mostly from the macrovasculature.

Gradient-echo and Spin-echo BOLD fMR Imaging

Important scan parameters for maximizing BOLD specificity include the spatial resolution (or voxel dimensions), TE, and the type of acquisition method: gradient-echo (GE) or spin-echo (SE) acquisition. For BOLD fMR imaging, the conventional acquisition method is GE because of its high sensitivity to changes in T_2*. However, GE measures from both the microvasculature and macrovasculature and, as a result, the specificity to active cortical regions can be reduced. An alternative is SE acquisition, which is characterized by a refocusing 180° radiofrequency pulse and is more sensitive to T_2 changes. In contrast, SE can be highly specific to the microvasculature at the cost of a reduced sensitivity to BOLD signal changes. At 7 T, the inherent increase in sensitivity, compared with lower B_0 field strength, makes SE BOLD fMR imaging advantageous. More importantly, SE BOLD fMR imaging at 7 T is weighted toward the microvasculature, making it a specific acquisition method.[27,51,53,54] The increased microvascular specificity of SE BOLD fMR imaging arises from the spatial dependency of the extravascular frequency offsets, as mentioned earlier, in combination with the diffusion of water protons around the blood vessels. The extent of the extravascular effects scales with the vessel size. For large vessels, the diffusing water protons experience a constant frequency offset within a certain diffusion time (ie, the TE). This phenomenon is called static dephasing.[46] However, for smaller vessels, such as the capillaries, the diffusing water protons experience a wider range of frequency offsets, known as dynamic dephasing.[49] The effect of an SE refocusing pulse is that it refocuses or cancels out any constant frequency offsets a diffusing proton experiences during a TE. However, the dynamic dephasing effects are time irreversible and thus cannot be refocused by the SE refocusing pulse. Hence, the SE acquisition method is not sensitive to extravascular signal changes around larger vessels, leaving only the extravascular signals of the microvasculature. Because signal changes with spatially constant frequency offsets are refocused the SE acquisition method has a reduced sensitivity compared with the GE method. Exploiting the increased specificity of SE BOLD fMR imaging at 7 T, Yacoub and colleagues[20] were able to robustly map the ocular dominance and orientation columns (spatial scale of ≈1 mm) in the visual cortex (**Fig. 2**). **Table 2** summarizes the dominant signal mechanisms and the specificity for GE and SE acquisitions methods across B_0 field strength

Table 1
Values of blood T_2 and gray matter T_2 for 1.5 T and 7 T

B_0	T_2 Blood (ms)	T_2 Gray Matter (ms)	T_2* Gray Matter (ms)
1.5 T	109[a]	77[b]	65[a]
7.0 T	7[a]	55[c]	25[a]

[a] *Data from* Ref.[49]
[b] *Data from* Ref.[50]
[c] *Data from* Ref.[51]

Dynamic Acquisition and Related Artifacts

Induced BOLD changes typically have a temporal resolution on the order of seconds (see **Fig. 1**

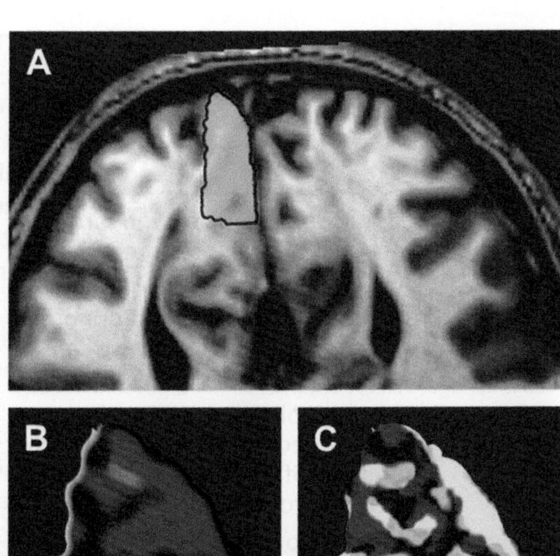

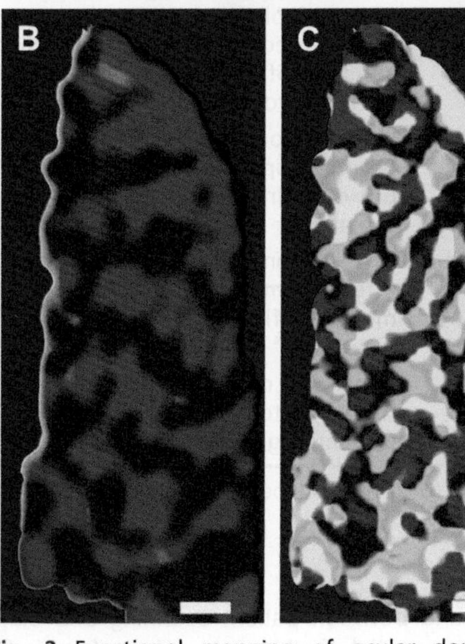

Fig. 2. Functional mapping of ocular dominance columns (ODC) and orientation columns in the primary visual cortex using ultra–high-field BOLD fMR imaging. (*A*) The region of interest (ROI) in green in the primary visual cortex from which columnar level BOLD fMR imaging maps of ODC (*B*) and orientation columns (*C*) are generated and characterized. The functional maps (*B, C*) are zoomed views of the ROI in (*A*). The red and blue colors in (*B*) indicate preferences to right or left eye stimulation, whereas the color distribution in (*C*) represents a given voxel's fMR imaging time course phase, which indicates its preferred visual stimulus orientation. Scale bar, 1.0 mm. (*Courtesy of* Rijlaarsdam AF, Jansma JM, Ramsey NF. University Medical Center Utrecht.)

(subsecond time differences in, for instance, the BOLD response onset time have been reported between functional brain regions or across the gray matter cortical depth[22,58,59])[43,60] and accurately tracking these changes over a large field of view requires a fast scanning technique. The workhorse in BOLD fMR imaging is the GE echo planar imaging (EPI) scanning technique, which is able to obtain a complete imaging volume with voxel dimensions on the order of millimeters in a matter of seconds. BOLD fMR imaging suffers from trade-offs (spatial vs temporal resolution) that must be considered depending on what results are desired. Higher spatial resolution reduces partial volume effects to allow a more accurate localization (higher specificity), but at the expense of temporal resolution. High-field MR systems offer increased SNR that can be used for increasing temporal or spatial resolution (or both).

A typical BOLD fMR imaging experiment involves dynamic EPI scans often taking upwards of 10 minutes to complete. For that reason, patient movement can be one of the largest confounds with respect to gathering reliable data. Furthermore, EPI-based BOLD fMR imaging experiments are subject to imaging artifacts prone to EPI. These artifacts mainly include ghosting, geometric distortion caused by inhomogeneous B_0, and susceptibility-related or signal dropout artifacts. Some examples are provided in **Fig. 3**.

Fig. 3A shows an example of image distortion. Image distortion is of particular importance with respect to clinical fMR imaging because many applications rely on precise structural localization (ie, functional or presurgical mapping). Using EPI, distortions (ie, pixel shifts) predominantly occur in the phase-encode direction because of phase accumulation between successive phase-encode steps (distortions in the readout direction are less because this step is fast, leading to less phase accumulation). The phase accumulation leading to image distortions are also caused by magnetic susceptibility effects (ie, inhomogeneous B_0). The susceptibility artifacts mentioned earlier all worsen at higher field strengths, which necessitates effective and elaborate shimming practices at high-B_0 field such as 7 T. **Fig. 3**B shows an example of signal dropout. Signal dropout is generally caused by inhomogeneities in the B_0 field caused by the object being scanned or by improper shimming. Signal loss is most prominent at air-tissue boundaries (eg, ear and nasal cavities) where large gradients in magnetic susceptibility exist. Also, metal and dental implants can cause major magnetic susceptibility effects leading to signal dropouts. These differences result in local field disturbances leading to dephasing of spins and increased T_2*-related signal loss. SE sequences are less sensitive to these effects. **Fig. 3**B shows an example of ghosting also called a Nyquist or N/2 ghost. Ghosting stems from a misalignment of odd and even echoes during the EPI readout and typically manifests as a ghost image that has been shifted by N/2 pixels in the phase-encode direction (where N is equal to the matrix size). Hardware timing

Table 2
Dominant BOLD signal mechanisms and specificity for GE and SE acquisitions methods across B_0 field strength

	SE	GE
Dominant BOLD signal mechanism $B_0 \geq 7$ T	EV. Dynamic dephasing. IV signal is suppressed[54,55]	EV. Static dephasing around large vessels. IV signal is suppressed[54,55]
Specificity $B_0 \geq 7$ T	Microvasculature with r<5–10 μm. Tight localization with active sites[48,53,54]	Predominantly venules and draining veins with r>10 μm. Downstream of activation[27]
Dominant BOLD signal mechanism 4 T $\leq B_0$>7 T	EV. Dynamic dephasing. IV signal caused by T_2>TE[27,54,55]	EV. Static dephasing. IV signal caused by increased T_2* with respect to TE Magnitude of relative contributions exhibits strong TE dependence[49,56]
Specificity 4 T $\leq B_0$>7 T	Microvasculature IV effects persist at long TE with potential for unlocalized signals from large downstream vessels[54]	EV effects around smaller vessels become apparent. Long TE and diffusion gradients can suppress IV signals[49]
Dominant BOLD signal mechanism $B_0 \leq 3$ T	IV effects from large vessels dominate[54,57]	EV effects dominate; however, IV effects from large vessels become more significant as field strength decreases[54]
Specificity $B_0 \leq 3$ T	IV. At low fields SE SNR is much lower than for GE (blood contributions downstream if SNR is sufficient)	Downstream of activation. High sensitivity to draining veins and pooling regions[56]

Relationships between IV and EV signal mechanisms, acquisition method (GE or SE), and specificity (vessel size, *r* denotes vessel radius) relative to field strength.
Abbreviations: EV, extravascular, IV, intravascular.

inconsistencies as well as spatially or temporally varying field inhomogeneities and patient motion can all worsen the artifact.[61]

In some cases, methods exist to correct for artifacts; however, these can be complicated, time consuming, and often require an experienced researcher to complete, which can limit the clinical viability of certain techniques because fast turnaround between patient scanning and diagnosis is essential. Furthermore, it is preferable for clinical applications to be stand-alone procedures that can be performed by technical staff without the need for extensive postprocessing or data analysis. It is also essential that technical staff be aware of common artifacts and the techniques used to avoid them.

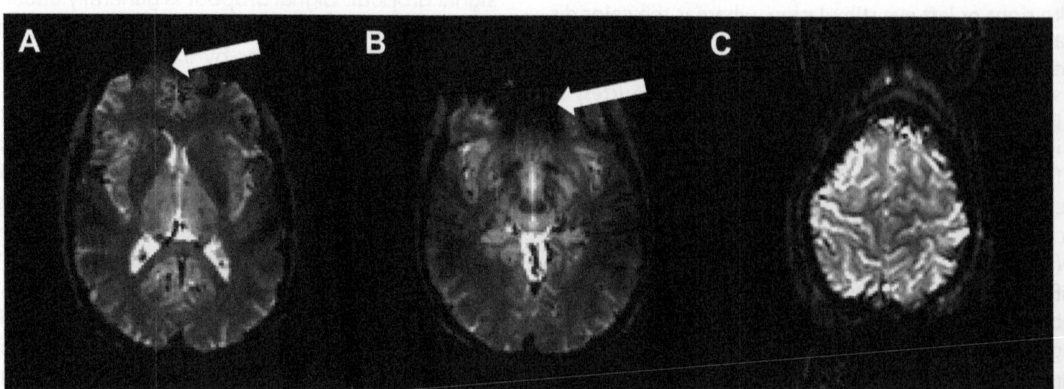

Fig. 3. (*A*) Distortion in EPI BOLD image, indicated by the white arrow, caused by magnetic susceptibility effects. (*B*) Signal dropout, as indicated by the white arrow, caused by high susceptibility gradient at tissue interfaces within the nasal canal. (*C*) Nyquist artifact shown by a ghost image that is shifted by N/2 pixels (N is matrix size in the phase-encoding direction).

EXPERIMENTAL DESIGNS AND ANALYSIS APPROACHES

There are several experimental designs and analysis methods for BOLD fMR imaging that all present different approaches to the challenge of the delayed BOLD fMR imaging signal response to neuronal activity. At the highest level it is possible to make a fundamental distinction between 2 approaches: task-based fMR imaging and resting-state fMR imaging. Both approaches apply fundamentally different analyses techniques and have different immediate goals. Although task-based fMR imaging seeks to understand function, resting-state fMR imaging searches for understanding of connections and organization.

Resting-state fMR Imaging

Resting-state fMR imaging is used to evaluate correlations between brain regions that occur when a subject is not performing a goal-oriented task and is provided with minimal external input (ie, the subject is at rest).[62,63] Because phasic changes in brain activity are always present, including in the absence of any external task or input, brain regions constantly show fluctuations in the BOLD signal. Resting-state fMR imaging is a technique that uses these fluctuations to explore regional correlations between brain regions.[18] In addition, it is used to examine potential alterations related to neurologic or psychiatric diseases.[64,65] Resting-state fMR imaging studies have revealed that the healthy brain has several consistent and reproducible resting-state networks.[66] One of the challenges of resting-state fMR imaging is to understand the relevance of the findings in terms of brain functionality and cognition. Important limiting factors in this challenge are the possible influence of nonneuronal effects such as the underlying brain physiology on BOLD fluctuations[67] as well as measurements being performed in the absence of any controlled cognitive activity.

Task-based fMR Imaging

Task-based BOLD fMR imaging experiments examine the functions of the brain as an input-output processing and a goal-oriented organ, which is accomplished by searching for changes in the BOLD fMR imaging signal that can be explained by the presented task. It is important to realize that the BOLD fMR imaging signal cannot be used as an absolute measurement of brain activity, but is only reliable as an indication of an increase or decrease in brain activity. It is thus impossible to measure the brain activity while a subject is performing a task, but it is possible to measure the change in brain activity in a subject between 2 or more tasks, or a task and rest, if these are alternated within a short time (ideally less than a minute, but there can be exceptions).

A task-based fMR imaging experiment is typically analyzed using a linear regression analysis. A linear regression analysis is a statistical technique that determines how much of the variation in a dependent variable (in this case the BOLD fMR imaging signal in a voxel) can be explained by a linear combination of dependent variables, or regressors. In an fMR imaging analysis, these dependent regressors include 1 or more task regressors that model the expected signal change based on the presented task. Furthermore, a set of nuisance regressors are included to model the expected signal drift over time. The nuisance regressors improve the overall fit, but are in general not of interest for the experimenter. Each regressor provides a beta value and a t score. The beta value represents the value that provides the best fit for that regressor, whereas the t score represents the explained variation. Two of the most popular experimental designs for task-based BOLD fMR imaging are the blocked design and the event-related design.

Blocked design

A blocked design is characterized by task conditions that are presented in long and fixed periods (~15–60 seconds), so-called blocks. For instance, a subject looks at a flickering checkerboard for 30 seconds, looks at 10 different pictures that are each presented for a couple of seconds, or performs several short trials of the same cognitive task. These tasks of interest are typically alternated with fixed periods of a baseline task that does not include the function of interest, or with a rest period (**Fig. 4**A). The blocked fMR imaging paradigm analysis is based on the assumption that the BOLD fMR imaging signal in regions that are involved in a task will show a constant signal over the task period, as the subject is performing 1 task during that period. Advantages of the blocked design are the high sensitivity, which is a result of all BOLD responses combining to create a high and stable signal change in the fixed block period. Further, a blocked design does not rely much on assumptions about the temporal characteristics of the BOLD fMR imaging signal. Most important disadvantages are a low temporal resolution, because each block provides only 1 BOLD fMR imaging signal value that represents the average signal change in that block. Further, the reliability of the results of a blocked design can be reduced because the assumption that the brain activity is constant over each block is not true, which can be a result of the high

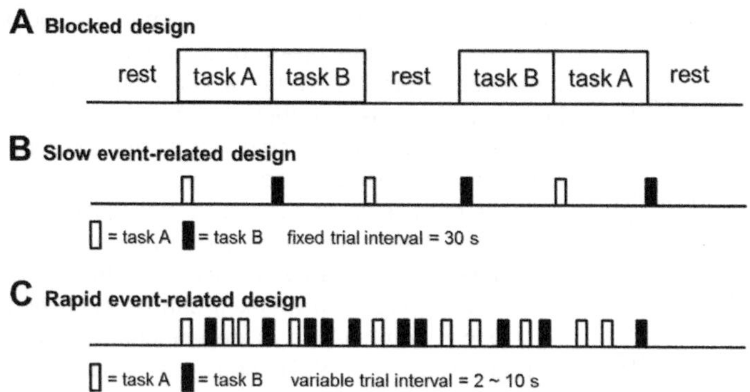

Fig. 4. Task-based BOLD fMR imaging approaches. (*A*) Blocked design: several trials using 1 or more different tasks (for example, task A and task B can be tapping the right or left index finger respectively). The tasks are performed for long periods of time (~15–60 seconds), alternating with periods of a control condition (rest). Advantage of the blocked design are the high sensitivity; a disadvantage is the low temporal resolution of the BOLD signal changes. (*B*) Slow event–related design: several trails are performed using 1 or more tasks with long periods of rest. An advantage of a slow event–related design is the possibility to measure the exact hemodynamic response function (HRF) to a single trial without the need for an a-priori model of the HRF. However, a slow event-related design has a low sensitivity and the overall experiment may become tedious because of long intertrial intervals. (*C*) Rapid event–related design: varying periods between trials of 1 or more tasks, which results in a higher sensitivity compared with the slow event–related design but at the small cost of reduced information that can be extracted. Because of the shorter intertrial intervals compared with the length of a BOLD response, it is necessary to use more complex analysis techniques.

predictability of the design, because subjects know they have to perform the same task for a longer period. This characteristic increases the chance of learning, adaptation, or attention effects that can influence brain activity within a block.

Event-related Design

An event-related fMR imaging (er-fMR imaging) design is characterized by single trials of 1 or more tasks being presented.[68,69] The least complicated approach of an er-fMR imaging is the slow er-fMR imaging design. In this design, trials are presented with a long and fixed interval to allow the BOLD fMR imaging signal to return to baseline (see **Fig. 4**B). Advantages of a slow event–related design are the possibility to measure the exact hemodynamic response function (HRF) to a single trial without the need for an a-priori model of the HRF. However, slow er-fMR imaging designs are not popular, because they suffer from low sensitivity, and from the task sometimes becoming tedious because of the long trial intervals. For instance, the subject may start to perform other uncontrollable tasks in the long periods between trials.

Because of these disadvantages, a rapid er-fMR imaging design is more popular. In a rapid er-fMR imaging design, trials are presented with short and varying intervals (see **Fig. 4**C). Because the intertrial intervals are shorter than the BOLD response, it is necessary to use more complex analysis techniques. A rapid er-fMR imaging design is typically analyzed using one of 2 approaches.[67,70] The first and most common approach is the canonical or signal detection analysis. Similar to a blocked design, this analysis applies a linear regression analysis with a single regressor for each task. However, in contrast with the blocked design, the shape of these regressors relies heavily on an a-priori defined model of the HRF (a canonical model) as well as the assumption that overlapping BOLD responses show a linear characteristic (ie, can simply be added). Because trials of each task have uniquely varying intertrial intervals, each task-regressor can only explain variation that belongs to 1 specific task. Advantages of the canonical approach are the high sensitivity, combined with the possibility of detecting trial-related activity. Disadvantages are the reliance on an a-priori HRF model, and the assumption of linear addition of overlapping BOLD fMR imaging responses, which may not always be correct.

Alternatively, a finite impulse response (FIR) or signal estimation analysis can be applied.[71,72] In this analysis, the full BOLD fMR imaging response is estimated by applying many impulse regressors per condition. Advantages of the FIR analysis are the high level of information, because the full HRF response can be estimated, combined with a good sensitivity. Disadvantages are the reduced sensitivity compared with canonical analysis, and the sensitivity to dependence between regressors, which can further lower statistical efficiency.

Historical Development

There is no ideal design or perfect analysis for BOLD fMR imaging. Depending on the specific research question and experiment requirements, each of the design and analysis approaches discussed earlier can be valuable (**Table 3**). However

Table 3
Feature comparison of task-based BOLD fMR imaging approaches

Type of Design	Analysis	Sensitivity	Information	Assumptions
Blocked	Canonical	++++	+	+++
Rapid event–related design	Canonical	+++	++	++++
Rapid event–related design	FIR	++	+++	++
Slow event–related design	Average	+	++++	+

over the last 20 years, there has been a slow shift from approaches that optimize sensitivity at the expense of information (blocked designs) to approaches that balance sensitivity with information (er-fMR imaging with canonical analysis). This development has progressed in parallel with the technical developments that have continuously increased SNR over the years. These developments include increases in field strength and the shift from single to parallel coils. If this trend is continued, it can be expected that, in the near future, the techniques that provide most information (slow er-fMR imaging and rapid er-fMR imaging in combination with FIR analysis) will become more popular.

CLINICAL APPLICATIONS OF FMR IMAGING

Because individual measurements have good spatial resolution and can easily be integrated with individual anatomic images, BOLD fMR imaging is frequently used for presurgical planning or as an adjunct to existing techniques for this purpose. At present, two important application fields for clinical BOLD fMR imaging are brain tumor and epilepsy surgery.

BOLD fMR Imaging in Epilepsy

In presurgical fMR imaging in epilepsy, fMR imaging is typically combined with electroencephalogram (EEG) recordings.[73–76] The presence of epileptic seizures during simultaneous recordings of EEG and fMR imaging is unlikely but also often detrimental to the measurements. Thus simultaneous EEG-fMR imaging in epilepsy typically focuses on identification of interictal epileptic discharges (IED), which are frequently observed, brief bursts of neuronal activity. The EEG recordings of these IED discharges are used as a regressor to analyze the fMR imaging data to determine the source location of the IEDs. **Fig. 5** shows an example of EEG-fMR imaging in epilepsy in which intracranial electrodes (electrocorticography [ECoG]) were used as a reference for evaluation of the technique.[73] Simultaneous EEG-fMR imaging has been proved clinically relevant because resection of tissue corresponding with the IED-related BOLD maximum has been associated

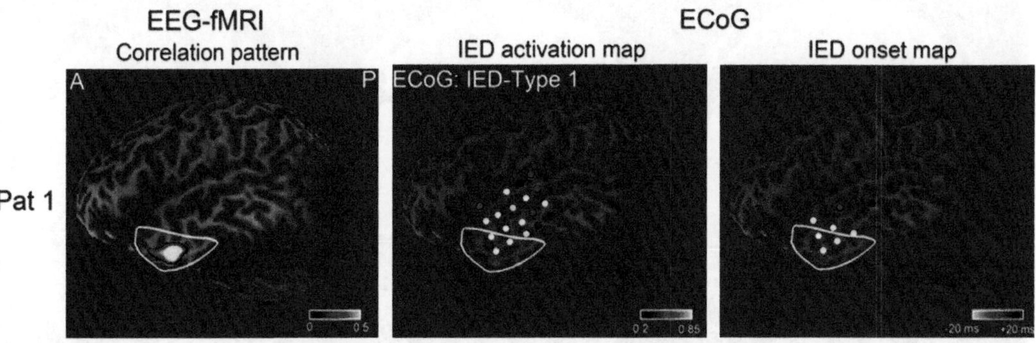

Fig. 5. Combined EEG-fMR imaging in epilepsy. EEG-fMR imaging correlation pattern (*left*) and electrocorticography (ECoG) results (*middle* and *right*) for a patient. The white contour line indicates the resected area. The color bars indicate the height of the correlation coefficient for the EEG-fMR imaging correlation pattern and for the ECoG activation map. For the ECoG onset map, the color bar indicates the delay of IED activity for a particular electrode relative to other electrodes. Early onset (ie, negative time values) is indicated with bright colors, whereas later time points are indicated with dark colors. A, anterior; P, posterior. (*Adapted from* van Houdt PJ, de Munck JC, Leijten FS, et al. EEG-fMRI correlation patterns in the presurgical evaluation of focal epilepsy: A comparison with electrocorticographic data and surgical outcome measures. Neuroimage 2013;75C:246–56; with permission.)

with a high chance of seizure freedom.[73,77] Although the advantages of simultaneous EEG-fMR imaging in epilepsy are undisputed, its application is limited by several practical and methodological challenges and limitations. The critical limiting factor in current methods of EEG-fMR imaging is the detection of enough clearly identifiable IED events to reach sufficient statistical power for fMR imaging. The main reasons for this EEG detection failure are (1) orientation, depth, or extent of the source; and (2) too many artifacts in the EEG caused by the MR imaging environment. A second important limiting factor of EEG-fMR imaging is the need for a specialized setup, which is only available at a few centers. However, current developments are shifting toward methods to detect IED in fMR imaging data without the need for simultaneous EEG measurements, which would greatly reduce both limitations.[78,79]

BOLD fMR Imaging in Brain Tumor Surgery

For patients with low-grade glioma, more extensive resection extends life expectancy and reduces the risk of recurrence.[80,81] With detailed knowledge of critical brain regions, the resection size can be increased while limiting functional damage. Thus, in brain tumor surgery, the localization of brain function is of critical importance. At present, direct cortical stimulation (DCS) is the gold standard for the localization of brain function and it has been proved to decrease the number of patients with permanent deficit after neurosurgery.[82] The application of BOLD fMR imaging for brain tumor surgery typically involves a standard task-based approach in which the task targets the functional area where the tumor is located.[83] **Fig. 6** shows the BOLD fMR imaging results for a patient with a low-grade glioma near the language

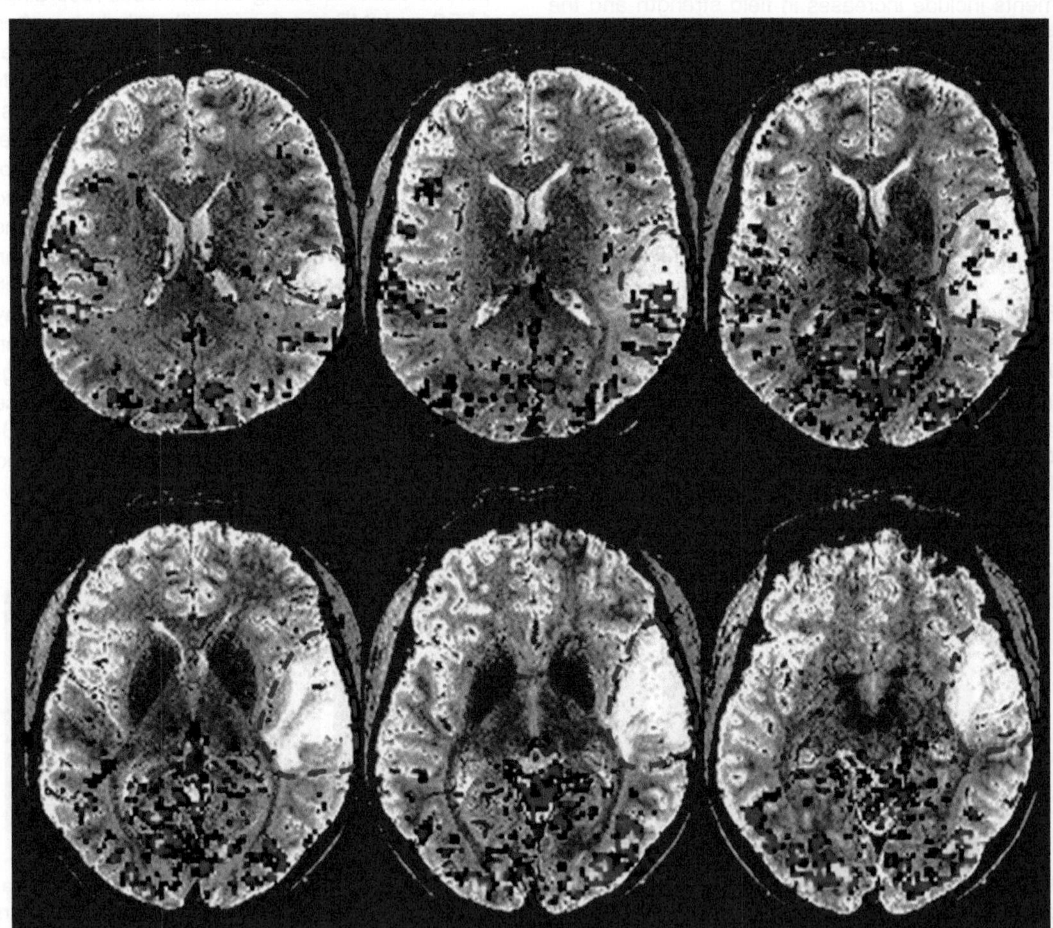

Fig. 6. BOLD fMR results for a 36-year-old man with a low-grade glioma near the language area in the left side of the brain, before surgical tumor removal. Scanning was performed at 7 T using an EPI protocol with a volume transmit coil and 16-channel receive coil. The tumor is indicated by the dashed red line. The highlighted areas are the areas activated during a language-related task (verb generation). Some activity is found inside the tumor area (P<.001). (*Courtesy of* A.F. Rijlaarsdam, J.M. Jansma, and N.F. Ramsey, University Medical Center Utrecht, Utrecht.)

area before surgical tumor removal. In contrast with DCS, BOLD fMR imaging can provide information before surgery, which can be used to improve surgical planning. One of the most important and reliable applications is the determination of language lateralization.[84] More spatially detailed information can also be used to improve the diagnosis and the decision process during surgery.[85]

Also, recent work by Remmele and colleagues[86] examined the use of BOLD MR imaging as a way to measure functional properties of brain tumor tissues during respiratory challenges. Dynamic acquisition of simultaneous T_1-weighted and T_2*-weighted images provides information on tissue oxygenation (via changes in T_1 relaxation) and also vascular reactivity because of BOLD-related signal changes (via changes in T_2* relaxation, relating to deoxyhemoglobin [dHb] concentration).[87] In combination with O_2 and CO_2 enhanced respiratory challenges, this technique has shown promising results with respect to classifying tissue-specific properties of intracranial tumors.[88]

Clinical fMR imaging: the effect of statistical analysis

Statistical analysis plays an important role in constructing an fMR imaging activation map. In contrast with standard MR imaging, an fMR imaging scan is not made up of a single measurement, but provides the results of a statistical analysis of a larger number of single scans.

A typical fMR imaging scan allows an assessment of the chance that a specific region is involved in a task. This information is projected on top of a background MR imaging scan that provides detailed information about the anatomy. If the chance is less than a certain threshold, a region is considered not to be related. Thus, determination of this threshold is crucial for understanding an fMR imaging scan. However, there is no perfect threshold. Using a low threshold results in higher sensitivity and detection of more active areas; however, this also results in more false-positives or localization of active voxels, caused by chance. Using a high threshold improves the reliability of the active regions, but also increases the number of false-negatives or the chance of missing an active region. In addition, individual signal strength and noise levels can vary between patients.

Comparison of fMR imaging and DCS

For evaluation of agreement between fMR imaging and the gold standard DCS, 2 measures are mostly used: sensitivity and specificity. To calculate these measures it is first necessary to calculate true-positive and true-negative stimulation points. A true-positive is a spatial area of the brain in which fMR imaging identifies language function (greater than a chosen threshold) and DCS confirms this, because stimulation of this spatial area results in language errors. A true-negative is a spatial area of the brain in which fMR imaging does not identify language function and neither does DCS. True-positives and true-negatives represent the overlap between fMR imaging and DCS (**Fig. 7**). Sensitivity is calculated by dividing the number of true-positives by the number of positive stimulation points. Specificity is calculated by dividing the number of true-negatives by the number of negative stimulation points. Disagreement between the two methods is represented by false-negatives (for which fMR imaging identifies no language function, whereas DCS results in language errors) and false-positives (for which fMR imaging identifies language function but DCS does not).

Studies comparing fMR imaging with DCS have shown that, for positive stimulation points (causing the patient to produce language errors), fMR imaging and DCS closely match,[89] up to 100% for language tasks (verb-generation tasks,

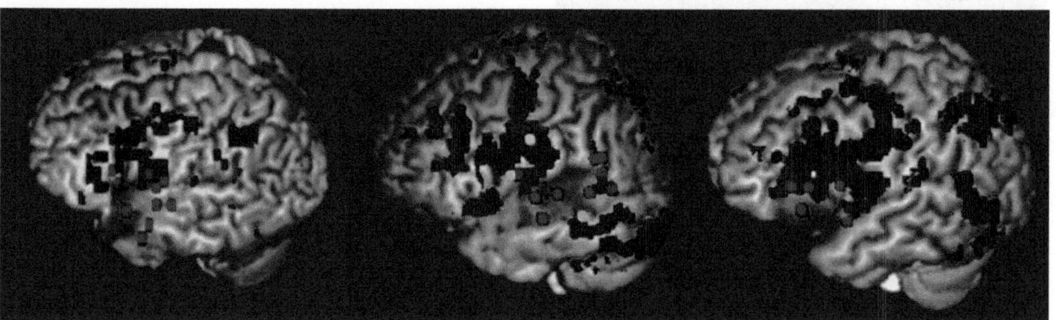

Fig. 7. BOLD fMR imaging activity maps for 3 patients with low-grade glioma, superimposed on DCS stimulation point measured at 3 T (threshold, t = 6.0). Patients performed a verb-generation language task. Green, positive DCS stimulation; light blue, true-positive; purple, true-negative; red, negative DCS stimulation. (*Courtesy of* A.F. Rijlaarsdam, J.M. Jansma, and N.F. Ramsey, University Medical Center Utrecht, Utrecht.)

picture-naming tasks, sentence comprehension). However, specificity was lower (62%), because fMR imaging also identified many areas that could not be confirmed by DCS. In line with these results, Bizzi and colleagues[90] showed a relationship between glioma grade and sensitivity versus specificity. The specificity was higher for patients with high-grade (IV) glioma, whereas patients with low-grade (II and III) glioma showed a high sensitivity (93%) but lower specificity (77% as compared to 93% for high-grade).

Cerebrovascular Reactivity Mapping Using BOLD

The standard clinical way to measure CVR is by measuring changes in blood flow velocity during carbogen inhalation using transcranial Doppler (TCD) ultrasonography. TCD provides a single value representing the reactivity of the whole brain and therefore may be insensitive to localized impairment. CVR can also be mapped using BOLD fMR imaging techniques,[91] which allow regional and even voxel-wise examination of vascular reactivity (**Fig. 8**).[92] Hypercapnic stimuli (ie, carbogen, rebreathing, feedback, or feed-forward targeting of arterial CO_2) cause cerebral vessels to dilate, resulting in increased CBV and CBF without a corresponding increase in $CMRo_2$ or OEF.[26] Increased CBF effectively washes out dHb, leading to an increase in the BOLD signal.

BOLD-CVR measurements performed on patients with carotid artery stenosis or occlusions have shown decreased reactivity in infarcted regions that was not apparent with TCD of the ipsilateral middle cerebral artery.[93] Reduced CVR has been linked to an increased risk of stroke[94] and has also been associated with severe depression.[95] Studies examining the change in vascular reactivity before and after corrective surgery have shown promising results with respect to clinical outcome. Patients with moyamoya disease undergoing surgical revascularization in hemodynamically impaired regions (as judged by preoperative CVR measurements) showed restored postoperative vascular reserve capacity.[96] Reversed CVR impairment was also seen in presurgical and postsurgical CVR mapping for patients who underwent carotid endarterectomy. Mikulis and colleagues[97] showed a restoration of collateral blood flow in regions that previously displayed vascular steal effects (caused by limited reactive capacity). A recent review by Zaca and colleagues[98] presented a case study in which mapping of CVR was used to identify neurovascular uncoupling for the purpose of presurgical planning in tumor resection. Vascular reactivity was used as a marker to identify functional tissue that might otherwise be removed. Thus, it is evident that BOLD-based CVR measurements provide a clinically viable way to assess surgical success as well as help in the evaluation of certain cerebrovascular disease states.

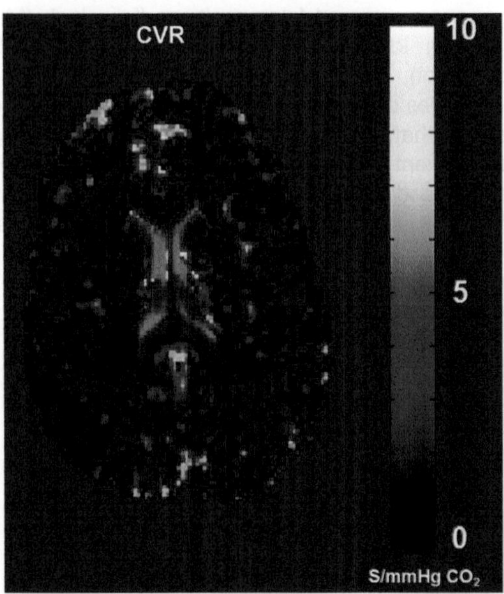

Fig. 8. CVR measured using BOLD MR imaging at 7 T using a targeted CO_2 ramp paradigm.[92] The slope of the signal change as a function of arterial CO_2 pressure can be used as a measure of cerebrovascular reactivity.

SUMMARY AND PERSPECTIVES

Presurgical function localization with fMR imaging can be an important tool in the clinic, because of its specific strengths. At present, important challenges remain that limit the role of BOLD fMR imaging in the clinic. In epilepsy, for example, the most important limitation seems to be the need to perform simultaneous EEG measurements. In tumor surgery, the most important limitation seems to be the low specificity. Nevertheless, emerging technical MR imaging developments as well as developments in analysis techniques are expected to reduce such limitations in the near future. Thus, it is likely that there will begin to be a larger role for fMR imaging in the clinic. For research applications (but not exclusively), cutting-edge scanning techniques are in development that will dramatically improve achievable temporal resolution. Some examples include inverse imaging, multiband and power independent of number of slices (PINS) acquisition for BOLD fMR imaging.[99–102] These methods will allow faster scanning but can also be used to increase the attainable brain coverage, which will create the possibility of investigating neurovascular coupling with high detail in larger regions and could be of interest when studying functional networks.[100] Furthermore, the increased SNR and chemical shift at ultrahigh fields (7 T) have prompted the development of MR spectroscopy (MRS) techniques that have shown potential to track metabolic fluctuations (eg, gamma-aminobutyric acid or glutamate) related to brain function.[103] It would be interesting to acquire high-fidelity MRS together with BOLD fMR imaging to obtain more information on the metabolic aspects of the neurovascular coupling equation.

REFERENCES

1. Roy CS, Sherrington CS. On the regulation of the blood-supply of the brain. J Physiol 1890;11(1–2): 85–158.17.
2. Duong TQ, Kim DS, Ugurbil K, et al. Localized cerebral blood flow response at submillimeter columnar resolution. Proc Natl Acad Sci U S A 2001;98(19):10904–9.
3. Duvernoy HM, Delon S, Vannson JL. Cortical blood vessels of the human brain. Brain Res Bull 1981; 7(5):519–79.
4. Gardner JL. Is cortical vasculature functionally organized? Neuroimage 2010;49(3):1953–6.
5. Woolsey TA, Rovainen CM, Cox SB, et al. Neuronal units linked to microvascular modules in cerebral cortex: response elements for imaging the brain. Cereb Cortex 1996;6(5):647–60.
6. Raichle ME, Grubb RL Jr, Gado MH, et al. Correlation between regional cerebral blood flow and oxidative metabolism. In vivo studies in man. Arch Neurol 1976;33(8):523–6.
7. Fox PT, Mintun MA. Noninvasive functional brain mapping by change-distribution analysis of averaged PET images of H215O tissue activity. J Nucl Med 1989;30(2):141–9.
8. Fox PT, Raichle ME. Focal physiological uncoupling of cerebral blood flow and oxidative metabolism during somatosensory stimulation in human subjects. Proc Natl Acad Sci U S A 1986;83(4): 1140–4.
9. Fox PT, Raichle ME, Mintun MA, et al. Nonoxidative glucose consumption during focal physiologic neural activity. Science 1988;241(4864):462–4.
10. Powers WJ, Hirsch IB, Cryer PE. Effect of stepped hypoglycemia on regional cerebral blood flow response to physiological brain activation. Am J Phys 1996;270(2 Pt 2):H554–9.
11. Bandettini PA, Wong EC, Hinks RS, et al. Time course EPI of human brain function during task activation. Magn Reson Med 1992;25(2):390–7.
12. Kwong KK, Belliveau JW, Chesler DA, et al. Dynamic magnetic resonance imaging of human brain activity during primary sensory stimulation. Proc Natl Acad Sci U S A 1992;89(12):5675–9.
13. Ogawa S, Tank DW, Menon R, et al. Intrinsic signal changes accompanying sensory stimulation: functional brain mapping with magnetic resonance imaging. Proc Natl Acad Sci U S A 1992;89(13): 5951–5.
14. Damoiseaux JS, Rombouts SA, Barkhof F, et al. Consistent resting-state networks across healthy subjects. Proc Natl Acad Sci U S A 2006;103(37): 13848–53.
15. Fox MD, Snyder AZ, Vincent JL, et al. The human brain is intrinsically organized into dynamic, anticorrelated functional networks. Proc Natl Acad Sci U S A 2005;102(27):9673–8.
16. Greicius MD, Menon V. Default-mode activity during a passive sensory task: uncoupled from deactivation but impacting activation. J Cogn Neurosci 2004;16(9):1484–92.
17. Shulman GL, Fiez JA, Corbetta M, et al. Common blood flow changes across visual tasks: II. Decreases in cerebral cortex. J Cogn Neurosci 1997;9:648–63.
18. van den Heuvel MP, Hulshoff Pol HE. Exploring the brain network: a review on resting-state fMRI functional connectivity. Eur Neuropsychopharmacol 2010;20(8):519–34.
19. Yacoub E, Shmuel A, Logothetis N, et al. Robust detection of ocular dominance columns in humans using Hahn Spin Echo BOLD functional MRI at 7 Tesla. Neuroimage 2007;37(4):1161–77.
20. Yacoub E, Harel N, Ugurbil K. High-field fMRI unveils orientation columns in humans. Proc Natl Acad Sci U S A 2008;105(30):10607–12.
21. Siero JC, Ramsey NF, Hoogduin H, et al. BOLD specificity and dynamics evaluated in humans at 7 T: comparing gradient-echo and spin-echo hemodynamic responses. PLoS One 2013;8(1): e54560.
22. Siero JC, Petridou N, Hoogduin H, et al. Cortical depth-dependent temporal dynamics of the BOLD response in the human brain. J Cereb Blood Flow Metab 2011;31(10):1999–2008.
23. Olman CA, Harel N, Feinberg DA, et al. Layer-specific fMRI reflects different neuronal computations at different depths in human V1. PLoS One 2012; 7(3):e32536.
24. Goense J, Merkle H, Logothetis NK. High-resolution fMRI reveals laminar differences in neurovascular coupling between positive and negative BOLD responses. Neuron 2012;76(3):629–39.
25. Cheng K, Waggoner RA, Tanaka K. Human ocular dominance columns as revealed by high-field functional magnetic resonance imaging. Neuron 2001; 32(2):359–74.
26. Blockley NP, Griffeth VE, Simon AB, et al. A review of calibrated blood oxygenation level-dependent

(BOLD) methods for the measurement of task-induced changes in brain oxygen metabolism. NMR Biomed 2012. [Epub ahead of print].

27. Uludag K, Müller-Bierl B, Ugurbil K. An integrative model for neuronal activity-induced signal changes for gradient and spin echo functional imaging. Neuroimage 2009;48(1):150–65.
28. Ogawa S, Menon RS, Tank DW, et al. Functional brain mapping by blood oxygenation level-dependent contrast magnetic resonance imaging. A comparison of signal characteristics with a biophysical model. Biophys J 1993;64(3):803–12.
29. Obata T, Liu TT, Miller KL, et al. Discrepancies between BOLD and flow dynamics in primary and supplementary motor areas: application of the balloon model to the interpretation of BOLD transients. Neuroimage 2004;21(1):144–53.
30. Mandeville JB, Marota JJ, Ayata C, et al. Evidence of a cerebrovascular postarteriole windkessel with delayed compliance. J Cereb Blood Flow Metab 1999;19(6):679–89.
31. Buxton RB, Uludag K, Dubowitz DJ, et al. Modeling the hemodynamic response to brain activation. Neuroimage 2004;23(Suppl 1):S220–33.
32. van Zijl PC, Hua J, Lu H. The BOLD post-stimulus undershoot, one of the most debated issues in fMRI. Neuroimage 2012;62(2):1092–102.
33. van Zijl PC, Eleff SM, Ulatowski JA, et al. Quantitative assessment of blood flow, blood volume and blood oxygenation effects in functional magnetic resonance imaging. Nat Med 1998;4(2):159–67.
34. Martindale J, Kennerley AJ, Johnston D, et al. Theory and generalization of Monte Carlo models of the BOLD signal source. Magn Reson Med 2008; 59(3):607–18.
35. Marques JP, Bowtell RW. Using forward calculations of the magnetic field perturbation due to a realistic vascular model to explore the BOLD effect. NMR Biomed 2008;21(6):553–65.
36. Attwell D, Buchan AM, Charpak S, et al. Glial and neuronal control of brain blood flow. Nature 2010; 468(7321):232–43.
37. Lauritzen M, Mathiesen C, Schaefer K, et al. Neuronal inhibition and excitation, and the dichotomic control of brain hemodynamic and oxygen responses. Neuroimage 2012;62(2):1040–50.
38. Hu X, Yacoub E. The story of the initial dip in fMRI. Neuroimage 2012;62(2):1103–8.
39. Yacoub E, Hu X. Detection of the early decrease in fMRI signal in the motor area. Magn Reson Med 2001;45(2):184–90.
40. Kim SG, Ogawa S. Biophysical and physiological origins of blood oxygenation level-dependent fMRI signals. J Cereb Blood Flow Metab 2012; 32(7):1188–206.
41. Donahue MJ, Stevens RD, de Boorder M, et al. Hemodynamic changes after visual stimulation and breath holding provide evidence for an uncoupling of cerebral blood flow and volume from oxygen metabolism. J Cereb Blood Flow Metab 2009; 29(1):176–85.
42. Dechent P, Schutze G, Helms G, et al. Basal cerebral blood volume during the poststimulation undershoot in BOLD MRI of the human brain. J Cereb Blood Flow Metab 2011;31(1):82–9.
43. de Zwart JA, Silva AC, van Gelderen P, et al. Temporal dynamics of the BOLD fMRI impulse response. Neuroimage 2005;24(3):667–77.
44. Handwerker DA, Ollinger JM, D'Esposito M. Variation of BOLD hemodynamic responses across subjects and brain regions and their effects on statistical analyses. Neuroimage 2004;21(4):1639–51.
45. Petridou N, Italiaander M, van de Bank B, et al. Pushing the limits of high resolution fMRI using a simple high density multi-element coil design. NMR Biomed 2013;26(1):65–73.
46. Yablonskiy DA, Haacke EM. Theory of NMR signal behavior in magnetically inhomogeneous tissues: the static dephasing regime. Magn Reson Med 1994;32(6):749–63.
47. Hoogenraad FG, Pouwels PJ, Hofman MB, et al. Quantitative differentiation between BOLD models in fMRI. Magn Reson Med 2001;45(2):233–46.
48. Boxerman JL, Hamberg LM, Rosen BR, et al. MR contrast due to intravascular magnetic susceptibility perturbations. Magn Reson Med 1995;34(4): 555–66.
49. Norris DG. Principles of magnetic resonance assessment of brain function. J Magn Reson Imaging 2006;23(6):794–807.
50. Georgiades CS, Itoh R, Golay X, et al. MR imaging of the human brain at 1.5 T: regional variations in transverse relaxation rates in the cerebral cortex. AJNR Am J Neuroradiol 2001;22(9):1732–7.
51. Yacoub E, Shmuel A, Pfeuffer J, et al. Imaging brain function in humans at 7 Tesla. Magn Reson Med 2001;45(4):588–94.
52. Posse S, Wiese S, Gembris D, et al. Enhancement of BOLD-contrast sensitivity by single-shot multi-echo functional MR imaging. Magn Reson Med 1999;42(1):87–97.
53. Yacoub E, Van De Moortele PF, Shmuel A, et al. Signal and noise characteristics of Hahn SE and GE BOLD fMRI at 7 T in humans. Neuroimage 2005;24(3):738–50.
54. Duong TQ, Yacoub E, Adriany G, et al. Microvascular BOLD contribution at 4 and 7 T in the human brain: gradient-echo and spin-echo fMRI with suppression of blood effects. Magn Reson Med 2003; 49(6):1019–27.
55. Thulborn KR, Waterton JC, Matthews PM, et al. Oxygenation dependence of the transverse relaxation time of water protons in whole blood at high field. Biochim Biophys Acta 1982;714(2):265–70.

56. Gati JS, Menon RS, Ugurbil K, et al. Experimental determination of the BOLD field strength dependence in vessels and tissue. Magn Reson Med 1997;38(2):296–302.
57. Jezzard P, Matthews PM, Smith SM. Functional MRI: an introduction to methods. Oxford, The United Kingdom: Oxford University Press; 2001.
58. Menon RS, Gati JS, Goodyear BG, et al. Spatial and temporal resolution of functional magnetic resonance imaging. Biochem Cell Biol 1998; 76(2–3):560–71.
59. Ogawa S, Lee TM, Stepnoski R, et al. An approach to probe some neural systems interaction by functional MRI at neural time scale down to milliseconds. Proc Natl Acad Sci U S A 2000;97(20): 11026–31.
60. Boynton GM, Engel SA, Glover GH, et al. Linear systems analysis of functional magnetic resonance imaging in human V1. J Neurosci 1996;16(13): 4207–21.
61. McRobbie DW, Moore EA, Graves MJ, et al. MRI from picture to proton. Cambridge, UK: Cambridge University Press; 2003.
62. Biswal B, Yetkin FZ, Haughton VM, et al. Functional connectivity in the motor cortex of resting human brain using echo-planar MRI. Magn Reson Med 1995;34:537–41.
63. Gusnard DA, Raichle ME. Searching for a baseline: functional imaging and the resting human brain. Nat Rev Neurosci 2001;2(10):685–94.
64. Fornito A, Bullmore ET. What can spontaneous fluctuations of the blood oxygenation-level-dependent signal tell us about psychiatric disorders? Curr Opin Psychiatry 2010;23(3):239–49.
65. Rosazza C, Minati L. Resting-state brain networks: literature review and clinical applications. Neurol Sci 2011;32(5):773–85.
66. Damoiseaux J. Regulatory T cells: back to the future. Neth J Med 2006;64(1):4–9.
67. Birn RM, Cox RW, Bandettini PA. Detection versus estimation in event-related fMRI: choosing the optimal stimulus timing. Neuroimage 2002;15: 252–64.
68. Burock MA, Buckner RL, Woldorff MG, et al. Randomized event-related experimental designs allow for extremely rapid presentation rates using functional MRI. Neuroreport 1998;9(16):3735–9.
69. Josephs O, Turner R, Friston K. Event-related fMRI. Hum Brain Mapp 1997;5(4):243–8.
70. Liu TT, Frank LR, Wong EC, et al. Detection power, estimation efficiency, and predictability in event-related fMRI. Neuroimage 2001;13(4):759–73.
71. Dale AM. Optimal experimental design for event-related fMRI. Hum Brain Mapp 1999;8(2–3):109–14.
72. Glover GH. Deconvolution of impulse response in event-related BOLD fMRI. Neuroimage 1999;9(4): 416–29.
73. van Houdt PJ, de Munck JC, Leijten FS, et al. EEG-fMRI correlation patterns in the presurgical evaluation of focal epilepsy: a comparison with electrocorticographic data and surgical outcome measures. Neuroimage 2013;75C:246–56.
74. Zijlmans M, Huiskamp G, Hersevoort M, et al. EEG-fMRI in the preoperative work-up for epilepsy surgery. Brain 2007;130:2343–53.
75. Vulliemoz S, Carmichael DW, Rosenkranz K, et al. Simultaneous intracranial EEG and fMRI of interictal epileptic discharges in humans. Neuroimage 2011;54:182–90.
76. Formaggio E, Storti SF, Bertoldo A, et al. Integrating EEG and fMRI in epilepsy. Neuroimage 2011;54:2719–31.
77. Ullsperger M, Debener S. Simultaneous EEG–fMRI: recording, analysis and application. New York: Oxford University Press; 2011.
78. Caballero Gaudes C, Petridou N, Francis ST, et al. Paradigm free mapping with sparse regression automatically detects single-trial functional magnetic resonance imaging blood oxygenation level dependent responses. Hum Brain Mapp 2011; 34(3):501–18.
79. Rodionov R, De Martino F, Laufs H, et al. Independent component analysis of interictal fMRI in focal epilepsy: comparison with general linear model-based EEG-correlated fMRI. Neuroimage 2007; 38:488–500.
80. Mikuni N, Miyamoto S. Surgical treatment for glioma: extent of resection applying functional neurosurgery. Neurol Med Chir (Tokyo) 2010; 50(9):720–6.
81. Duffau H. Surgery of low-grade gliomas: towards a 'functional neurooncology'. Curr Opin Oncol 2009; 21(6):543–9.
82. Duffau H, Lopes M, Arthuis F, et al. Contribution of intraoperative electrical stimulations in surgery of low grade gliomas: a comparative study between two series without (1985-96) and with (1996-2003) functional mapping in the same institution. J Neurol Neurosurg Psychiatr 2005;76(6):845–51.
83. Rutten GJ, Ramsey NF. The role of functional magnetic resonance imaging in brain surgery. Neurosurg Focus 2010;28(2):E4.
84. Binder JR. Preoperative prediction of verbal episodic memory outcome using FMRI. Neurosurg Clin North Am 2011;22(2):219–32, ix.
85. Wengenroth M, Blatow M, Guenther J, et al. Diagnostic benefits of presurgical fMRI in patients with brain tumours in the primary sensorimotor cortex. Eur Radiol 2011;21(7):1517–25.
86. Remmele S, Dahnke H, Flacke S, et al. Quantification of the magnetic resonance signal response to dynamic (C)O(2)-enhanced imaging in the brain at 3 T: R*(2) BOLD vs. balanced SSFP. J Magn Reson Imaging 2010;31(6):1300–10.

87. Muller A, Remmele S, Wenningmann I, et al. Analysing the response in R2* relaxation rate of intracranial tumours to hyperoxic and hypercapnic respiratory challenges: initial results. Eur Radiol 2011;21(4):786–98.
88. Remmele S, Sprinkart AM, Muller A, et al. Dynamic and simultaneous MR measurement of R(1) and R(2)* changes during respiratory challenges for the assessment of blood and tissue oxygenation. Magn Reson Med 2012. [Epub ahead of print].
89. Rutten G. fMRI-determined language lateralization in patients with unilateral or mixed language dominance according to the Wada test. Neuroimage 2002;17:447–60.
90. Bizzi A, Blasi V, Falini A, et al. Presurgical functional MR imaging of language and motor functions: validation with intraoperative electrocortical mapping. Radiology 2008;248(2):579–89.
91. Lythgoe DJ, Williams SC, Cullinane M, et al. Mapping of cerebrovascular reactivity using BOLD magnetic resonance imaging. Magn Reson Imaging 1999;17(4):495–502.
92. Bhogal A, Philippens M, Fisher JA, et al. Cerebrovascular reactivity (CVR) measured using targeted hypo/hypercapnia BOLD imaging at 7 T. Paper presented at the annual meeting of the International Society for Magnetic Resonance Imaging, April 26 2013, Salt Lake City.
93. Ziyeh S, Rick J, Reinhard M, et al. Blood oxygen level-dependent MRI of cerebral CO_2 reactivity in severe carotid stenosis and occlusion. Stroke 2005;36(4):751–6.
94. Gupta A, Chazen JL, Hartman M, et al. Cerebrovascular reserve and stroke risk in patients with carotid stenosis or occlusion: a systematic review and meta-analysis. Stroke 2012;43(11): 2884–91.
95. Lemke H, de Castro AG, Schlattmann P, et al. Cerebrovascular reactivity over time-course - from major depressive episode to remission. J Psychiatr Res 2010;44(3):132–6.
96. Han JS, Abou-Hamden A, Mandell DM, et al. Impact of extracranial-intracranial bypass on cerebrovascular reactivity and clinical outcome in patients with symptomatic moyamoya vasculopathy. Stroke 2011;42(11):3047–54.
97. Mikulis DJ, Krolczyk G, Desal H, et al. Preoperative and postoperative mapping of cerebrovascular reactivity in moyamoya disease by using blood oxygen level-dependent magnetic resonance imaging. J Neurosurg 2005;103(2):347–55.
98. Zaca D, Hua J, Pillai JJ. Cerebrovascular reactivity mapping for brain tumor presurgical planning. World J Clin Oncol 2011;2(7):289–98.
99. Feinberg DA, Moeller S, Smith SM, et al. Multiplexed echo planar imaging for sub-second whole brain FMRI and fast diffusion imaging. PLoS One 2010;5(12):e15710.
100. Koopmans PJ, Boyacioglu R, Barth M, et al. Whole brain, high resolution spin-echo resting state fMRI using PINS multiplexing at 7 T. Neuroimage 2012; 62(3):1939–46.
101. Lin FH, Witzel T, Mandeville JB, et al. Event-related single-shot volumetric functional magnetic resonance inverse imaging of visual processing. Neuroimage 2008;42(1):230–47.
102. Norris DG, Koopmans PJ, Boyacioglu R, et al. Power independent of number of slices (PINS) radiofrequency pulses for low-power simultaneous multislice excitation. Magn Reson Med 2011; 66(5):1234–40.
103. Andreychenko A, Boer VO, Arteaga de Castro CS, et al. Efficient spectral editing at 7 T: GABA detection with MEGA-sLASER. Magn Reson Med 2012; 68(4):1018–25.

Toward Noninvasive Characterization of Breast Cancer and Cancer Metabolism with Diffuse Optics

David R. Busch, PhD[a,b,*], Regine Choe, PhD[c], Turgut Durduran, PhD[d], Arjun G. Yodh, PhD[b]

KEYWORDS

• Diffuse optical tomography • Diffuse optical spectroscopy • Metabolic imaging • Blood flow • Breast cancer • Neoadjuvant chemotherapy

KEY POINTS

- Diffuse optical spectroscopies provide noninvasive, nonionizing, serial measurements of tissue blood flow, oxygenation, and concentration.
- These physiologic parameters provide a window into tissue metabolism without necessitating the use of ionizing radiation or transport to imaging suites.
- Current clinical investigations of diffuse optical mammography include applications of diffuse optical tomography and monitoring to neoadjuvant chemotherapy, contrast agent discovery, computer-aided detection, and measurement of breast oxygen metabolism.
- Diffuse optical measurements hold significant promise for commercialization and clinical integration.

A.G.Y. gratefully acknowledges partial support from the National Institutes of Health through grants CA087971, NS060653, EB002109, and EB015893.

T.D. gratefully acknowledges partial support by Fundació Cellex Barcelona, Marie Curie IRG (FP7, RPTAMON), Institute de Salud Carlos III (DOM-MON, FIS), Ministerio de Ciencia e Innovación (MICINN), Ministerio de Economía y Comepetitividad, Institució CERCA (DOCNEURO, PROVAT-002-11), Generalitat de Catalunya, European Regional Development Fund (FEDER/ERDF) and LASERLAB (FP7) and Photonics4Life (FP7) consortia.

R.C. gratefully acknowledges support from the National Institutes of Health through K99/R00-CA126187.

D.R.B. gratefully acknowledges partial support from the Thrasher Research Fund and National Institutes of Health through grant NS072338.

The authors (T.D., R.C., and A.G.Y.) are coinventors in various patents about diffuse optical technologies, but they do not currently receive any royalties. There are no other conflicting financial or ethical issues to disclose.

[a] Division of Neurology, Department of Pediatrics, Children's Hospital of Philadelphia, 3615 Civic Center Boulevard, Philadelphia, PA 19104, USA; [b] Department of Physics and Astronomy, University of Pennsylvania, 3231 Walnut Street, Philadelphia, PA 19104, USA; [c] Department of Biomedical Engineering, University of Rochester, Goergen Hall, Intercampus Drive, Rochester, NY 14620, USA; [d] Medical Optics Department, ICFO - Institut de Ciències Fotòniques, Mediterranean Technology Park Avenue Carl Friedrich Gauss, 3 08860 Castelldefels (Barcelona), Spain

* Corresponding author. Division of Neurology, Department of Pediatrics, Children's Hospital of Philadelphia, Philadelphia, PA 19104.

E-mail address: drbusch@sdf.org

PET Clin 8 (2013) 345–365
http://dx.doi.org/10.1016/j.cpet.2013.04.004
1556-8598/13/$ – see front matter

Acronyms and symbols utilized in this manuscript

ACRONYMS	Description
ASL-MRI	Arterial-Spin Labeling MRI
BF	Blood Flow
CAD	Computer Aided Detection
CT (X-Ray)	Computed Tomography
DCS	Diffuse Correlation Spectroscopy
DCT	Diffuse Correlation Tomography
DOS	Diffuse Optical Spectroscopy
DOT	Diffuse Optical Tomography
DOT-CAD	Diffuse Optical Tomography - Computer Aided Detection
FDG-PET	Fluoro-deoxyglucose Positron Emission Tomography
Hb	Deoxygenated Hemoglobin Concentration
HbO_2	Oxygenated Hemoglobin Concentration
Hb_t	Total Hemoglobin Concentration
H_2O	Water Concentration
l^*	Photon Random Walk Step
l_a	Photon Absorption Length
Lipid	Lipid Concentration
M	Malignancy Parameter
μ_a	Absorption Coefficient
μ_{eff}	Overall Optical Attenuation Coefficient
$MMRO_2$	Mammary Metabolic Rate of Oxygen consumption
μ_s'	Reduced Scattering Coefficient
MRI	Magnetic Resonance Imaging
NIR	Near Infra-Red Spectral Range, 650-950 nm
NIRS	Near Infra-Red Spectroscopy (a.k.a. DOS)
OEF	Oxygen Extraction Fraction
PET	Positron Emission Tomography
$P(M)$	Probability of Malignancy
RBCs	Red Blood Cells
StO_2	Blood Oxygen Saturation
TOI	Tissue Optical Index

CONTINUOUS, NONINVASIVE MONITORING OF BLOOD VOLUME, FLOW, AND OXYGENATION

Despite major advances in diagnosis and preventive medicine, breast cancer remains among the principal causes of death in women. In the United States, for example, in 2012 approximately 230,000 new cases of breast cancer were diagnosed and roughly 40,000 died of the disease.[1] At present, clinical recommendations are focused on the early detection of cancer and risk stratification, with screening techniques ranging from breast self-examinations and clinical palpation, to serial x-ray mammographic imaging, to genetic testing. Ultrasonography and magnetic resonance (MR) imaging are frequently used in conjunction with the traditional techniques, for example, to confirm a diagnosis. Modern screening of breast cancer depends heavily on x-ray mammography, which is especially sensitive to microcalcifications. However, this structural imaging modality can suffer from low sensitivity and specificity, especially in younger women.[2]

Ultrasonographic breast imaging is highly effective in identifying classes of cysts,[3,4] but is not yet widely used for whole breast imaging. Contrast-enhanced MR imaging can be highly sensitive and some studies have reported high specificity, but it is generally applied only to high-risk populations because of its cost and limited availability.[5–7] Thus, the ideal screening modality has yet to be found, and multimodal approaches, including genetic testing, are gaining popularity.

This article is primarily concerned with the potential role of optics in clinical management of breast cancer and (possibly) screening based on the local tissue metabolism. Indeed, the enhanced glucose metabolism of cancer tissues is the basis for the success of ^{18}F-fluorodeoxyglucose (FDG) Positron Emission Tomography (PET) cancer imaging which, in breast cancer, is primarily used to identify metastases and to stage disease.[8] Measurements of the local metabolism provide insights into aggressiveness of the cancer and response to the treatments.

Significant recent research in breast cancer has been oriented toward identifying and using the potential of hemodynamic parameters such as blood flow; for example, as a means to access tissue metabolism. This reasoning is based on the fact that cancers are frequently hypermetabolic and have associated formation of angiogenic vessels, therefore local blood flow may provide a cancer contrast. Doppler-ultrasound imaging of blood flow in breast cancer has been extensively explored over the past three decades, both with and without contrast agents.[4] In MR imaging, uptake and kinetics of gadolinium chelate contrast agent provide clinicians with information on perfusion of breast cancer, and is part of the current clinical standard of care.[5] An alternative MR imaging method, arterial spin-labeling MR imaging (ASL-MRI), has proved to be very useful in probing brain blood flow without the injection of contrast agents. However, its use in the breast[9] is hampered by the low absolute blood flow in the breast tissue. Of note, none of these techniques provides information about tumor blood oxygenation; this technical limitation makes it harder to gain insights about oxidative metabolism in cancer.

Diffuse optical measurements can probe blood flow, oxygenation, and concentration, permitting calculation of tissue oxygen delivery, and perhaps offering a method to complement PET. Measurement of these important physiologic parameters has been one of the driving reasons for the continued interest in diffuse optical mammography, despite its bumpy history dating from the 1920s.[10] These methods were attractive because of their noninvasive nature, relative low cost, and other features. The photons used for clinical diffuse optical measurements are nonionizing (~1.5 eV), permitting repeated measurements without significant risk to the subjects.[11,12] Indeed, pulse-oximeters using similar wavelengths and light power are ubiquitous in hospital settings for long-term care.

Diffuse optical spectroscopy (DOS) provides a localized measurement of optical properties. In the most basic form of imaging, an array of DOS measurements can be taken and the results projected onto a two-dimensional (2D) map of tissue properties.[13,14] More sophisticated imaging strategies rely on tomographic reconstruction, in which volumetric three-dimensional (3D) maps of optical properties are reconstructed from light fluence measurements on the tissue surface. Human use of diffuse optical tomography (DOT) is most advanced in imaging of breast cancer, due in part to technical (low optical absorption and malleability of breast tissue) and logistical (public awareness of breast cancer, accessibility) factors. DOS is also sometimes referred to as near-infrared spectroscopy (NIRS).

To date, both DOS and DOT technologies have been applied to quantify the optical properties of healthy human breast tissue[15–22] and its correlation with cancer risk prediction.[23–26] Several reviews of DOT imaging of and contrast in breast cancer are also available[20,27,28]; exogenous contrast agents can also be used and are discussed later in this article. DOT has been the focus of much effort in both academic[15,29–35] and industrial[36–41] settings. More details about the DOT reconstruction process may be found in the recent review by Arridge and Schotland.[42]

Table 1 illustrates some of the broad characteristics of current imaging techniques and the niche which the authors believe diffuse optics can fill; for example, for provision of continuous metabolic measurements without the use of ionizing radiation.

One of the obvious applications of optical metabolic monitoring of tumors arises during therapy. This monitoring is of particular interest in the case of neoadjuvant chemotherapy, which is an increasingly popular treatment protocol for breast cancer. For neoadjuvant chemotherapy, drugs are administered before surgical excision[43] to reduce the tumor size and eliminate or reduce micrometastases before the surgery. **Fig. 1** delineates a potential timeline for DOS/DOT to assist in judging the efficacy of therapy planning. This sequence permits the early observation of the clinical effects of specific drug regimens which, in turn, could potentially permit early determination of the chemotherapy's effectiveness and inform clinical decisions on continuing a particular therapy. Monitoring the efficacy of neoadjuvant chemotherapy is an active area of research in clinical medicine,[44–46] including optical imaging and monitoring.[47–67]

It is not the intention of this review to cover clinical applications of diffuse optics exhaustively; rather, the aim is to provide a snapshot of recent diffuse optics–based efforts to noninvasively quantify oxygen metabolism in breast tissue, with an emphasis (though not exclusively) on research from the authors' laboratories. For more extensive discussion on these issues, the reader is encouraged to peruse the primary articles cited, as well as recent reviews about diffuse optical imaging/spectroscopy[68,69] and diffuse correlation spectroscopy.[61,68,70–72]

The review is organized as follows. The initial focus is on the use of statistical analysis of diffuse optical data to derive a probability of malignancy for cancer localization and therapy tracking. The promise of diffuse optical data in metabolic

Table 1
Characteristics of several imaging modalities

	Radiography	PET	Ultrasonography	MR Imaging	Diffuse Optics
Ionizing radiation	Yes	Yes	No	No	No
Tissue structure	Yes	No	Yes	Yes	No
Tissue metabolism	No	Yes	No	No	Yes
Clinician's office	No	No	Yes	No	Yes
Frequent measurements	No	No	Yes	No	Yes

Note that diffuse optics permits convenient, nonionizing, and frequent measurement of tissue metabolism.

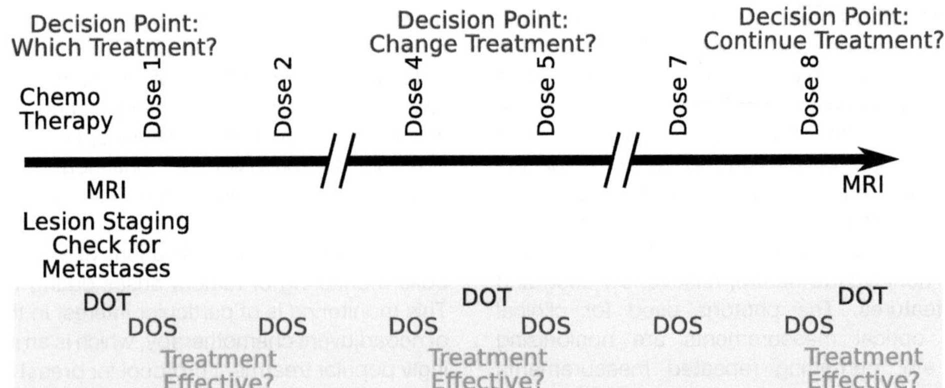

Fig. 1. A proposed timeline for including diffuse optical spectroscopy (DOS) and diffuse optical tomography (DOT) in the planning of neoadjuvant chemotherapy (*yellow box*). DOS provides rapid measurements, integrable into each patient visit. More time-consuming volumetric imaging with DOT provides more detailed information. Together, these frequent measurements of tissue metabolic state may permit clinicians to more rapidly shift to more efficacious treatment regimens or even identify a complete response before completion of all scheduled doses.

imaging is then examined. This is followed by a comparison study between endogenous DOT and FDG PET imaging, an all-optical metabolism measurement, and the use of external perturbations to probe tissue metabolism. Finally, the use of exogenous contrast agents in optical breast cancer imaging is reviewed.

THE PROPAGATION OF PHOTONS IN TISSUES

Physics of Diffuse Optics

Light in the Near Infra Red (NIR) spectral window (650–950 nm) is weakly absorbed but strongly scattered by tissue. **Fig. 2** depicts this scenario in a model turbid medium. **Fig. 2**B shows the propagation of laser light through a clear, nonscattering medium (tap water). Note that the light propagates straight across the bath, with minimal dispersion of the columnated beam. Scatterers are then added to the medium; with a small amount of scattering agent, the beam is broadened in a manner akin to the visibility on a "foggy day" (see **Fig. 2**C), and with a large amount of scattering agent the photon transport is diffusive as is NIR light in tissue (see **Fig. 2**D). Two length scales are important: (1) a photon random walk step (l^*) and (2) a photon absorption length (l_a). The random walk step (l^*), or photon transport mean free path, corresponds to the typical distance traveled by a typical photon before its initial propagation direction becomes randomized ($l^* \sim 1$ mm). For example, most of the photons shown in **Fig. 2**D have had their initial direction randomized, and the directionality of the laser

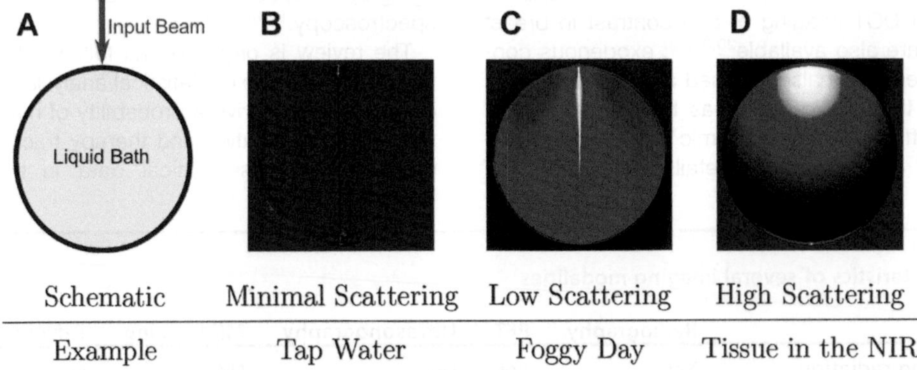

Fig. 2. Illustration of photon migration in turbid media. (*A*) A schematic of the experiment. (*B*) Container filled with tap water, with minimal scattering from air bubbles and tank walls. The columnated laser beam propagates straight across the liquid bath. (*C*) Container filled with a low scattering liquid (a dilute mixture of soy emulsion and water). The light beam is somewhat dispersed. (*D*) Container filled with a high scattering liquid (a more concentrated soy emulsion mixture). These optical properties are similar to tissue in the near-infrared (NIR) spectral region. Note that the light spreads almost isotropically from the point where the beam enters the scattering medium. Photos are in false color. (*Courtesy of* Han Ban, MS, University of Pennsylvania, Philadelphia, PA.)

beam is lost; by contrast, in **Fig. 2**C many photons are still traveling in a straight line through the medium. A wavelength (λ)-dependent reduced scattering coefficient ($\mu'_s(\lambda)=1/l^*$) denotes the reciprocal of this photon transport mean free path, and is often the term of choice to describe tissue scattering. The absorption length (l_a) corresponds to the typical distance traveled by a photon before it is absorbed; it is also wavelength dependent. In the NIR range, this absorption length in tissue is typically much longer (~200 mm) than scattering length. Its reciprocal is denoted by the absorption coefficient ($\mu_a(\lambda)$).

The first incarnation of optical mammography in the 1920s[10,73] simply relied on the transmission of lamp light through the breast and its observation in a dark room. Unfortunately, as the authors of the original articles admit, this technique was highly qualitative and unreliable. In the early 1980s the technique was revisited, this time using wide-beam transillumination; however, it was not successful clinically, due (in part) to limited projection information and lack of separation of tissue absorption from tissue-scattering effects.[74–85]

The key to the reemergence of optical techniques for the imaging of breast cancer was the realization that light transport through tissue is a diffusive process and the subsequent development of accurate physical/mathematical models for photon propagation that separated tissue absorption from tissue-scattering effects. This mathematical approach enabled researchers to accurately quantify both tissue absorber (or chromophore) concentrations and tissue-scattering coefficients. By the mid-1990s the acceptance of this physical model, alongside the advances in the algorithms and technologies, reignited interest in the field.[86,87]

Once a paradigm was developed to separate tissue absorption from tissue scattering, the use of multiple optical wavelengths enabled experimenters to quantitatively determine the concentrations of various tissue chromophores (and contrast agents). For example, because oxyhemoglobin has an optical spectrum markedly different from that of deoxyhemoglobin (Hb) in the NIR (**Fig. 3**), it is readily possible to use absorption coefficient data at multiple wavelengths to recover absolute values of the concentrations of the hemoglobin species. Similar information about other chromophores, such as water and lipid content, and the scattering components of the tissue can be derived from the wavelength-dependent absorption and scattering data.

Fig. 4 illustrates two geometries frequently used in optical mammography. Parallel-plate transmission (left) and reemission (right) geometries for measurements are shown. Other geometries include rings, and combinations of transmission and reemission measurements. In all instruments, one or more light (e.g., laser) sources inject light into the tissue, and the light transmitted through

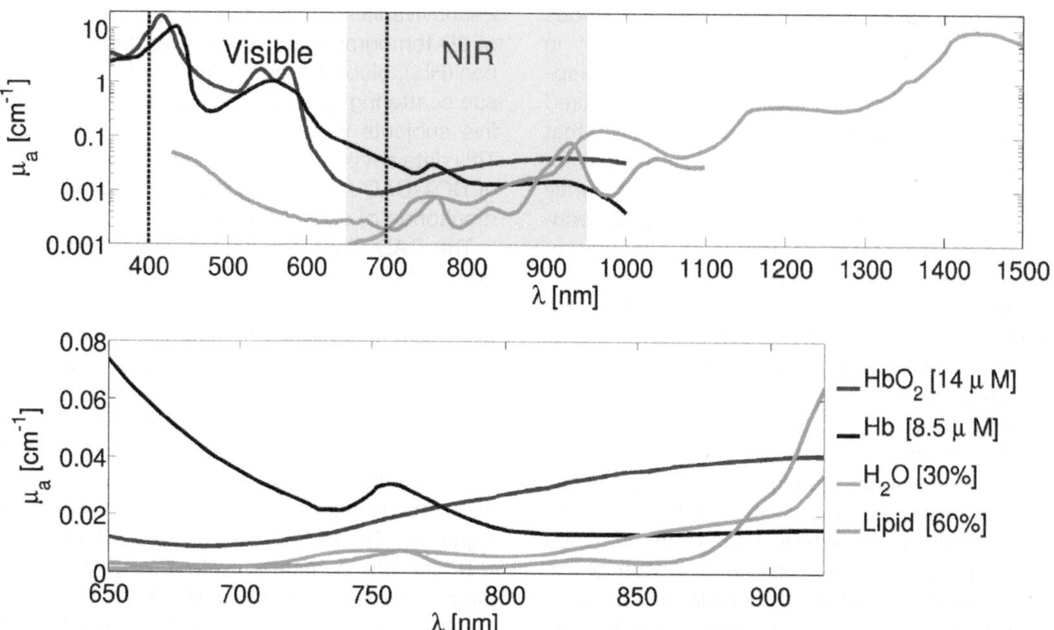

Fig. 3. Spectra of major tissue chromophores. (*Top*) the visible and NIR windows overlap somewhat; note the much lower absorption in the NIR. (*Bottom*) Expanded view of chromophores in the NIR spectral region at approximate concentrations found in human breast tissue.

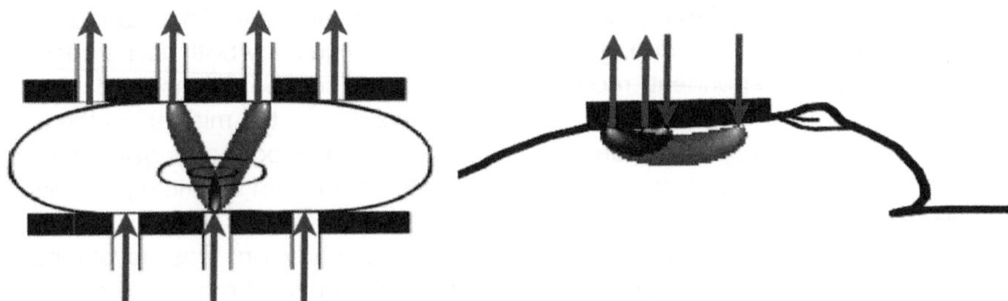

Fig. 4. Example transmission (*left*) and reemission (*right*) geometry measurements in optical mammography. One or more lasers typically inject light into the tissue (*maroon arrows*), and the light transmitted through the tissue is collected by one or more detectors (*red arrows*). Typical representations of the most probable trajectories of the detected photons are superimposed in gray scale.

the tissue is collected by one or more detectors. In **Fig. 4**, representations of the most probable trajectories of the detected photons are superimposed in gray scale; these trajectories are derived from analytical solutions of the photon diffusion equation in the relevant geometry.

PROBABILITY OF MALIGNANCY OPTICAL INDICES BASED ON DOT OF BREAST

Most current work in DOT focuses on the metabolically dependent physiologic variables, without explicitly calculating tissue metabolism. This section discusses DOT imaging of total hemoglobin concentration (Hb_t), blood oxygen saturation (StO_2), and tissue scattering (μ_s'), and the subsequent development of malignancy indices. Several researchers have pushed diffuse optical methods to add additional specificity for diagnosis; in some cases, this research has led to the development of useful combinations of the measured physiologic parameters or composite indices that better distinguish malignant from benign lesions.[13,35,51,88,89] Here the focus is on a recently developed computer-aided detection (CAD) technique that builds on ideas from the x-ray community to improve interpretation of radiologic data.[90] These CAD techniques are quite versatile; for example, besides use of multidimensional optical data, they permit simultaneous use of multiparameter data; for example, combining FDG uptake measured with PET and Gd contrast agent kinetics with MR imaging.[91]

DOT offers a fertile testing ground to apply these ideas in detection, diagnosis, and therapy monitoring of cancer. In general, each of the detected optical parameters is sensitive to tissue physiology, but interpretation of multiple 3D images is challenging. CAD offers a simple paradigm to develop composite indices, taking into account all parameters and their heterogeneities while deriving a single "probability of malignancy" tomogram. To date, several groups have applied statistical analysis techniques to multiparameter optical measurements to derive risk factors. Applications have included arthritic joints,[92] high-risk[93] or high-mammographic-density[23,24] breast tissue, and various "endoscopic" measurements or excised tissues.[94] However, these data sets have limited spatial information and orders of magnitude fewer measurements per subject than, for example, the breast tomograms to be discussed herein. Other researchers have implemented automated DOT image analysis techniques to identify lesions in a particular subject[95–97]; however, this analysis neglects information about the common signatures of cancer across a population.

Here the authors present illustrative results drawn from work conducted at the University of Pennsylvania.[35,66,98] The work is based on a set of 3D tomograms of total hemoglobin concentration (Hb_t), blood oxygen saturation (StO_2), and tissue scattering (μ_s') that were obtained from thirty five subjects with biopsy-confirmed lesions.[34,35] This data set permitted exploration of the potential of DOT-CAD for both cancer localization and the monitoring of cancer therapy.

The CAD algorithm requires identification of a group of subjects with data from both the modality under consideration (DOT) and a gold-standard diagnosis. Essentially, training-set data from this group is used to derive a common malignancy signature, from the combination of optical parameters that best reproduces the gold-standard diagnosis. As a test, the signature is then examined in additional subjects (the test set), who were not included in developing the diagnostic signature. Finally, the diagnostic results from the test set are compared with the gold-standard diagnosis to evaluate the utility of the test.

Regarding diffuse optical properties of breast, the authors[35] and others[20,51,99] have observed that the intersubject variation of physiologic parameters (Hb_t, StO_2, μ_s') can be quite large

Therefore, the first technical strategy introduced was to adopt an intrasubject normalization scheme that reduces this intersubject variation. Specifically, all data are log-transformed, then the mean value of each parameter in healthy tissue for each subject is subtracted; finally, this result is divided by the standard deviation of the parameter in healthy tissue. Thus a "Z-score" normalized variable for each optical parameter is obtained. This *intrasubject* normalization spectacularly reduces the *intersubject* variation in all of the optically measured parameters, as shown in **Fig. 5**A.

With these new Z-score normalized tissue parameters one can sensibly combine the Hb_t, StO_2, and μ_s' data from the tissue volume elements (voxels) of multiple subjects (training set) to generate a single statistically derived malignancy parameter (M). M is a weighted linear combination of physiologic parameters from the training population of cancers. The weighting vectors, $\vec{\beta}$, are optimized using data from each voxel of each patient and logistic regression. The extracted weighting factors (or weighting vector) is then applied to an additional subject (test set); thus the M of each voxel in the subject is computed and a probability of malignancy ($P(M)$) for each volume element in the breast can be assigned. A threshold probability is then used to define a binary mask for cancer location (see **Fig. 5**B). Example results are shown in **Fig. 6**. Note that the blood oxygen saturation (StO_2) images (see **Fig. 6**B) have the least lesion contrast; the weighting factor of StO_2 is significantly smaller than Hb_t and μ_s'. Of interest, one of the authors' subjects with an *in situ* lesion (see **Fig. 6**, left column) exhibited a probability of malignancy that was significantly lower than the threshold cutoff obtained for malignant tissue. This observation suggests the potential for future versions of the metric to distinguish between types of lesions, as well as between healthy and malignant tissue.

The authors have recently extended the DOT-CAD results to monitor the efficacy of neoadjuvant chemotherapy.[66] The $P(M)$ calculation brings together several physiologic parameters to identify changes. In contrast to the composite probability of malignancy signature, significant differences were not observed in the responses of both absolute and relative values of the *individual* physiologic parameters (Hb_t, StO_2, μ_s'). Although this pilot study was limited to three subjects, two of whom responded completely to chemotherapy and one who had a partial response, the dynamics of changes in $P(M)$ between these two groups were significantly different (**Fig. 7**). The observations shown in **Figs. 6** and **7** demonstrate potential for extraction of a simple, clinically relevant metric for cancer staging and therapy monitoring from diffuse optical images. Promising early results[64] suggest that these optical techniques

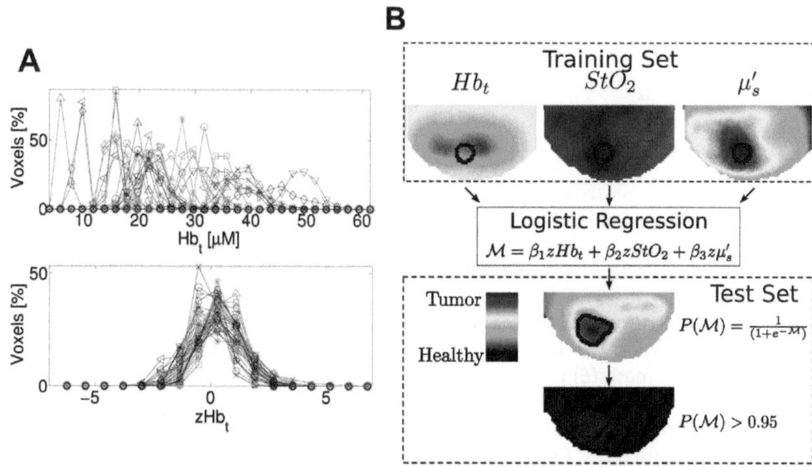

Fig. 5. (*A*) Intrasubject data normalization brings intersubject data distributions close to a normal distribution in the healthy tissue of thirty five breasts with biopsy-confirmed malignant lesions.[98] The top row shows, for the full population, absolute values of Hb_t, and the bottom row shows the population distribution of Z-transformed variables after intrasubject normalization (zHb_t). Each trace/color represents the healthy region of one subject. For clarity of presentation, the vertical axis is normalized to the total number of voxels in each subject. (*B*) Schematic of probability of malignancy calculation. Weighting coefficients ($\vec{\beta}$) are calculated from normalized data in a population of known cancers (training set); this same weighting vector is then applied to data from an additional subject (test set) to calculate a probability of malignancy ($P(M)$) and a binary mask of tumor location. (*From* Busch DR, Guo W, Choe R, et al. Computer aided automatic detection of malignant lesions in diffuse optical mammography. Med Phys 2010;37(4):1843; with permission.)

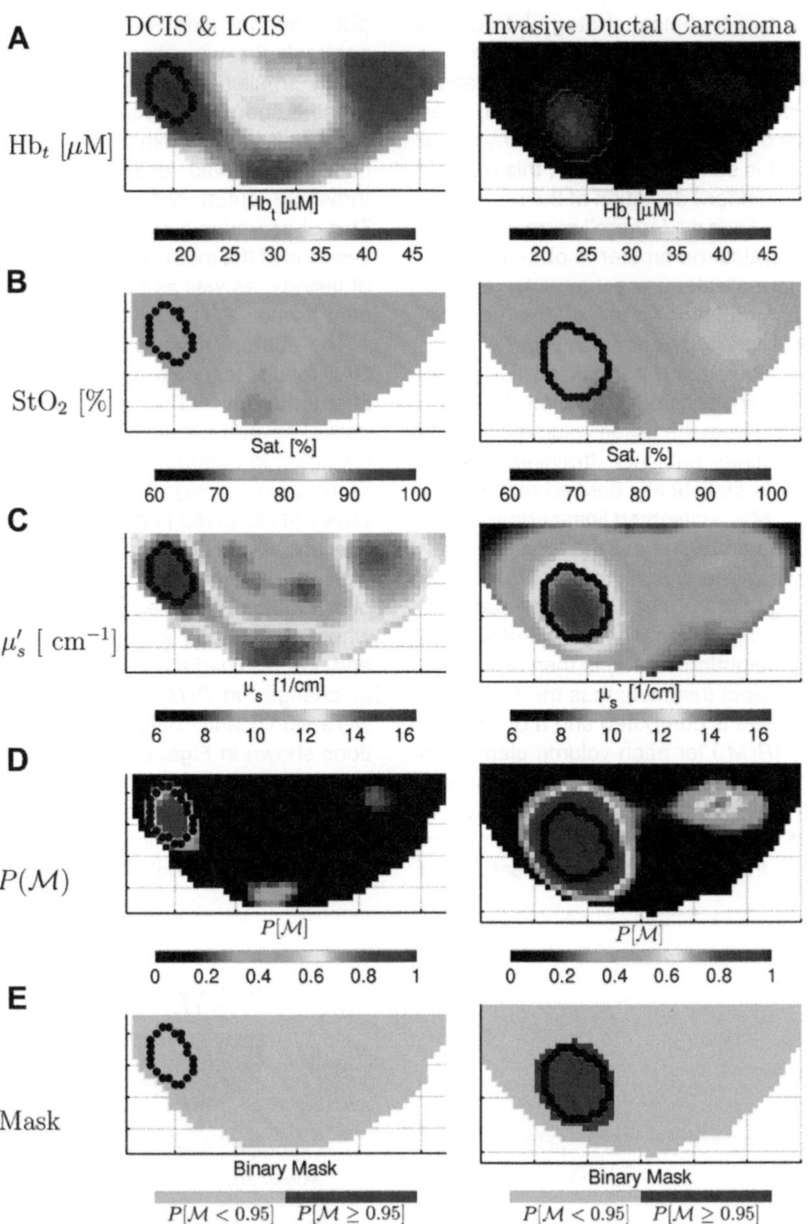

Fig. 6. Slices from three-dimensional (3D) images of two subjects, showing total hemoglobin concentration (*A*, Hb_t), blood oxygen saturation (*B*, StO_2), reduced scattering coefficient (*C*, μ_s'), probability of malignancy (*D*, $P(M)$), and a binary cancer mask (*E*) using a cutoff of $P(M) = 0.95$. The DCIS & LCIS (ductal and lobular carcinoma *in situ*) lesion in the left column provides an interesting case study, with the $P(M)$ falling between the malignant lesions and the healthy regions. The invasive ductal carcinoma in the right column shows a typical result from invasive cancers. (*From* Busch DR. Computer-aided, multi-modal, and compression diffuse optical studies of breast tissue [PhD thesis]. University of Pennsylvania; 2011; with permission.)

could be used to determine the efficacy of particular neoadjuvant chemotherapy regimens well before tumor changes are revealed by structural imaging.

Overall the results of this study are encouraging, suggesting that statistical analysis of the metabolically dependent, optically measured physiologic parameters of cancer tissue can yield a useful signature of cancer location and response to treatment. The study described here was derived from a limited population (thirty five subjects), and the chemotherapy monitoring is only at the pilot stage (three subjects). A more expansive study is now needed.

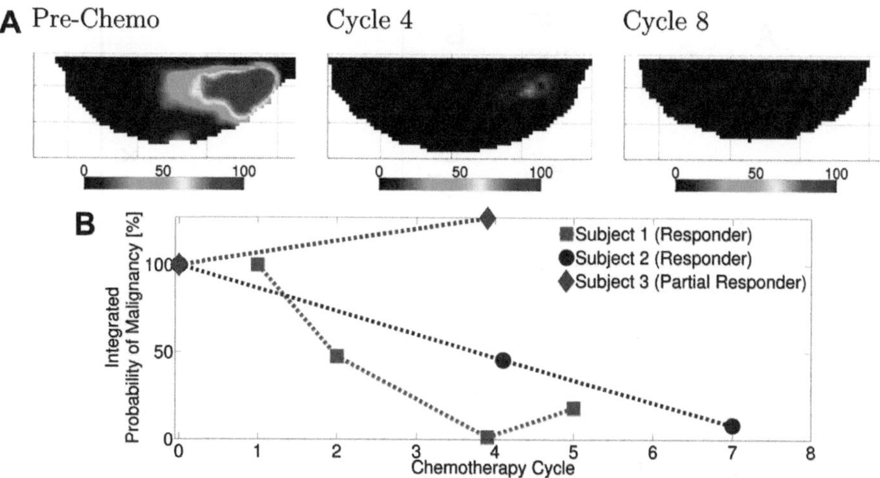

Fig. 7. Pilot study of monitoring chemotherapy using DOT with computer-aided detection in 3 subjects. (*A*) Example images of $P(M)$ changing during the course of chemotherapy (subject 2). (*B*) Integrated probability of malignancy in tumor regions, normalized to first time point in subjects with complete (subjects 1 and 2) and partial (subject 3) response to chemotherapy. (*From* Busch DR, Choe R, Rosen MA, et al. Optical malignancy parameters for monitoring progression of breast cancer neoadjuvant chemotherapy. Biomed Opt Express 2013;4(1):105–21.)

TOWARD METABOLIC IMAGING

Endogenous DOT Versus PET Glucose Imaging

It is difficult to validate the hemodynamic parameters measured by DOT directly against other diagnostic modalities, because none is able to noninvasively measure all of the same parameters. However, correlation of parameters such as the total hemoglobin concentration measured by DOT with microvessel density measured by histopathology has been carried out.[54,63,100,101] To date, two major approaches have been explored for direct correlation/comparison of DOT with other imaging modalities: (1) image correlation based on the stand-alone images taken independently, and (2) correlation based on concurrent image acquisition. The deformability of breast tissue makes the former approach challenging. Nonetheless, research along these lines has demonstrated that the high tumor-to-background ratio detected by DOT corresponds to the tumor locations identified by MR imaging[50,52,102] and PET.[89] These and other works have led to the development of advanced software suites that permit researchers to transform the volumetric information between imaging modalities.

Regarding concurrent acquisition, it is challenging but possible to integrate DOT source and detector systems into other medical imaging modalities. This development has led to interesting multimodal imaging instrumentation, for example, DOT and MR imaging,[103–106] DOT and tomosynthesis,[107,108] and, DOT and ultrasonographic imaging.[109–111] The primary disadvantage of the multimodal approach is that hardware constraints limit the total number of DOT measurements to values less than typical for stand-alone DOT systems. Most efforts to date have focused on use of anatomic information from MR imaging, tomosynthesis, and ultrasonography to derive spatial priors for DOT reconstructions; this concept has been shown to improve DOT quantification. Furthermore, concurrent multimodal imaging offers a great opportunity for DOT validation. In this vein, the combination of PET and DOT (and/or diffuse correlation spectroscopy) is interesting for validation of mechanisms of oxidative metabolism, and for consideration of DOT as a surrogate to PET when frequent measurements are desirable.

Although concurrent PET and DOT have not yet been demonstrated in humans, the coregistration and correlation of nonconcurrent DOT and PET has been performed.[89] **Fig. 8**A shows a qualitative correlation between FDG and DOT signals in axial, sagittal, and coronal views of patients' breasts. Note that PET imaged the whole body in this comparison, whereas DOT imaged a single breast. The dotted square in PET indicates the same breast imaged by DOT. Because image coregistration between breast images taken in supine and prone positions is difficult, each 3D image was analyzed independently for quantifying tumor-to-background ratio for each parameter. **Fig. 8**B shows a selected example from correlation between FDG and DOT-derived parameters. Positive correlations ($P<.05$) were found between FDG uptake and Hb_t, and FDG uptake and μ_s'. The positive correlation between FDG and Hb_t might be

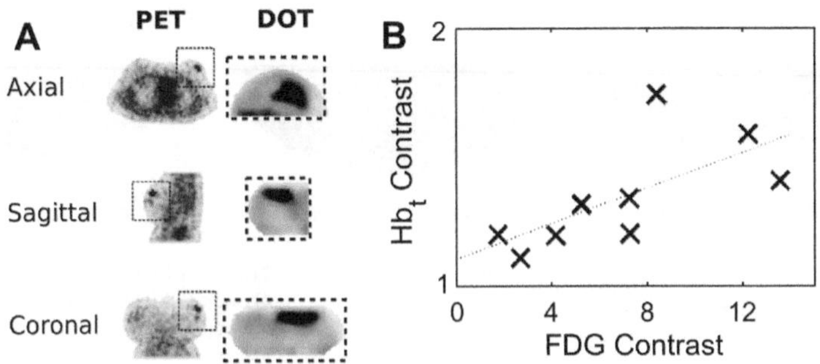

Fig. 8. (*A*) Axial, sagittal, and coronal slices from the whole-body FDG PET and DOT images of overall optical attenuation coefficient: μ_{eff}. Note the whole-body PET image is of the whole torso with both breasts, whereas DOT shows the left breast only. The rectangular dotted box in each image denotes the breast corresponding to the DOT image. (*B*) Correlation between contrast ratios in FDG uptake and Hb_t for the 9 patients with tumors visible to both DOT and PET. (*Adapted from* Konecky SD, Choe R, Corlu A, et al. Comparison of diffuse optical tomography of human breast with whole-body and breast-only positron emission tomography. Med Phys 2008;35(2):446–55; with permission.)

expected, because increases in glucose metabolism of breast cancer require more blood for glucose and oxygen delivery which, in turn, is typically accompanied by an increased total hemoglobin concentration.

For three patients, PET imaging was performed using a dedicated breast-imaging PET scanner.[112,113] Then, a coregistration algorithm based on rigid body motion (translation and rotation) and linear scaling[102] was used to transform the DOT image space into the PET image space as DOT was measured with axial compression whereas PET was measured without compression. A caudal-cranial slice from a 3D DOT image encompassing the suspicious mass for each parameter (Hb_t, StO_2, μ_s') is presented along with the FDG image slice in **Fig. 9**. Subject A had a ductal carcinoma *in situ*, subject B had a palpable mass that turned out to be a seroma caused by biopsy-induced hemorrhage in the center, and subject C had invasive ductal carcinoma. Increases in Hb_t and μ_s' contrast showed correspondence with similar high-FDG regions in the PET images. In sum, these results demonstrate that DOT is indeed sensitive to the local metabolism and may provide information complementary to PET.

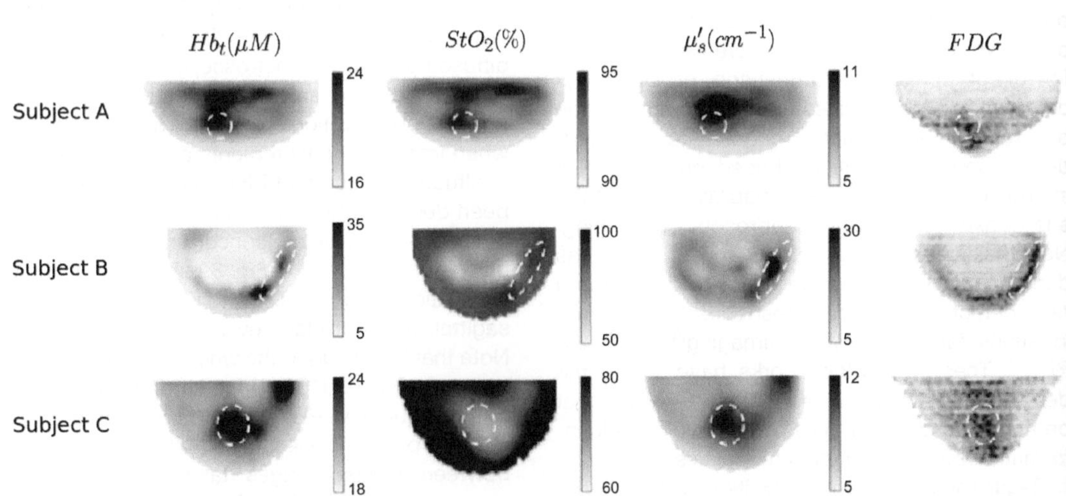

Fig. 9. Images of the breasts of three women imaged with DOT and with a dedicated breast-imaging PET. A representative caudal-cranial slice taken from the 3D reconstruction of a breast is presented for each parameter and patient. The DOT images have been transformed, using a coregistration algorithm, to be in the same uncompressed state as PET. The rows correspond to each patient with suspicious lesions. The columns correspond to Hb_t, StO_2, μ_s' measured by DOT, and FDG uptake measured by PET. The dashed white ellipses enclose regions with suspicious lesions. (*Adapted from* Konecky SD, Choe R, Corlu A, et al. Comparison of diffuse optical tomography of human breast with whole-body and breast-only positron emission tomography. Med Phys 2008;35(2):446–55; with permission.)

All-Optical Measurement of Oxygen Extraction Fraction and Metabolism

Another approach uses diffuse light to noninvasively measure microvascular, local blood flow (*BF*). The measurement uses a technique referred to as diffuse correlation spectroscopy (DCS) in the biomedical optics community.[61,68,114,115] DCS uses coherent laser sources and the temporal statistics of light speckles emerging from tissue. These statistics reveal quantitative information about the motion of red blood cells (RBCs) in the interrogated tissues. *BF* is characterized by an index derived from the temporal decay rate of the diffusing light field temporal intensity autocorrelation function.

Optical mammography, or breast tumor monitoring, with DCS was first introduced in 2005.[116] In that study, the investigators observed a significant increase of the DCS *BF* index in tumors in comparison with the normal tissue. Later, the investigators demonstrated that early changes in tumor physiology can also be discerned by DCS flow measurements and that the relative changes were comparable with relative changes measured by DOS/DOT.[53] Most recently, these approaches have shown potential to differentiate responders from nonresponders among patients on neoadjuvant chemotherapy, and potential for use in drug-development schemes.[61] For recent reviews, see Refs.[61,68]

DCS information can readily be combined with information from DOS/DOT to gain access to tissue oxygen metabolism. This combination is attractive for several reasons: (1) DCS and DOS/DOT probe very similar tissue volumes for the same source-detector positions, so the results are easily combined and compared; (2) the ability to collectively measure blood flow, blood volume, and blood oxygenation enables researchers to estimate the oxygen extraction fraction and the tissue metabolic rate of oxygen extraction.[53,68,117]

To illustrate this latter point, two composite "optical indices" are introduced, which indicate the tissue physiology. The tissue optical index (*TOI*) suggested by the Tromberg group at the University of California, Irvine is a multiparameter contrast function created to maximize both the contrast and the specificity of the optical measurement. *TOI* is defined as[13,51]

$$\mathrm{TOI} = \frac{\mathrm{Hb}\cdot\mathrm{H_2O}}{\mathrm{Lipid}}. \tag{1}$$

TOI is empirically constructed from the concentrations of deoxyhemoglobin (*Hb*), water (H_2O), and lipids (*Lipid*). Increased *TOI* has been found to reflect a higher chance of tumor malignancy, and *TOI* is also related to metabolic activity, because increases in deoxyhemoglobin are often a symptom of unmet metabolic demand.

Inclusion of DCS in the arsenal of diffuse optical tools for optical mammography enables one to derive a direct estimate of tissue oxygen metabolism by combining information about blood flow (delivery of oxygen) with the chromophore concentration information such as blood oxygen saturation (ie, oxygen availability). This approach has most often been employed in neurologic applications with hybrid diffuse optics,[68] but these ideas are readily translated to other tissues, albeit without a robust validation. Here, a simple model and index is described, which offers a new means to define tumor contrast based on mammary metabolic rate of oxygen consumption ($MMRO_2$) following Zhou.[53,117] We define

$$\mathrm{MMRO_2} = \gamma\cdot\frac{\mathrm{Hb}}{\mathrm{Hb_t}}\cdot\mathrm{BF} \tag{2}$$

where $\gamma = \frac{Hb_v/Hb_{tv}}{Hb/Hb_t}$, the ratio of deoxyhemoglobin (*Hb*) to total hemoglobin (Hb_t) in the venous compartment (*v*) compared with the ratio of deoxyhemoglobin to total hemoglobin in the total vasculature. Here, the relative rates of oxygen metabolism between tumor ("*T*") and normal ("*N*") breast tissues $\left(rMMRO_{2(T/N)} = \frac{MMRO_{2(T)}}{MMRO_{2(N)}}\right)$ are defined as

$$\mathrm{rMMRO_{2(T/N)}} = \frac{\gamma_T}{\gamma_N}\cdot\frac{\mathrm{Hb_{(T)}}}{\mathrm{Hb_{(N)}}}\cdot\left(\frac{\mathrm{Hb_{t(T)}}}{\mathrm{Hb_{t(N)}}}\right)^{-1}\cdot\frac{\mathrm{BF_{(T)}}}{\mathrm{BF_{(N)}}} \tag{3}$$

$$= \frac{\gamma_T}{\gamma_N}\cdot\mathrm{rHb_{(T/N)}}\cdot\left(\mathrm{rHb_{t(T/N)}}\right)^{-1}\cdot\mathrm{rBF_{(T/N)}}. \tag{4}$$

In Eqn. 4, the relative values of a parameter between tumor and normal tissue are abbreviated as $rX_{(T/N)} = X_T/X_N$. If it is assumed that the ratio of γ_T/γ_N is unity and constant over time, Eqn. 4 reduces to

$$\mathrm{rMMRO_{2(T/N)}} = \frac{\mathrm{rHb_{(T/N)}}}{\mathrm{rHb_{t(T/N)}}}\cdot\mathrm{rBF_{(T/N)}} \tag{5}$$

or alternatively

$$\mathrm{rMMRO_{2(T/N)}} = \frac{1-\mathrm{StO_{2(T)}}}{1-\mathrm{StO_{2(N)}}}\cdot\mathrm{rBF_{(T/N)}} \tag{6}$$

where StO_2 is the tissue oxygen saturation.

$rMMRO_{2(T/N)}$ is thus the relative oxygen extraction multiplied by the relative blood flow in the tumor compared with the normal tissue; that is, $MMRO_2$ relates the local blood flow and the local oxygen extraction fraction to each other in a manner that is presumably proportional to the extraction of oxygen derived from the local oxygen metabolism. $rMMRO_{2(T/N)}$ is an attempt to quantify the tumor oxygen metabolism with respect to the healthy surrounding tissue.

Fig. 10 shows how one can use these data and these new indices in monitoring cancer therapy. **Fig. 10** shows data from a 45-year-old pre-menopausal woman undergoing neoadjuvant chemotherapy treatment for an invasive ductal carcinoma in the left breast.[53,117] The patient was treated with neoadjuvant chemotherapy delivered in multiple stages. The initial treatment stage consisted of doxorubicin and cyclophosphamide. Further details are provided by Zhou and colleagues.[53,117]

The data shown in **Fig. 10** indicate the richness of the parameters measurable with the hybrid diffuse optical instrumentation. Both hemodynamic and structural information about the tumor are assessed over time. These parameters all show varying degrees of change as the therapy progresses at a very early stage, that is, as early as three days after the start of the therapy. In particular, *BF* measured with DCS increased initially on day three after the start of therapy, and then decreased sharply and in a sustained manner during days four, five, and seven. This type of behavior, in response to therapy, was

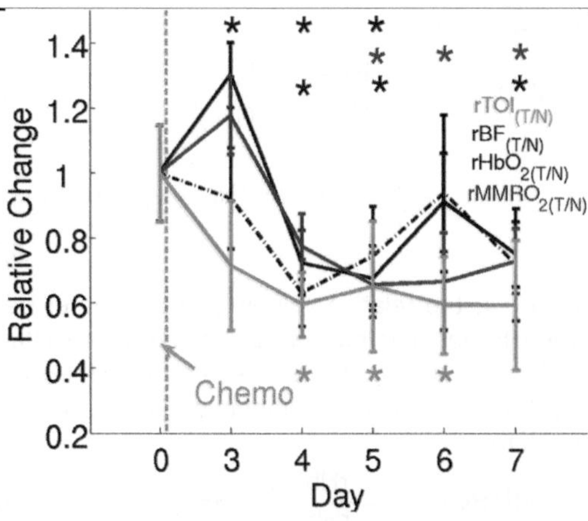

Fig. 10. Relative tumor/normal oxyhemoglobin ($rHbO_{2(T/N)}$), blood flow index ($rBF_{(T/N)}$), optical index ($rTOI_{(T/N)}$), and mammary metabolic rate of oxygen consumption ($rMMRO_{2(T/N)}$). Contrasts in response to chemotherapy are shown. The optical indices were calculated as the ratio of the average tumor value to the average value of the normal tissue on the same side of the breast. These indices were then normalized to the prechemotherapy values to reflect relative changes. Asterisk denotes statistically significant (at $P<.05$) difference from prechemotherapy values. (*Courtesy of* Chao Zhou, PhD, Lehigh University, Bethlehem, PA.)

found again in later studies and was suggested to indicate therapy response.[61]

Fig. 10 shows the evolution of the two composite indices $rMMRO_{2(T/N)}$ and $rTOI_{(T/N)}$ ($rTOI_{(T/N)} = TOI_T/TOI_N$). Note that they have diverged from one another by day three, wherein $rTOI_{(T/N)}$ showed an initial drop and $rMMRO_{2(T/N)}$ showed an initial increase. After day four, both metabolic indices dropped significantly and then stabilized until the end of the monitoring period. The authors of this work have speculated that although both $rTOI_{(T/N)}$ and $rMMRO_{2(T/N)}$ are related to tumor metabolic responses, $rTOI_{(T/N)}$ provides information about tumor cellular metabolic activities, whereas $rMMRO_{2(T/N)}$ provides information about tumor oxygen metabolic changes. At this time it is too early to say whether these composite parameters will prove to be useful in therapy monitoring or diagnostics in optical mammography, but they do provide a new approach to direct probing of the tissue physiology.

In principle, DCS can be used to carry out tomographic optical mammography of blood flow, that is, diffuse correlation tomography (DCT). At this time, however, DCT has only been demonstrated in tissue phantoms and in rat brain.[118] The authors expect that with increased parallelization and improved technologies, DCT might soon be used for breast imaging. In fact, some spectroscopic results in the transmission geometry have been published,[119] which suggest that with a better dynamic range it should be possible to construct a stand-alone breast DCT system.

Dynamic Imaging of Physiologic Perturbations

This section highlights a different approach to optical mammography, which uses physiologic perturbations to generate contrast in human breast tissue.[119–125] For example, internal or external applied pressure can alter tissue optical properties in a predictable manner, and thus provide the experimenter with additional metabolic/hemodynamic tissue information and contrast. Specifically, Carp and colleagues[126] have used mild cyclical perturbations of the applied load to derive an estimate for the baseline metabolism of breast tissue. Their experiment consisted of placing the breast between two parallel plates, similar to the geometry of an axial mammogram. Then frequency-domain optical data (DOS) was collected in the remission geometry from the inferior plate as a stepper motor applied force (up to 6 lb/2.7 kg) to the superior plate for ninty seconds (repeating the cycle three times). The underlying idea of this approach is that the changes in total hemoglobin concentration in response to partial vessel occlusion serve as a proxy for net, bulk blood flow. This notion is essentially borrowed from other areas such as venous cuff-occlusion photoplethysmography. The derived flow information is combined with measured changes in tissue oxygen saturation, in a manner similar to the aforementioned $MMRO_2$, to calculate the bulk tissue oxygen consumption. When compared with values reported in the literature (**Table 2**), their measurements appear to underestimate these quantities. However, in the remission geometry one might also expect the measurements to be much more sensitive to the outer fatty region of breast rather than the central fibroglandular region. Thus, the underestimation may be due to low blood flow and oxygen consumption in the fatty region. Despite this limitation, this approach represents a step forward regarding extraction of absolute numbers for oxygen consumption and blood flow.

Similarly, while not explicitly extracting metabolic parameters, other scientists have used compression schemes to create differential images based on the variation of the compressibility and/or the vascular resistance of the tumors by comparison with surrounding healthy tissue.[17,38,120–122] Xu and colleagues[124] have developed a hand-held pressure modulation device, and Dixit and colleagues[129,130] have used inhaled gasses to generate vascular contrast.[131] Overall, these dynamic methods demonstrate the versatility of the diffuse optical techniques in seeking different physiologic contrasts.

EXOGENOUS CONTRAST AGENTS

Like other conventional imaging modalities, the capabilities of diffuse optics can be enhanced with the use of exogenous contrast agents. With the increase in contrast by use of a contrast agent, image resolution and fidelity can be improved. In a different vein and perhaps more interestingly, DOT could be used to access numerous parameters related to tumor pathology (e.g. pH, tumor-specific receptors, glucose metabolism) with optimized tumor-targeting optical contrast agents.[132] Such agents are commonly used in animal models, and are expected to become more widely available for human use in the near future.

At present, the metabolic sensitivity and the spatial resolution of DOT are analogous to that of PET before the advent of PET/computed tomography (CT) systems. As noted earlier, several research groups are exploring potential multimodal combinations of DOT with other techniques that are sensitive to tissue structure. This multimodal approach, analogous to that of PET/CT, could open a new chapter for the field. An interesting advantage to DOT, for example, in comparison with some modalities is its potential for simultaneous imaging of multiple contrast agents. This capability provides opportunities for simultaneous monitoring of several tumor characteristics.[106,133]

Indocyanine green (ICG, sold under the brand name Cardio-Green[134]) is currently the only agent approved by the Food and Drug Administration for use as an absorption-enhancing or a fluorescence agent in the NIR spectral region. In this case, the absorption/excitation (peak ~800 nm) and emission (peak ~820 nm) wavelengths have low absorption in tissue, permitting highly sensitive detection. ICG is used routinely in the clinic for measurement of cardiac output, in hepatology for evaluation of liver function, in ophthalmology for choroidal angiography, and in neurology for detection of cerebral artery infarction.[135] In plasma, rapid binding of ICG to macromolecules such as lipoproteins and albumin causes ICG to act as a blood-pooling agent. ICG is eliminated by the liver with a half-life of a few minutes.[136] In malignant tumors, new blood vessels tend to be hyperpermeable, enabling large molecules such as albumin to extravasate into the interstitium.[137] Thus, there is a good probability that ICG bound to macromolecules could leak out of vasculature and therefore serve as a marker for vascular permeability.

Table 2
Comparison of metabolic parameters (oxygen consumption and blood flow) reported in the PET literature and estimated using DOS

Method	Breast	N	Oxygen Consumption (μmol/100 mL/min)	Blood Flow (mL/100 mL/min)
PET, ^{15}O inhalation[127]	Normal	9	19.8	3.96
PET, ^{15}O inhalation[128]	Normal	20	N/A	5.6 ± 1.4
DOS[126]	Healthy	28	1.9 ± 1.3	2.8 ± 1.7

PET literature included both tumor and normal breast values, but only normal values are presented in this table for comparison.

The first uses of ICG in diffuse optics were as an absorption and fluorescence contrast agent for optical mammography. With a concurrent MR imaging/DOT device, absorption enhancement due to ICG at 830 nm was used to highlight different degrees of enhancement in three cases: one with an invasive ductal carcinoma, one with fibroadenoma, and another with no disease.[103] The highest tumor-to-normal contrast was found in the invasive ductal carcinoma in 2D DOT, and its location was confirmed with simultaneous MR imaging.

The first 3D reconstruction of ICG **fluorescence** in human breast has since been demonstrated in three subjects with malignant breast tumors.[138] High ICG concentration was found in the same region, exhibiting high endogenous contrast (ie, Hb_t, μ_s'); the fluorescence concentration contrast even for this blood-pool agent was significantly higher than endogenous contrast based on absorption/scattering. Of note, the contrast enhancement attributable to ICG was even more dramatic in the heterogeneously dense breast than in the entirely fatty breast. In addition to static imaging, some attempts at differentiating benign from malignant tumors have been performed, based on the different pharmacokinetics of ICG-based absorption contrast. These results have been mixed and to date have only been investigated in a limited number of subjects.[139–142] The mixed results could be attributed to the fact that these measurements were taken within 10 minutes after bolus ICG injection when the signal was dominated by ICG contained in the blood, but not by ICG in the extravascular space.

Researchers at Physikalisch-Technische Bundesanstalt (PTB) and Charité Hospital in Berlin have imaged ICG in vascular and extravascular phases using a combination of ICG bolus injection and continuous infusion (**Fig. 11**).[143] The fluorescence-to-absorption ratio image taken during the extravascular phase showed enhancement corresponding to the location of an invasive ductal carcinoma. This lesion was detected using contrast-enhanced MR imaging but was not detected in an x-ray mammogram. In the case of fibroadenoma, fluorescence-to-absorption ratio images were similar to those of surrounding healthy tissue. Charité has extended this study to twenty women with twenty one breast lesions (eight benign and thirteen malignant lesions) yielding mean sensitivity of 92% and specificity of 75%. Compared with the approximately 100% sensitivity and 25% specificity of conventional mammography alone, this fluorescence technique demonstrated improvement in specificity.[144]

Recently, Bayer Schering Healthcare (Berlin, Germany) has attempted to translate a new NIR fluorescent optical contrast agent, Omocianine, to human use. Omocianine is an ICG derivative with a plasma half-life of approximately fifteen hours in humans and with superior quantum efficiency compared with ICG (ie, higher florescence). However, absorption and fluorescence measurements did not differentiate between benign and malignant tumors with this particular agent.[135,145]

In summary, several research groups have demonstrated that quantification of in vivo fluorescent dye concentration in breast is feasible in humans. One can simply enhance vascular contrast for DOT with bolus ICG during the vascular phase and/or access an additional parameter, vascular leakiness, with a carefully designed ICG injection protocol in the extravascular phase. The latter parameter may be an especially powerful tool to differentiate benign and malignant lesions. Although Omocianine failed to show improvement over ICG in imaging of breast cancer, other researchers have found multiple applications for ICG fluorescent imaging in translational research.[146] When new fluorescent dyes with higher quantum efficiency than ICG, or moieties targeting particular cellular markers, finally are transitioned into the clinic, the arsenal of optically available tumor characteristics will increase, and optical imaging and monitoring should emerge as a powerful tool.

SUMMARY AND OUTLOOK

This article discusses the recent trends in optical mammography as the field moves toward metabolic imaging and monitoring. The discussion is oriented toward diffuse optics technologies, with attention to composite signatures of malignancy, metabolic information from blood flow and hemoglobin concentration parameters, exogenous contrast agents, and dynamic contrast. Indeed, the American Cancer Society 2003 guidelines for the screening of breast cancer recognized diffuse optical mammography as a promising technology worthy of future study.[147] Since these guidelines were published a decade ago the field has advanced significantly, with several studies incorporating larger patient populations.[20,33,148–150] Researchers have focused on niche applications, for example, monitoring of neoadjuvant chemotherapy,[61,151] with perhaps the most exciting recent development, in terms of its translation to routine clinical use, being an ongoing trial sponsored by the American College of Radiology Imaging Network (ACRIN), in which patients on neoadjuvant chemotherapy are enrolled in a seven-site trial with identical instrumentation (ACRIN 6691).

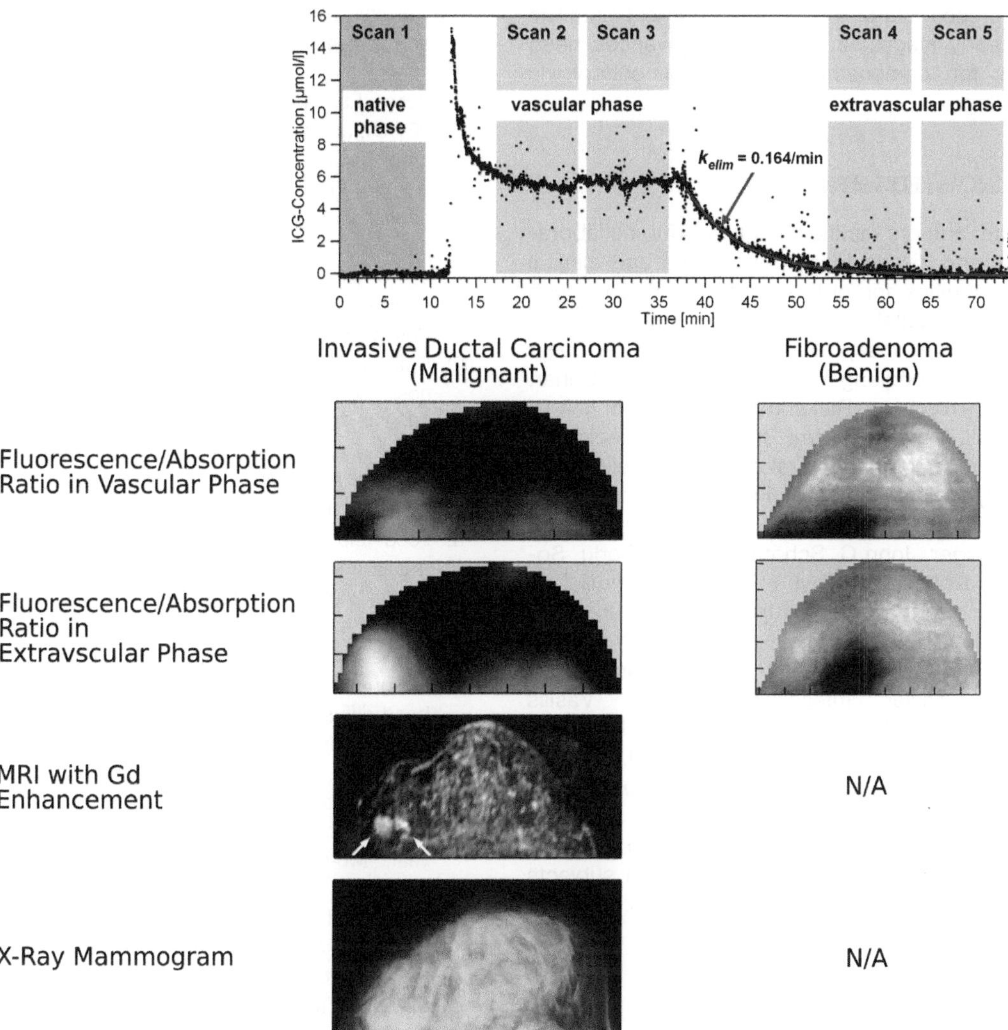

Fig. 11. (*Upper panel*) Time course of molar indocyanine green (ICG) concentration in arterial blood, recorded by transcutaneous pulse densitometry. Optical mammogram measurements were performed during the native phase (ie, before ICG injection, *gray shading*), vascular phase (ie, after ICG bolus injection followed by continuous infusion, *light salmon shading*), and extravascular phase (ie, more than 20 minutes after termination of infusion, *blue shading*). (*Lower panels*) Images of an invasive ductal carcinoma (malignant lesion, *center column*) and a fibroadenoma (benign lesion, *right column*). In the fluorescent/absorption ratio images, the malignant lesion lacks contrast in the vascular phase (*top row*), but is clearly visible in the extravascular phase (*second row*), whereas the benign lesion is much less distinct at both time points. Gadolinium-enhanced MR imaging (*third row*) shows the malignant lesion clearly, although this lesion is difficult to locate in the x-ray mammogram (*bottom row*).

In addition to the deep-tissue applications of diffuse optics, there has been considerable effort focused on intraoperative measurements of cancer margins and biopsy samples.[152–160] Fluorescence planar imaging through thin tissue for sentinel lymph nodes may also offer an alternative to radioscintigraphy.[161–163] Other notable recent developments not reviewed here include novel multimodal instrumentation combining diffuse optics with ultrasonography (photoacoustic tomography), taking advantage of hemoglobin absorption to selectively induce photothermal expansion. This rapid expansion produces a pressure wave detectable with ultrasound transducers,[164] a technique that has been demonstrated in the breast.[165–167]

It is hoped that the reader is able to discern that the diffuse optical technologies offer potential applications over a wide range of areas in the screening, detection, staging, and therapy monitoring of breast cancer. Indeed, in many ways the present stage of DOT development parallels the early stages of PET. More advances need time for demonstration, but the outlook is exciting.

ACKNOWLEDGMENTS

The authors acknowledge fruitful collaborations and discussions about optics and clinical opportunities for optics over many years with numerous outstanding scientists including Britton Chance, Joseph P. Culver, Xingde Li, David A. Boas, Guoqiang Yu, Chao Zhou, Ulas Sunar, Bruce Tromberg, Rickson Mesquita, Mitchell D. Schnall, Mark A. Rosen, Brian J. Czerniecki, Julia Tchou, Douglas L. Fraker, Angela DeMichele, Carolyn Mies, Michael D. Feldman, Mary E. Putt, Wensheng Guo, Simon R. Arridge, Martin Schweiger, John C. Schotland, Alper Corlu, Soren D. Konecky, So Hyun Chung, Wesley Baker, Ashwin Parthasarathy, Kijoon Lee, Saurav Pathak, Han Y. Ban, Malavika Chandra, Yu Chen, Jonathan Fisher, Joe Giammarco, Monica Holboke, Xavier Intes, Xingde Li, Vasilis Ntziachristos, Maureen O'Leary, Yalin Ti, Hsing-Wen Wang, Guoqiang Yu, Udo Weigel, Peyman Zirak, Parisa Farzam, Johannes Johansson, Ki Won Jung, and Leonid Zubkov.

This research would not have been possible without the generosity of the research subjects who participated in the authors' studies.

REFERENCES

1. Siegel R, Naishadham D, Jemal A. Cancer statistics, 2012. CA Cancer J Clin 2012;62(1):10–29.
2. Kriege M, Brekelmans CT, Boetes C, et al. Efficacy of MRI and mammography for breast-cancer screening in women with a familial or genetic predisposition. N Engl J Med 2004;351(5):427–37.
3. Boyd J, Jellins J, Reeve T, et al. Ultrasound examination of the breast. In: Jellins J, Kobayashi T, editors. Doppler examination of the breast. New York: John Wiley and Sons; 1983. p. 385–6.
4. Sehgal CM, Weinstein SP, Arger PH, et al. A review of breast ultrasound. J Mammary Gland Biol Neoplasia 2006;11(2):113–23.
5. Saslow D, Boetes C, Burke W, et al. American Cancer Society guidelines for breast screening with MRI as an adjunct to mammography. CA Cancer J Clin 2007;57(2):75–89.
6. Lord S, Lei W, Craft P, et al. A systematic review of the effectiveness of magnetic resonance imaging (MRI) as an addition to mammography and ultrasound in screening young women at high risk of breast cancer. Eur J Cancer 2007;43(13):1905–17.
7. Weinstein SP, Localio AR, Conant EF, et al. Multimodality screening of high-risk women: a prospective cohort study. J Clin Oncol 2009;27(36):6124–8.
8. Rosen EL, Eubank WB, Mankoff DA. FDG PET, PET/CT, and breast cancer imaging. Radiographics 2007;27(Suppl 1):S215–29.
9. Wu WC, Englander S, Schnall, et al. Feasibility of arterial spin labeling in the measurement of breast perfusion. In: Proceedings of the International Society for Magnetic Resonance in Medicine. vol. 13. Berkeley, USA: International Society of Magnetic Resonance in Medicine; 2007. p. 2801.
10. Cutler M. Transillumination as an aid in the diagnosis of breast lesions. Surg Gynecol Obstet 1929;48:721–9.
11. Laser Institute of America. American national standard for the safe use of lasers: Ansi z136.1-2007. Orlando (FL): Laser Institute of America; 2007.
12. Food and Drug Administration. Code of federal regulations, title 21, vol. 8. US government Printing Office; 2003. 21CFR1040.10.
13. Cerussi A, Shah N, Hsiang D, et al. In vivo absorption, scattering, and physiologic properties of 58 malignant breast tumors determined by broadband diffuse optical spectroscopy. J Biomed Opt 2006;11:044005 (16pp).
14. Chance B, Nioka S, Zhang J, et al. Breast cancer detection based on incremental biochemical and physiological properties of breast cancers a six-year, two-site study. Acad Radiol 2005;12(8): 925–33.
15. Durduran T, Choe R, Culver JP, et al. Bulk optical properties of healthy female breast tissue. Phys Med Biol 2002;47:2847–61.
16. Spinelli L, Torricelli A, Pifferi A, et al. Bulk optical properties and tissue components in the female breast from multiwavelength time-resolved optical mammography. J Biomed Opt 2004;9(6):1137–42.
17. Fang Q, Carp SA, Selb J, et al. Combined optical imaging and mammography of the healthy breast: optical contrast derived from breast structure and compression. IEEE Trans Med Imaging 2009; 28(1):30–42.
18. Taroni P, Bassi A, Comelli D, et al. Diffuse optical spectroscopy of breast tissue extended to 1100 nm. J Biomed Opt 2009;14(5):054030.
19. Taroni P, Pifferi A, Salvagnini E, et al. Seven-wavelength time-resolved optical mammography extending beyond 1000 nm for breast collagen quantification. Opt Express 2009;17(18):15932–46.
20. Leff DR, Warren OJ, Enfield LC, et al. Diffuse optical imaging of the healthy and diseased breast: a systematic review. Breast Cancer Res Treat 2008; 108(1):9–22.
21. Srinivasan S, Pogue BW, Carpenter C, et al. Developments in quantitative oxygen-saturation imaging of breast tissue in vivo using multispectra

near-infrared tomography. Antioxid Redox Signal 2007;9(8):1143–56.

22. Shah N, Cerussi AE, Jakubowski D, et al. Spatial variations in optical and physiological properties of healthy breast tissue. J Biomed Opt 2004;9(3): 534–40.
23. Blyschak K, Simick M, Jong R, et al. Classification of breast tissue density by optical transillumination spectroscopy: optical and physiological effects governing predictive value. Med Phys 2004;31(6): 1398–414.
24. Blackmore KM, Knight JA, Jong R, et al. Assessing breast tissue density by transillumination breast spectroscopy (TIBS): an intermediate indicator of cancer risk. Br J Radiol 2007;80(955):545–56.
25. Blackmore KM, Knight JA, Lilge L. Association between transillumination breast spectroscopy and quantitative mammographic features of the breast. Cancer Epidemiol Biomarkers Prev 2008;17(5): 1043.
26. Taroni P, Pifferi A, Quarto G, et al. Noninvasive assessment of breast cancer risk using time-resolved diffuse optical spectroscopy. J Biomed Opt 2010; 15:060501.
27. Nioka S, Chance B. NIR spectroscopic detection of breast cancer. Technol Cancer Res Treat 2005; 4(5):497–512.
28. Ntziachristos V, Chance B. Probing physiology and molecular function using optical imaging applications to breast cancer. Breast Cancer Res 2001;3: 41–6.
29. Enfield LC, Gibson AP, Everdell NL, et al. Three-dimensional time-resolved optical mammography of the uncompressed breast. Appl Opt 2007; 46(17):3628–38.
30. Poplack SP, Tosteson TD, Wells WA, et al. Electromagnetic breast imaging: results of a pilot study in women with abnormal mammograms. Radiology 2007;243(2):350–9.
31. Nioka S, Yung Y, Shnall M, et al. Optical imaging of breast tumor by means of continuous waves. Adv Exp Med Biol 1997;411:227–32.
32. Grosenick D, Wabnitz H, Rinneberg HH, et al. Development of a time-domain optical mammograph and first in vivo applications. Appl Opt 1999;38(13):2927–43.
33. Spinelli L, Torricelli A, Pifferi A, et al. Characterization of female breast lesions from multi-wavelength time-resolved optical mammography. Phys Med Biol 2005;50(11):2489–502.
34. Culver JP, Choe R, Holboke MJ, et al. Three-dimensional diffuse optical tomography in the parallel plane transmission geometry: evaluation of a hybrid frequency domain/continuous wave clinical system for breast imaging. Med Phys 2003;30:235–47.
35. Choe R, Konecky SD, Corlu A, et al. Differentiation of benign and malignant breast tumors by in-vivo three-dimensional parallel-plate diffuse optical tomography. J Biomed Opt 2009;14(2):024020 (18pp).
36. Hoogenraad JH, van der Mark MB, Colak SB, et al. First results from the Philips Optical Mammoscope. Photon Propagation in Tissues III 1998; 3194:184–90.
37. Nielsen T, Brendel B, Ziegler R, et al. Linear image reconstruction for a diffuse optical mammography system in a noncompressed geometry using scattering fluid. Appl Opt 2009;48(10):D1–13.
38. Schmitz CH, Klemer DP, Hardin R, et al. Design and implementation of dynamic near-infrared optical tomographic imaging instrumentation for simultaneous dual-breast measurements. Appl Opt 2005;44(11):2140–53.
39. Intes X, Djeziri S, Ichalalene Z, et al. Time-domain optical mammography Softscan: initial results. Acad Radiol 2005;12(8):934–47.
40. Athanasiou A, Vanel D, Fournier L, et al. Optical mammography: a new technique for visualizing breast lesions in women presenting non palpable BIRADS 4-5 imaging findings: preliminary results with radiologic-pathologic correlation. Cancer Imaging 2007;7(1):34.
41. Fournier LS, Vanel D, Athanasiou A, et al. Dynamic optical breast imaging: a novel technique to detect and characterize tumor vessels. Eur J Radiol 2009; 69(1):43–9.
42. Arridge S, Schotland J. Optical tomography: forward and inverse problems. Inverse Probl 2009; 25(12):123010 (59pp).
43. Kaufmann M, von Minckwitz G, Bear HD, et al. Recommendations from an international expert panel on the use of neoadjuvant (primary) systemic treatment of operable breast cancer: new perspectives 2006. Ann Oncol 2007;18(12):1927–34.
44. Arlinghaus LR, Li X, Levy M, et al. Current and future trends in magnetic resonance imaging assessments of the response of breast tumors to neoadjuvant chemotherapy. J Oncol 2010;2010. pii: 919620. 1–17.
45. Esserman L, Berry D, Cheang M, et al. Chemotherapy response and recurrence-free survival in neoadjuvant breast cancer depends on biomarker profiles: results from the I-SPY 1 TRIAL (CALGB 150007/150012; ACRIN 6657). Breast Cancer Res Treat 2011;30:3242–9.
46. McGuire K, Toro-Burguete J, Dang H, et al. MRI staging after neoadjuvant chemotherapy for breast cancer: does tumor biology affect accuracy? Ann Surg Oncol 2011;18(11):3149–54.
47. Falou O, Soliman H, Sadeghi-Naini A, et al. Diffuse optical spectroscopy evaluation of treatment response in women with locally advanced breast cancer receiving neoadjuvant chemotherapy. Transl Oncol 2012;5(4):238–46.

48. Tromberg BJ, Pogue BW, Paulsen KD, et al. Assessing the future of diffuse optical imaging technologies for breast cancer management. Med Phys 2008;35(6):2443–51.
49. Jakubowski DB, Cerussi AE, Bevilacqua F, et al. Monitoring neoadjuvant chemotherapy in breast cancer using quantitative diffuse optical spectroscopy: a case study. J Biomed Opt 2004;9(1):230–8.
50. Shah N, Gibbs J, Wolverton D, et al. Combined diffuse optical spectroscopy and contrast-enhanced magnetic resonance imaging for monitoring breast cancer neoadjuvant chemotherapy: a case study. J Biomed Opt 2005;10(5):051503.
51. Tromberg BJ, Cerussi A, Shah N, et al. Imaging in breast cancer: diffuse optics in breast cancer: detecting tumors in pre-menopausal women and monitoring neoadjuvant chemotherapy. Breast Cancer Res 2005;7(6):279–85.
52. Choe R, Corlu A, Lee K, et al. Diffuse optical tomography of breast cancer during neoadjuvant chemotherapy: a case study with comparison to MRI. Med Phys 2005;32:1128–39.
53. Zhou C, Choe R, Shah N, et al. Diffuse optical monitoring of blood flow and oxygenation in human breast cancer during early stages of neoadjuvant chemotherapy. J Biomed Opt 2007;12:051903.
54. Zhu Q, Tannenbaum S, Hegde P, et al. Noninvasive monitoring of breast cancer during neoadjuvant chemotherapy using optical tomography with ultrasound localization. Neoplasia 2008;10(10):1028–40.
55. Cerussi A, Hsiang D, Shah N, et al. Predicting response to breast cancer neoadjuvant chemotherapy using diffuse optical spectroscopy. Proc Natl Acad Sci U S A 2007;104(10):4014–9.
56. Tanamai W, Chen C, Siavoshi S, et al. Diffuse optical spectroscopy measurements of healing in breast tissue after core biopsy: case study. J Biomed Opt 2009;14(1):014024.
57. Jiang S, Pogue BW, Carpenter CM, et al. Evaluation of breast tumor response to neoadjuvant chemotherapy with tomographic diffuse optical spectroscopy: case studies of tumor region-of-interest changes. Radiology 2009;252:551–60.
58. Cerussi AE, Tanamai VW, Mehta RS, et al. Frequent optical imaging during breast cancer neoadjuvant chemotherapy reveals dynamic tumor physiology in an individual patient. Acad Radiol 2010;17(8):1031–9.
59. Soliman H, Gunasekara A, Rycroft M, et al. Functional imaging using diffuse optical spectroscopy of neoadjuvant chemotherapy response in women with locally advanced breast cancer. Clin Cancer Res 2010;16(9):2605–14.
60. Cerussi AE, Tanamai VW, Hsiang D, et al. Diffuse optical spectroscopic imaging correlates with final pathological response in breast cancer neoadjuvant chemotherapy. Philos Trans A Math Phys Eng Sci 2011;369(1955):4512–30.
61. Choe R, Durduran T. Diffuse optical monitoring of the neoadjuvant breast cancer therapy. IEEE J Sel Top Quantum Electron 2012;18(99):1367–86.
62. Enfield LC, Cantanhede G, Westbroek D, et al. Monitoring the response to primary medical therapy for breast cancer using three-dimensional time-resolved optical mammography. Technol Cancer Res Treat 2011;10(6):533–47.
63. Pakalniskis MG, Wells WA, Schwab MC, et al. Tumor angiogenesis change estimated by using diffuse optical spectroscopic tomography: demonstrated correlation in women undergoing neoadjuvant chemotherapy for invasive breast cancer? Radiology 2011;259(2):365–74.
64. Roblyer D, Ueda S, Cerussi A, et al. Optical imaging of breast cancer oxyhemoglobin flare correlates with neoadjuvant chemotherapy response one day after starting treatment. Proc Natl Acad Sci U S A 2011;108(35):14626–31.
65. Santoro Y, Leproux A, Cerussi A, et al. Breast cancer spatial heterogeneity in near-infrared spectra and the prediction of neoadjuvant chemotherapy response. J Biomed Opt 2011;16: 097007.
66. Busch DR, Choe R, Rosen MA, et al. Optical malignancy parameters for monitoring progression of breast cancer neoadjuvant chemotherapy. Biomed Opt Express 2013;4(1):105–21.
67. Chung SH, Mehta R, Tromberg BJ, et al. Non-invasive measurement of deep tissue temperature changes caused by apoptosis during breast cancer neoadjuvant chemotherapy: a case study. J Innov Opt Health Sci 2011;4(4):361–72.
68. Durduran T, Choe R, Baker WB, et al. Diffuse optics for tissue monitoring and tomography. Rep Prog Phys 2010;73(7):076701.
69. Jacques SL, Pogue BW. Tutorial on diffuse light transport. J Biomed Opt 2008;13(4). 041302–1:19.
70. Mesquita R, Durduran T, Yu G, et al. Direct measurement of tissue blood flow and metabolism with diffuse optics. Philos Trans A Math Phys Eng Sci 2011;369(1955):4390–406.
71. Yu G. Near-infrared diffuse correlation spectroscopy in cancer diagnosis and therapy monitoring. J Biomed Opt 2012;17(1). 010901–19.
72. Yu G. Diffuse correlation spectroscopy (DCS): a diagnostic tool for assessing tissue blood flow in vascular-related diseases and therapies. Curr Med Imaging Rev 2012;8(3):194–210.
73. Cutler M. Transillumination of the breast. Ann Surg 1931;93(1):223–34.
74. Homer MJ. Breast imaging: pitfalls, controversies and some practical thoughts. Radiol Clin North Am 1985;23:459–72.
75. Watmough DJ. Transillumination of breast tissues: factors governing optimal imaging of lesions. Radiology 1983;147:89–92.

76. Sickles EA. Breast cancer detection with transillumination and mammography. Am J Roentgenol 1984;142:841–4.
77. Wallberg H, Alveryd A, Bergvall U, et al. Diaphanography in breast carcinoma. Acta Radiol Diagn 1985;26:33–44.
78. Profio AE, Navarro GA. Scientific basis of breast diaphanography. Med Phys 1989;16:60–5.
79. Pera A, Freimanis AK. The choice of radiologic procedures in the diagnosis of breast disease. Obstet Gynecol Clin North Am 1987;14(3):635–50.
80. Carlsen EN. Transillumination light scanning. Diagn Imaging 1982;4:28–34.
81. Marshall V, Williams DC, Smith KD. Diaphanography as a means of detecting breast cancer. Radiology 1984;150:339–43.
82. Monsees B, Destouet JM, Totty WG. Light scanning versus mammography in breast cancer detection. Radiology 1987;163:463–5.
83. Gisvold JJ, Brown LR, Swee RG, et al. Comparison of mammography and transillumination light scanning in the detection of breast lesions. AJR Am J Roentgenol 1986;147(1):191–4.
84. Bartrum RJ Jr, Crow HC. Transillumination light scanning to diagnose breast cancer: a feasibility study. AJR Am J Roentgenol 1984;142:409–14.
85. Alveryd A, Andersson I, Aspegren K, et al. Lights canning versus mammography for the detection of breast cancer in screening and clinical practice. A Swedish multicenter study. Cancer 1990;65(8): 1671–7.
86. Hebden J, Arridge S, Delpy D. Optical imaging in medicine: I. Experimental techniques. Phys Med Biol 1997;42:825–40.
87. Arridge SR, Hebden JC. Optical imaging in medicine: II. Modelling and reconstruction. Phys Med Biol 1997;42(5):841–53.
88. Zhu Q, Hegde PU, Ricci A, et al. Early-stage invasive breast cancers: potential role of optical tomography with us localization in assisting diagnosis. Radiology 2010;256(2):367–78.
89. Konecky SD, Choe R, Corlu A, et al. Comparison of diffuse optical tomography of human breast with whole-body and breast-only positron emission tomography. Med Phys 2008;35(2):446–55.
90. Doi K. Computer-aided diagnosis in medical imaging: historical review, current status and future potential. Comput Med Imaging Graph 2007;31(4–5):198.
91. Pichler BJ, Kolb A, Nägele T, et al. PET/MRI: paving the way for the next generation of clinical multimodality imaging applications. J Nucl Med 2010; 51(3):333–6.
92. Klose CD, Klose AD, Netz U, et al. Multiparameter classifications of optical tomographic images. J Biomed Opt 2008;13(5):050503.
93. Simick MK, Jong R, Wilson B, et al. Non-ionizing near-infrared radiation transillumination spectroscopy for breast tissue density and assessment of breast cancer risk. J Biomed Opt 2004;9(4):794–803.
94. Zhu C, Breslin TM, Harter J, et al. Model based and empirical spectral analysis for the diagnosis of breast cancer. Opt Express 2008;16(19):14961–78.
95. Song X, Pogue BW, Jiang S, et al. Automated region detection based on the contrast-to-noise ratio in near-infrared tomography. Appl Opt 2004;43(5): 1053–62.
96. Pogue BW, Davis SC, Song X, et al. Image analysis methods for diffuse optical tomography. J Biomed Opt 2006;11(3):033001 (16pp).
97. Wang JZ, Liang X, Zhang Q, et al. Automated breast cancer classification using near-infrared optical tomographic images. J Biomed Opt 2008;13: 044001 (10pp).
98. Busch DR, Guo W, Choe R, et al. Computer aided automatic detection of malignant lesions in diffuse optical mammography. Med Phys 2010;37(4): 1840–9.
99. Pogue BW, Jiang S, Dehghani H, et al. Characterization of hemoglobin, water, and NIR scattering in breast tissue: analysis of intersubject variability and menstrual cycle changes. J Biomed Opt 2004;9:541.
100. Pogue BW, Poplack SP, McBride TO, et al. Quantitative hemoglobin tomography with diffuse near-infrared spectroscopy: pilot results in the breast. Radiology 2001;218(1):261.
101. Srinivasan S, Pogue BW, Brooksby B, et al. Near-infrared characterization of breast tumors in vivo using spectrally-constrained reconstruction. Technol Cancer Res Treat 2005;4(5):513–26.
102. Azar FS, Lee K, Khamene A, et al. Standardized platform for coregistration of nonconcurrent diffuse optical and magnetic resonance breast images obtained in different geometries. J Biomed Opt 2007; 12(5):051902.
103. Ntziachristos V, Yodh AG, Schnall M, et al. Concurrent MRI and diffuse optical tomography of breast after indocyanine green enhancement. Proc Natl Acad Sci U S A 2000;97:2767–72.
104. Ntziachristos V, Yodh AG, Schnall MD, et al. MRI-guided diffuse optical spectroscopy of malignant and benign breast lesions. Neoplasia 2002;4:347–54.
105. Carpenter CM, Srinivasan S, Pogue BW, et al. Methodology development for three-dimensional MR-guided near infrared spectroscopy of breast tumors. Opt Express 2008;16(22):17903–14.
106. Pogue BW, Leblond F, Krishnaswamy V, et al. Radiologic and near-infrared/optical spectroscopic imaging: where is the synergy? AJR Am J Roentgenol 2010;195:321–32.
107. Li A, Miller EL, Kilmer ME, et al. Tomographic optical breast imaging guided by three-dimensional mammography, guided by three-dimensional mammography. Appl Opt 2003;42(25):5181–90.

108. Boverman G, Miller EL, Li A, et al. Quantitative spectroscopic diffuse optical tomography of the breast guided by imperfect a priori structural information. Phys Med Biol 2005;50(17):3941–56.
109. Zhu Q, Durduran T, Ntziachristos V, et al. Imager that combines near-infrared diffusive light and ultrasound. Opt Lett 1999;24:1050–2.
110. Holboke MJ, Tromberg BJ, Li X, et al. Three-dimensional diffuse optical mammography with ultrasound localization in a human subject. J Biomed Opt 2000;5:237–47.
111. Zhu Q, Tannenbaum S, Kurtzman SH. Optical tomography with ultrasound localization for breast cancer diagnosis and treatment monitoring. Surg Oncol Clin N Am 2007;16:307–21.
112. Freifelder R, Karp JS. Dedicated PET scanners for breast imaging. Phys Med Biol 1997;42:2453–80.
113. Freifelder R, Cardi C, Grigoras I, et al. First results of a dedicated breast PET imager, BPET, using NaI(Tl) curve plate detectors. IEEE Nucl Sci Symp Conf Rec 2001;3:1241–5.
114. Boas DA, Campbell LE, Yodh AG. Scattering and imaging with diffusing temporal field correlations. Phys Rev Lett 1995;75(9):1855–8.
115. Boas DA, Yodh AG. Spatially varying dynamical properties of turbid media probed with diffusing temporal light correlation. J Opt Soc Am A Opt Image Sci Vis 1997;14(1):192–215.
116. Durduran T, Choe R, Yu GQ, et al. Diffuse optical measurement of blood flow in breast tumors. Opt Lett 2005;30:2915–7.
117. Zhou C. In-vivo optical imaging and spectroscopy of cerebral hemodynamics [PhD thesis]. Philadelphia: University of Pennsylvania; 2007.
118. Zhou C, Yu G, Daisuke F, et al. Diffuse optical correlation tomography of cerebral blood flow during cortical spreading depression in rat brain. Opt Express 2006;14:1125–44.
119. Busch DR. Computer-aided, multi-modal, and compression diffuse optical studies of breast tissue [PhD thesis]. University of Pennsylvania; 2011.
120. Flexman M, Khalil M, Al Abdi R, et al. Digital optical tomography system for dynamic breast imaging. J Biomed Opt 2011;16:076014.
121. Al abdi R, Graber HL, Xu Y, et al. Optomechanical imaging system for breast cancer detection. J Opt Soc Am A Opt Image Sci Vis 2011;28(12):2473–93.
122. Jiang S, Pogue BW, Paulsen KD, et al. In vivo near-infrared spectral detection of pressure-induced changes in breast tissue. Opt Lett 2003;28(14):1212–4.
123. Jiang SD, Pogue BW, Laughney AM. Measurement of pressure-displacement kinetics of hemoglobin in normal breast tissue with near-infrared spectral imaging. Appl Opt 2009;48(10).
124. Xu RX, Qiang B, Mao JJ, et al. Development of a handheld near-infrared imager for dynamic characterization of in vivo biological tissue systems. Appl Opt 2007;46(30):7442–51.
125. Carp SA, Kauffman T, Fang Q, et al. Compression-induced changes in the physiological state of the breast as observed through frequency domain photon migration measurements. J Biomed Opt 2006;11(6):064016.
126. Carp SA, Selb J, Fang Q, et al. Dynamic functional and mechanical response of breast tissue to compression. Opt Express 2008;16(20):16064–78.
127. Beaney RP, Lammertsma AA, Jones T, et al. Positron emission tomography for in-vivo measurement of regional blood flow, oxygen utilisation, and blood volume in patients with breast carcinoma. Lancet 1984;1:131–4.
128. Wilson CB, Lammertsma AA, McKenzie CG, et al. Measurements of blood flow and exchanging water space in breast tumors using positron emission tomography: a rapid and noninvasive dynamic method. Cancer Res 1992;52:1592–7.
129. Dixit SS, Kim H, Comstock C, et al. Near infrared transillumination imaging of breast cancer with vasoactive inhalation contrast. Biomed Opt Express 2010;1(1):295–309.
130. Dixit SS, Kim H, Visser B, et al. Development of a transillumination infrared modality for differential vasoactive optical imaging. Appl Opt 2009;48:100949.
131. Kotz KT, Dixit SS, Gibbs AD, et al. Inspiratory contrast for in vivo optical imaging. Opt Express 2008;16(1):19–31.
132. Weissleder R, Ntziachristos V. Shedding light onto live molecular targets. Nat Med 2003;9(1):123–8.
133. Tichauer KM, Holt RW, El-Ghussein F, et al. Dual-tracer background subtraction approach for fluorescent molecular tomography. J Biomed Opt 2013;18(1):16003.
134. Akorn Inc. IC-Green™ Sterile Indocyanine Green [Drug Packaging Insert]. Version: 6-DCGN-01 2006.
135. Poellinger A. Near-infrared imaging of breast cancer using optical contrast agents. J Biophotonics 2012;5(11–12):815–26.
136. Ott P. Hepatic elimination of indocyanine green with special reference to distribution kinetics and the influence of plasma protein binding. Pharmacol Toxicol 1998;83(S2):1–48.
137. Carmeliet P, Jain RK. Angiogenesis in cancer and other diseases. Nature 2000;407:249–57.
138. Corlu A, Choe R, Durduran T, et al. Three-dimensional in vivo fluorescence diffuse optical tomography of breast cancer in humans. Opt Express 2007;15(11):6696–716.
139. Intes X, Ripoll J, Chen Y, et al. In vivo continuous-wave optical breast imaging enhanced with indocyanine green. Med Phys 2003;30(6):1039–47.

140. Alacam B, Yazici B, Intes X, et al. Pharmacokinetic-rate images of indocyanine green for breast tumors using near-infrared optical methods. Phys Med Biol 2008;53:837–59.
141. Rinneberg H, Grosenick D, Moesta KT, et al. Detection and characterization of breast tumours by time-domain scanning optical mammography. Opto-Electronics Review 2008;16(2):147–62.
142. Schneider P, Piper S, Schmitz CH, et al. Fast 3D near-infrared breast imaging using indocyanine green for detection and characterization of breast lesions. Rofo 2011;183(10):956–63.
143. Hagen A, Grosenick D, Macdonald R, et al. Late-fluorescence mammography assesses tumor capillary permeability and differentiates malignant from benign lesions. Opt Express 2009;17(19):17016–33.
144. Poellinger A, Burock S, Grosenick D, et al. Breast cancer: early- and late-fluorescence near-infrared imaging with indocyanine green—preliminary study. Radiology 2011;258(2):409.
145. Poellinger A, Persigehl T, Mahler M, et al. Near-infrared imaging of the breast using omocianine as a fluorescent dye: results of a placebo-controlled, clinical, multicenter trial. Invest Radiol 2011;46(11):697–704.
146. Sevick-Muraca E. Translation of near-infrared fluorescence imaging technologies: emerging clinical applications. Annu Rev Med 2012;63:217–31.
147. Smith RA, Saslow D, Sawyer KA, et al. American Cancer Society guidelines for breast cancer screening: update 2003. CA Cancer J Clin 2003; 53(3):141–69.
148. Grosenick D, Wabnitz H, Moesta KT, et al. Time-domain scanning optical mammography: II. Optical properties and tissue parameters of 87 carcinomas. Phys Med Biol 2005;50(11): 2451–68.
149. Grosenick D, Moesta KT, Mller M, et al. Time-domain scanning optical mammography: I. Recording and assessment of mammograms of 154 patients. Phys Med Biol 2005;50(11):2429–49.
150. Taroni P, Danesini G, Torricelli A, et al. Clinical trial of time-resolved scanning optical mammography at 4 wavelengths between 683 and 975 nm. J Biomed Opt 2004;9(3):464–73.
151. Enfield LC, Gibson AP, Hebden JC, et al. Optical tomography of breast cancer-monitoring response to primary medical therapy. Target Oncol 2009;4: 219–33.
152. Bigio IJ, Brown SG, Briggs G, et al. Diagnosis of breast cancer using elastic-scattering spectroscopy: preliminary clinical results. J Biomed Opt 2000;5:221–8.
153. Keller MD, Majumder SK, Mahadevan-Lansen A. Spatially offset Raman spectroscopy of layered soft tissues. Opt Lett 2009;34:926–8.
154. Haka AS, Volynskaya Z, Gardecki JA, et al. Diagnosing breast cancer using Raman spectroscopy: prospective analysis. J Biomed Opt 2009;14: 054023.
155. Nguyen FT, Zysk AM, Chaney EJ, et al. Intraoperative evaluation of breast tumor margins with optical coherence tomography. Cancer Res 2009;69: 8790–6.
156. Nachabé R, Evers DJ, Hendriks BH, et al. Diagnosis of breast cancer using diffuse optical spectroscopy from 500 to 1600 nm: comparison of classification methods. J Biomed Opt 2011;16:087010.
157. Wilke LG, Brown JQ, Bydlon TM, et al. Rapid noninvasive optical imaging of tissue composition in breast tumor margins. Am J Surg 2009;198:566–74.
158. Brown JQ, Bydlon TM, Richards LM, et al. Optical assessment of tumor resection margins in the breast. IEEE J Sel Top Quantum Electron 2010; 16(3):530–44.
159. Bydlon TM, Barry WT, Kennedy SA, et al. Advancing optical imaging for breast margin assessment: an analysis of excisional time, cautery, and patent blue dye on underlying sources of contrast. PLoS One 2012;7:e51418.
160. McLaughlin RA, Quirk BC, Kirk RW, et al. Imaging of breast cancer with optical coherence tomography needle probes: feasibility and initial results. IEEE J Sel Top Quantum Electron 2012; 18:1184–91.
161. Tanaka E, Choi HS, Fujii H, et al. Image-guided oncologic surgery using invisible light: completed pre-clinical development for sentinel lymph node mapping. Ann Surg Oncol 2006;13:1671–81.
162. Sevick-Muraca EM, Sharma R, Rasmussen JC, et al. Imaging of lymph flow in breast cancer patients after microdose administration of a near-infrared fluorophore: feasibility study. Radiology 2008;246(3):734–41.
163. Hutteman M, Mieog JS, van der Vorst JR, et al. Randomized, double-blind comparison of indocyanine green with or without albumin premixing for near-infrared fluorescence imaging of sentinel lymph nodes in breast cancer patients. Breast Cancer Res Treat 2011;127(1):163–70.
164. Li C, Wang LV. Photoacoustic tomography and sensing in biomedicine. Phys Med Biol 2009; 54(19):R59.
165. Oraevsky AA, Jacques SL, Tittel FK. Measurement of tissue optical properties by time-resolved detection of laser-induced transient stress. Appl Opt 1997;36(1):402–15.
166. Ermilov SA, Khamapirad T, Conjusteau A, et al. Laser optoacoustic imaging system for detection of breast cancer. J Biomed Opt 2009;14(2):024007.
167. Kruger RA, Lam RB, Reinecke DR, et al. Photoacoustic angiography of the breast. Med Phys 2010;37(11):6096.

Potential Clinical Applications of PET/Magnetic Resonance Imaging

Annemieke S. Littooij, MD[a,*], Drew A. Torigian, MD, MA[b], Thomas C. Kwee, MD, PhD[a], Bart de Keizer, MD, PhD[a,d], Abass Alavi, MD, PhD[c], Rutger A.J. Nievelstein, MD, PhD[a]

KEYWORDS

• Hybrid imaging • Magnetic resonance imaging • PET/MR imaging

OBJECTIVES

- Review potential clinical indications of hybrid PET/magnetic resonance (MR) imaging whereby simultaneous morphologic and functional imaging is expected to improve diagnostic performance.
- Discuss advantages, disadvantages, and limitations of hybrid PET/MR imaging.
- Highlight the importance of further research to assess the incremental benefit of multiparametric MR imaging with PET using different radiotracers in a variety of disease conditions.

INTRODUCTION

Recently, the first integrated PET/magnetic resonance (MR) imaging technique has been introduced in clinical practice. This new technology has potential advantages over PET/computed tomography (CT) and potential synergetic value in comparison with separate acquisition of PET and MR imaging. The major advantage consists of combining excellent anatomic information and functional MR imaging parameters with the metabolic and molecular information obtained with PET. Besides the superior soft-tissue contrast of MR imaging relative to CT, the lack of ionizing radiation is highly appealing, which is particularly important when children, young adults, or pregnant women are to be imaged. Simultaneous acquisition of MR imaging and PET data can be used to improve the accuracy of PET images and minimize the artifacts caused by motion and partial volume errors. In addition, the patient is not required to undergo separate examinations that may increase stress, costs, and potentially lead to a delay in diagnosis and staging. Of course, hybrid PET/MR imaging is not without its limitations. Attenuation correction, quantification of radiotracer uptake, and whole-body imaging with MR are still technically challenging. Moreover, the high costs associated with current PET/MR imaging may limit general acceptance of this method for clinical purposes.[1]

An integrated PET/MR imaging system for simultaneous morphologic and functional imaging carries great potential for improving diagnostic performance in oncologic, cardiovascular, neurologic, and musculoskeletal disease conditions. The first experiences and preliminary data are being reported, but little has yet been published on the incremental benefit of PET/MR imaging over PET/CT for individual clinical indications. The purpose of this review is to highlight potential clinical

[a] Department of Radiology, University Medical Center Utrecht, Heidelberglaan 100, Utrecht 3584 CX, The Netherlands; [b] Department of Radiology, Hospital of the University of Pennsylvania, 3400 Spruce Street, Philadelphia, PA 19104, USA; [c] Division of Nuclear Medicine, Hospital of the University of Pennsylvania, 3400 Spuce Street, Philadelphia, PA 19104, USA; [d] Department of Nuclear Medicine, University Medical Center Utrecht, Heidelberglaan 100, Utrecht 3584 CX, The Netherlands
* Corresponding author.
E-mail addresses: alittooij@hotmail.com; A.S.Littooij-2@umcutrecht.nl

PET Clin 8 (2013) 367–384
http://dx.doi.org/10.1016/j.cpet.2013.03.005
1556-8598/13/$ – see front matter

applications in neurologic, cardiovascular, and musculoskeletal disease conditions, with special attention to applications in oncologic imaging.

IMAGING TECHNIQUE

The introduction of avalanche photodiode PET detectors, which are not affected by strong magnetic fields, allows acquisition of PET and MR imaging data in a single scanner. At present, sequential and concurrent approaches are available. In the sequential approach, two separate examinations are integrated into one data set. The patient is transported between the modalities either in the same room with a rotating patient table or on a detachable patient table with scanners in 2 separate rooms. Sequential PET/MR imaging acquisition faces some additional challenges, such as the length of the 2 combined studies and accuracy of fusion. In the concurrent approach, data from PET and MR imaging can be acquired nearly simultaneously, which is advantageous for limiting the length of study and allowing for excellent coregistration.[2] Technical issues in both techniques are related to interference of MR surface array coils with gamma rays from PET, obtaining an appropriate MR imaging–based attenuation correction of PET data, and reproducible semiquantitative measurements of radiotracer uptake.[3,4]

Problems to be Solved

One of the technical issues of interest is related to obtaining an adequate MR imaging–based attenuation correction of PET data. In conventional PET/CT scanners, attenuation correction is derived from transformation of the CT Hounsfield units into attenuation factors at 511 keV. However, because MR imaging signal intensity is not related to radiodensity of the tissue, an MR imaging signal cannot directly be used. The main challenge in using MR data for attenuation correction of PET data is to locate bone, the major attenuating structure of the body. Bone is intrinsically not detectable with conventional MR sequences because of its low proton density.[3,4] Several approaches have been described, including anatomically based attenuation maps or automated atlas-based pattern recognition. Hoffman and colleagues[5] compared these 2 methods in 11 patients and found a better performance of automated atlas-based pattern recognition.

Furthermore, in PET/MR imaging, anatomic information for image reconstruction, partial volume correction, and motion correction needs to be performed with MR imaging, which is generally more time-consuming in comparison with CT.

In view of these basic technical differences between PET/CT and PET/MR imaging, quantification of radiotracer uptake (such as with standardized uptake value [SUV] measurement), which is especially important in oncologic applications, is another topic for further research. First clinical experiences report a high correlation between SUVs measured with PET/CT and those measured with PET/MR imaging in suspicious lesions, despite different technologies and methods of attenuation correction.[6,7] Drzezga and colleagues[7] suggest that PET/MR imaging is suitable for quantitative evaluation in longitudinal studies such as for therapy response assessment, but that comparison between different types of scan is currently unreliable.

Advanced MR Imaging Techniques that can be Combined with PET

MR imaging is based on the interaction between radio waves and hydrogen nuclei in the presence of a strong external magnetic field. In MR imaging, the image is influenced by the molecular environment in which hydrogen nuclei are located. Therefore, MR imaging can provide information such as the local chemical environment (via MR spectroscopy) or the translational motion of water molecules in tissues (via diffusion-weighted [DW] imaging) (**Table 1**).[1,8]

Special PET Radiotracers

Molecular imaging with PET can be performed with other radiotracers beyond ^{18}F-2-fluorodeoxyglucose (FDG). A major strength of PET is that important biomolecules of interest can be radiolabeled with positron-emitting isotopes for potential study and measurement in vivo (**Table 2**).[1]

NEUROLOGIC DISEASE

Intracranial Masses

Conventional, structural MR imaging is the first-line method for assessing brain tumors, although there are still some limitations. First, it may be difficult to ascertain the full extent of infiltrating glioma along white matter tracts, which may extend beyond the regions of signal change present on MR images. Second, contrast enhancement appears to be suboptimal for defining tumor grade and guiding biopsies. Third, differentiation between residual/recurrent tumor and post-therapy changes is often limited on conventional MR imaging.[9]

Metabolic imaging with PET can be of significant additive value through use of amino acid radiotracers such as ^{18}F-fluorethyl-L-tyrosine (FET),

Table 1
Summary of available advanced MR imaging techniques

MR Imaging Method	Characteristics	Potential Applications
Diffusion-weighted imaging	Measures diffusivity of water molecules	Detection of acute ischemia Staging, response prediction, and treatment monitoring in oncology Detection of inflammatory disease activity, eg, inflammatory bowel disease, cystic fibrosis
Diffusion tensor imaging	Measures directionality of water diffusion	Assessment of white matter tracts Assessment of peripheral nerves
Magnetic resonance spectroscopy	Measures chemical composition	Characterization of lesions
Functional magnetic resonance imaging	Sensitive either to blood oxygenation level dependent (BOLD) change sequences or to perfusion changes via arterial spin labeling contrast	Characterization of functional anatomy in the brain
Magnetic resonance elastography	Quantitative assessment of shear modulus of tissues	Assessment of hepatic fibrosis Assessment of tumors

Table 2
Summary of molecular imaging targets and possible PET radiotracers

Biological Process/Molecular Target of Interest	PET Radiotracer
Glucose metabolism	^{18}F-2-Fluoro-2-deoxy-D-glucose (FDG)
Cell proliferation	^{11}C-Thymidine 3′-Deoxy-3′-^{18}F-fluorothymidine (FLT)
Choline kinase activity-synthesis of membrane phospholipids	^{11}C-Choline ^{18}F-Fluorocholine
Amino acid metabolism	L-[methyl-^{11}C]Methionine (MET) *O*-(2-^{18}F-Fluoroethyl)-L-tyrosine (FET) ^{18}F-6-Fluorodihydroxyphemylalanine (FDOPA)
Hypoxia	^{18}F-Fluoromisonidazole (FMISO) ^{64}Cu(II)-Diacetyl-bis(N4-methylthiosemicarbazone) (^{64}Cu-ATSM) ^{18}F-2-(2-Nitro-^{1}H-imidazol-1-yl)-N-(2,2,3,3,3-pentafluoropropyl)-acetamide (^{18}F-EF5)
Angiogenesis	^{18}F-Galacto-arginine-glycine-aspartate (RGD)
Apoptosis	4-^{18}F-Fluorobenzoyl-annexin V
Myocardial oxidative metabolism	^{11}C-Acetate
Myocardial fatty acid metabolism	^{11}C-Palmitate
Blood flow	^{13}N-Ammonia ^{15}O-Water
Myocardial perfusion	^{82}Rb
Bone metabolism/calcification	^{18}F-Sodium fluoride (^{18}F-NaF)
Somatostatin receptors	^{68}Ga-DOTA-Tyr^{3}-Thr^{8}-octreotide (^{68}Ga-DOTATATE) ^{68}Ga-DOTA-1-Nal^{3}-octreotide(^{68}Ga-DOTANOC) ^{68}Ga-DOTA-Phe^{1}-Tyr^{3}-octreotide (DOTATOC)
Estrogen receptors	16α-^{18}F-fluoroestradiol-17β (FES)
Catecholamine analogs	^{11}C-Hydroxyephedrine ^{124}I-Metaiodobenzylguanidine (^{124}I-MIBG)

and ^{11}C-L-methionine (MET). In primary diagnosis, additional information provided by such studies can improve biopsy targeting in heterogeneous processes and improve the determination of tumor extent.[10] After treatment, amino acid PET imaging can help to delineate post-therapy changes from tumor recurrence.[11]

Advanced functional MR imaging techniques, such as proton MR spectroscopy, perfusion MR imaging, DW imaging, and diffusion tensor (DT) imaging can add valuable information as well. MR spectroscopy enables assessment of the chemical composition of tissue. DW imaging can be applied to detect, characterize, and monitor changes in brain tumors following treatment. DT imaging provides additional information on white matter integrity and fiber tracts, and can be particularly useful for pretreatment planning by localizing major fiber tracts to decrease the chance of injury to normal tissues. Furthermore, functional MR imaging could influence neurosurgical intervention by identifying eloquent brain areas close to the tumor.[11] Thus, the combination of PET and MR imaging potentially increases the diagnostic accuracy in comparison with single modalities.

Recent studies showed that structural, functional, and molecular imaging of patients with brain tumors is feasible with diagnostic image quality using simultaneous PET/MR imaging.[9,12,13] Besides its potential additional value for improved diagnosis, integrated PET/MR imaging may be beneficial for target volume definition in individualized radiotherapy planning for brain lesions.[14]

Seizure Foci

PET/MR imaging is a promising technique for presurgical evaluation of medically refractory epilepsy. Salamon and colleagues[15] reported that multimodality presurgical evaluation including PET/MR imaging coregistration enhances noninvasive identification of subtle cortical dysplasia, with subsequent successful surgical treatment.

Neurodegenerative Diseases

FDG-PET is an established technique in demonstrating regional functional impairment in neurodegenerative diseases. For example, a reduction in cerebral glucose metabolism in neocortical association areas is found in Alzheimer dementia. Impairment of this glucose metabolism may be seen before clinical symptoms are apparent.[16] Early diagnosis of dementia and cognitive impairment has become more clinically relevant since potential treatment to decelerate Alzheimer disease has recently been introduced.[17] Kawachi and colleagues[18] found that in very mild Alzheimer dementia, both MR imaging and FDG-PET showed a high diagnostic accuracy, and suggested a potential benefit from complementary information of structural and functional images with hybrid PET/MR imaging.

Glucose Metabolism

Cho and colleagues[19,20] showed in several publications the evolving possibilities of exploring the detailed structure and function of substructures of the brain that are important in human behavior and memory. These investigators were able to measure glucose metabolism in hippocampal substructures by sequential FDG-PET and 7.0-T MR imaging, and demonstrated that measurement of glucose metabolism in individual thalamic nuclei is feasible. Moreover, they were able to visualize individual raphe nucleus groups within the brainstem and quantify their glucose metabolism, which in the past were only visible through in vitro histologic studies.

CARDIOVASCULAR DISEASE

PET/MR imaging has potential for a wide range of clinical applications in cardiovascular disease conditions such as myocardial infarction, cardiomyopathy, myocarditis, atherosclerosis, vasculitis, and cardiac/pericardiac tumors. Besides providing a wide array of available sequences, MR imaging could be useful in improving the image quality of PET by providing kinetic information on breathing and cardiac activity.

Diagnosis of Coronary Artery Disease

In coronary artery disease (CAD), it is important to assess the presence of significant coronary artery stenoses as well as to demonstrate their hemodynamic relevance by means of myocardial perfusion imaging. Two well-established nuclear medicine techniques are available for myocardial perfusion imaging: single-photon emission CT and PET. Available evidence indicates that myocardial perfusion imaging with PET provides the most sensitive noninvasive method for diagnosing obstructive CAD.[21,22] The role of MR perfusion imaging in the detection of CAD is still not fully elucidated.[23] MR imaging allows for characterization of the morphology of atherosclerotic plaques. Despite the small size of the coronary artery walls, a reported study indicated the feasibility of visualization of increased wall thickness in patients with atherosclerosis using 3-dimensional (3D) black blood sequences.[24]

Myocardial infarction and sudden cardiac death result from rupture of atherosclerotic plaques.

Before rupture, these vulnerable plaques may not be associated with significant flow limitation.[25] Identification of these plaques could be a new application for hybrid PET/MR imaging, as it can simultaneously provide information about vascular wall thickness, wall inflammation, plaque vulnerability, and degree of luminal narrowing.[26]

Assessment of Heart Failure

Ischemic myocardium that is dysfunctional but viable has the potential to recover after revascularization. Although there are limited data on the combined use of PET and MR imaging in the assessment of myocardial viability, potential additional value lies in accurate classification of ischemic segments as clinically viable or nonviable.[27,28]

Several PET radiotracers, such as the catecholamine analogue ^{11}C-hydroxyephedrine, can be used to visualize defects in cardiac innervation caused by various conditions such as CAD, heart failure, and arrhythmogenic disorders. A hybrid PET/MR imaging study could provide important information in patients with heart failure by combined assessment of the cardiac innervation defects together with left ventricular function by means of MR imaging. Bengel and colleagues[29] showed that ^{11}C-hydroxyephedrine PET with separate acquisition of structural and wall motion imaging by MR can be useful in delineating regional reinnervation and control mechanisms in cardiac transplantation or dilated cardiomyopathy.

MUSCULOSKELETAL DISEASE

True hybrid PET/MR imaging might present a milestone of diagnostic assessment in a wide array of musculoskeletal applications (**Fig. 1**) because MR imaging provides excellent soft-tissue contrast, which is especially relevant in the musculoskeletal system.

For example, FDG-PET can assess the metabolic activity in synovitis and can measure disease activity in rheumatoid arthritis. In 2011, Miese and colleagues[30] published a case of hybrid PET/MR imaging of the hand in early rheumatoid arthritis, and concluded that PET/MR imaging is technically feasible and is a potential tool for the study of different aspects of inflammatory arthritis.

Nawaz and colleagues[31] tested the diagnostic performance of FDG-PET and MR imaging in assessing osteomyelitis in the diabetic foot, and demonstrated that FDG-PET and MR imaging are complementary for the evaluation of osteomyelitis and Charcot neuropathy in such feet. For the diagnosis of osteomyelitis, FDG-PET had sensitivity and specificity of 81% and 93%, respectively, compared with 91% and 78%, respectively, for MR imaging.

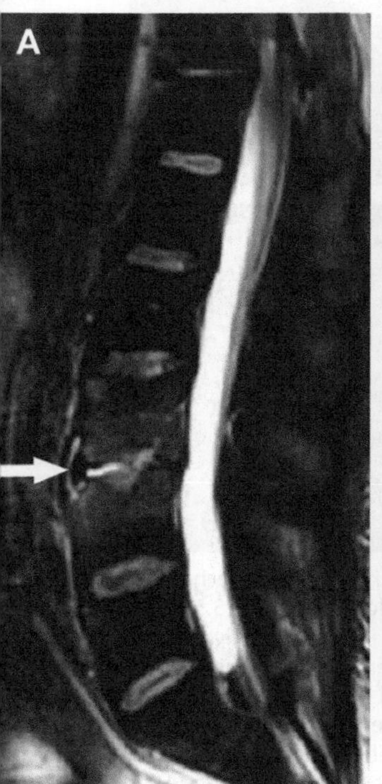

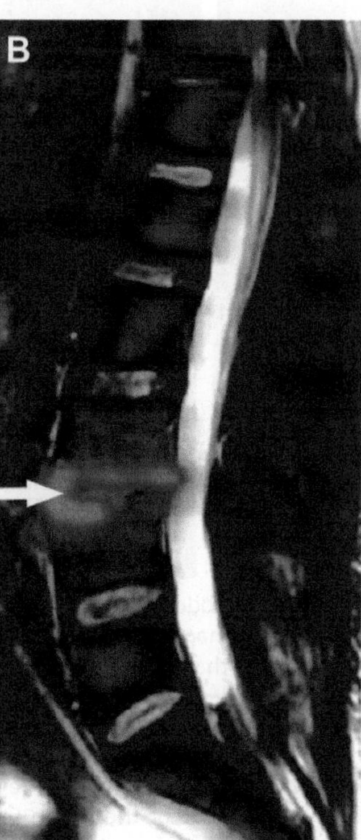

Fig. 1. A 46-year-old man with recent onset of intractable back pain, fever, and rigors. (*A*) Sagittal fat-suppressed T2-weighted image through the lumbar spine shows decreased intervertebral disc height, increased high signal-intensity fluid within disc space, and increased signal intensity within subjacent vertebral endplates at the L3-L4 level (*arrow*). (*B*) Sagittal fused PET/MR image at the same level demonstrates avid FDG uptake within the L3-L4 intervertebral disc space and surrounding vertebral endplates (*arrow*). These findings are diagnostic for discitis/osteomyelitis.

Warmann and colleagues[32] studied FDG-PET/CT and MR imaging in 6 children treated for osteomyelitis. PET/CT was superior to MR imaging in distinguishing between infection and reparative activity after acute osteomyelitis. Hybrid PET/MR imaging may become a future alternative for this young population.

ONCOLOGIC DISEASE

Staging in oncology using the standardized TNM cancer staging system, forms the basis for appropriate treatment planning and determination of individual prognosis. Imaging plays a key role in the evaluation of the local tumor extent (T), detection of locoregional lymph nodes (N), and detection of distant metastases (M). The recently introduced integrated whole-body PET/MR imaging can compete with PET/CT in oncologic imaging, particularly for indications that require superior soft-tissue contrast, such as tumors in the head and neck region, abdominal/pelvic region (**Fig. 2**), and in soft tissues, or for assessment of systemic diseases such as lymphomas. In comparison with PET/CT, a fully integrated PET/MR imaging system allows for near simultaneous acquisition of metabolic, functional, and anatomic information, minimizing mismatch. Another advantage of PET/MR imaging could lie in additional functional information, including that from DW imaging, being obtained. This additional information may improve detection and characterization of tumors and their spatial extent, which may influence biopsy and pretreatment planning.[33,34] Furthermore, DW imaging could play a role in early response assessment by detecting improvement of restricted diffusion before morphologic changes become apparent.[34] An advantage of DW imaging over FDG-PET is its superior ability in evaluating the urinary tract, where normal FDG accumulation may obscure pathologic appearance. However, DW imaging shows impeded diffusion in some normal structures, and apparent diffusion coefficient (ADC) measurements of benign and malignant lesions may overlap, leading to nonspecificity.[34] Therefore, FDG-PET and MR imaging (including DW imaging) may compensate for their weaknesses such that the combination may outperform either one of them alone.

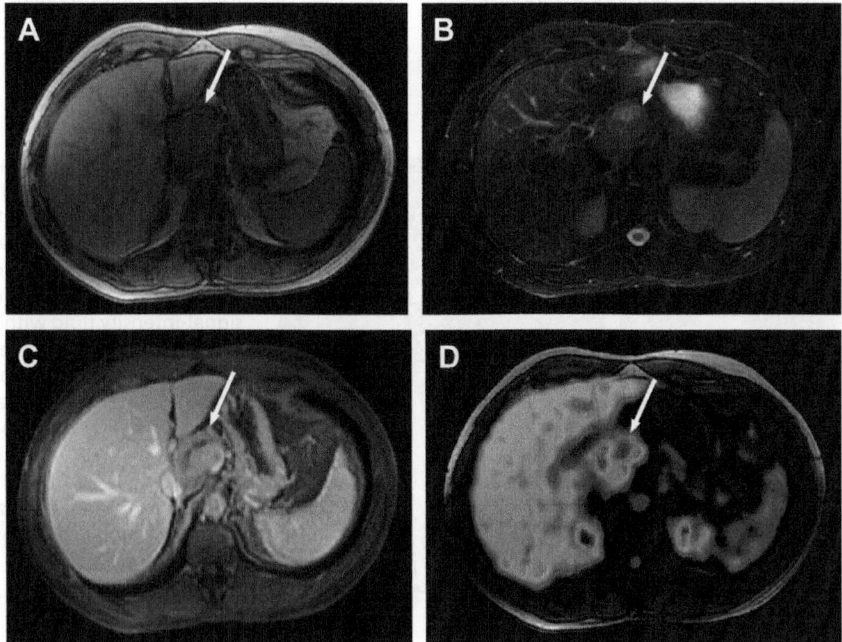

Fig. 2. A 49-year-old man undergoing evaluation of abdominal mass identified on prior echocardiography. (*A*) Axial opposed-phase T1-weighted gradient-echo MR image through the abdomen shows a 5.5 × 4.9-cm retroperitoneal mass (*arrow*) in the gastrohepatic ligament with intermediate signal intensity relative to muscle. (*B*) Axial fat-suppressed T2-weighted image at the same level demonstrates heterogeneously increased signal intensity of the mass (*arrow*) relative to muscle, located just anterior to the flow void of the inferior vena cava. (*C*) Axial delayed-phase postcontrast fat-suppressed T1-weighted image at the same level reveals heterogeneous enhancement of the mass (*arrow*). (*D*) Axial fused PET/MR image at the same level shows heterogeneous FDG uptake within the mass (*arrow*). Surgical resection was performed; the lesion was due to high-grade retroperitoneal leiomyosarcoma.

This section addresses potential indications for PET/MR imaging, classified according to tumor type (T-staging).

Head and Neck Cancer

Accurate staging of tumor extent and regional lymph node involvement is usually performed by morphologic imaging with MR imaging. There is increasing evidence that additional metabolic information using FDG-PET significantly enhances the diagnostic accuracy in staging, restaging, and assessment of response to therapy.[35]

Boss and colleagues[36] prospectively studied 8 patients with head and neck malignancies with simultaneous PET/MR imaging after FDG-PET/CT, and demonstrated superior tumor delineation and good correlation between the metabolic ratios using PET/MR imaging and PET/CT. Platzek and colleagues[6] studied 20 patients with squamous cell carcinoma of the head and neck, and demonstrated that PET/MR imaging is feasible without impairment of PET or MR imaging image quality. In a prospective study, 48 patients with head and neck cancer underwent MR imaging and FDG-PET scans with a reported sensitivity for T-staging of 100% for post hoc fused PET/MR images, compared with 98% for MR imaging alone.[37] Huang and colleagues[38] evaluated the diagnostic value of fused PET/MR imaging, PET/CT, MR imaging, and CT in assessing surrounding tissue invasion of advanced buccal squamous cell carcinoma in 17 patients. Fused PET/MR imaging appeared to be more reliable for local invasion assessment and tumor size delineation in advanced buccal squamous cell carcinoma.

Thyroid Cancer

Patients with differentiated thyroid carcinoma will undergo radioiodine therapy after initial thyroidectomy for ablation of remnant thyroid tissue and treatment of possible lymph node metastases. Pretherapeutic dosimetry with ^{124}I-PET can be used to estimate the individual dose of ^{131}I. At present, CT is used to assess lesion volume, which is necessary for calculation of this dose. Unfortunately, often no corresponding morphologic abnormality can be detected, as CT needs to be performed without intravenous contrast to avoid iodine exposure. Nagarajah and colleagues[39] prospectively compared ^{124}I-PET/CT with software coregistered ^{124}I-PET/MR imaging for the diagnosis and dosimetry of thyroid remnant tissue and lymph node metastasis in 33 patients with differentiated thyroid carcinoma. One hundred six lesions were detected with PET. In total, 23 lesions were not discernible with CT but were visible on MR imaging, 15 of which were smaller than 10 mm. Recalculation of dosimetry based on MR imaging findings for these small lesions would have changed therapy in 5 patients. It was concluded that PET/MR imaging enhances diagnostic certainty for lesions smaller than 10 mm and improves pretherapeutic lesion dosimetry in differentiated thyroid carcinoma.[39]

Pulmonary Tumors

Recently the first prospective study on pulmonary lesion assessment reported similar lesion characterization and tumor stage based on FDG-PET/CT and PET/MR images in 7 of 10 patients.[40] The investigators indicated a potential superiority of PET/MR imaging in determining chest wall and mediastinal infiltration. The superior role of MR imaging in assessing brachial plexus involvement in superior sulcus tumors has already been shown.[41] Therefore, PET/MR imaging is a promising tool for initial staging of superior sulcus tumors.

Breast Cancer

For the detection of breast carcinoma, breast MR imaging has proved to be a sensitive tool but has limited specificity. A prospective study of 36 patients suggested a significant increase in specificity from 53% to 97% with the addition of prone FDG-PET for the detection of malignant breast lesions.[42] However, Heusner and colleagues[43] demonstrated in a prospective study on 27 patients a minimal improvement of specificity from 60% to 73%, and concluded that FDG-PET cannot be recommended as an adjunct to breast MR imaging because in their group of patients, only surgical treatment in 1 patient would have changed. The potential additional value of PET in the initial assessment of breast cancer could lie in the reported relevant prognostic information of SUV measurements in patients who are candidates for breast-conserving therapy.[44]

Abdominopelvic Tumors

Hepatocellular carcinoma

For the detection of hepatocellular carcinoma, FDG-PET generally has limited sensitivity. Buchbender and colleagues[45] reported that when compared with PET/CT, hybrid PET/MR imaging improves therapeutic response assessment and early diagnosis of tumor recurrence in patients treated with ^{90}Y-loaded particles.

Malignant pheochromocytoma

In malignant pheochromocytoma, tumor dosimetry with ^{124}I-metaiodobenzylguanidine (MIBG)-PET is performed for dose calculation in treatment planning with ^{131}I-MIBG. Recently the first case report of hybrid ^{124}I-MIBG PET/MR imaging in pretreatment dosimetry of malignant pheochromocytoma has been published. The investigators reported a more accurate volumetry of tumor than with ^{124}I-MIBG PET/CT, with a subsequent reduction of dose in the surrounding tissues.[46]

Pancreatic cancer

Patients with pancreatic cancer generally have a poor prognosis, with a 5-year survival rate of less than 5%.[47] As surgery is the only treatment that can offer potential cure, determination of resectability is the principal goal of staging assessment. In most institutions staging is performed using cross-sectional imaging, with good diagnostic performances reported. For example, Birchard and colleagues[47] reported 97.7% sensitivity and 85.1% specificity for dynamic contrast-enhanced 3D MR imaging in the detection of pancreatic cancer. Tatsumi and colleagues[48] retrospectively compared FDG-PET/CT with fused PET/MR imaging in 47 patients with suspected or known pancreatic cancer, and reported significantly higher confidence scores of tumor visibility on T1-weighted MR imaging than with CT. The diagnostic accuracy of PET/T1-weighted MR imaging (93%) was better than that of PET/CT (88.4%), though nonsignificant.

Epelbaum and colleagues[49] recently demonstrated that dynamic contrast-enhanced FDG-PET/CT in newly diagnosed pancreatic cancer correlated with aggressiveness of disease. Quantitative FDG influx was the most significant variable for overall survival in patients with localized disease, whether resectable or not.

Therefore, combining prognostic information from PET with morphologic information about tumor resectability from MR imaging may provide the optimal staging method for pancreatic cancer.

Gynecologic tumors

Nakajo and colleagues[50] retrospectively compared the diagnostic performance of FDG-PET/CT with fused PET/MR imaging in 31 patients with gynecologic malignancies, and concluded that PET/T2-weighted images are superior for the detection and localization of uterine and ovarian cancer.

For staging purposes, MR imaging provides the best visualization of the primary tumor in gynecologic malignancies, whereas FDG-PET is as good as, or better, for assessing nodal involvement and distant metastases (**Fig. 3**).[50–52] Combined

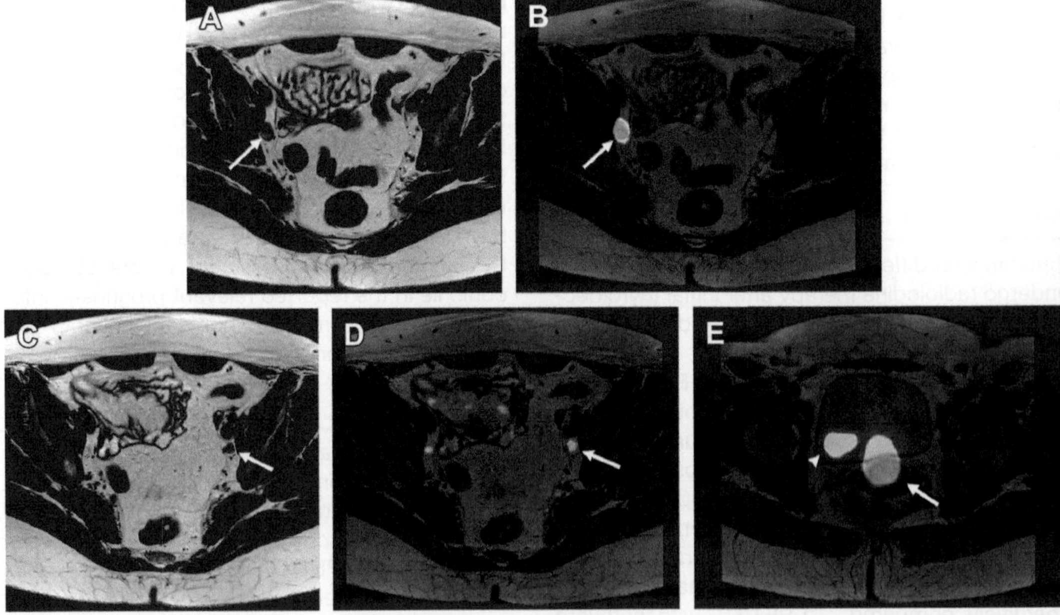

Fig. 3. A 52-year-old-woman undergoing staging for cervical carcinoma. (*A*) Axial T2-weighted image shows an enlarged right external iliac lymph node (*arrow*). (*B*) Axial fused PET/MR image at the same level demonstrates avid FDG uptake within this lymph node (*arrow*). (*C*) Axial T2-weighted image shows a round, but not enlarged left external iliac lymph node (*arrow*). (*D*) Axial fused PET/MR image at the same level reveals avid FDG uptake within this lymph node (*arrow*). (*E*) Axial fused PET/MR image demonstrates mismatch of the avid FDG uptake of the primary tumor (*arrow*) and the anatomic substrate on MR imaging, owing to a different amount of bladder filling. Intense FDG activity is noted in the bladder (*arrowhead*).

PET/MR imaging may provide a 1-step staging method with superior diagnostic accuracy.

Endometrial cancer

It is essential to perform appropriate patient selection for primary lymphadenectomy at the time of hysterectomy. In patients with endometrial cancer, histologic tumor grade and depth of myometrial invasion strongly correlate with the presence of lymph node metastasis and patient survival. The accuracy of MR imaging for the assessment of myometrial invasion has been reported to be about 91%.[53] Park and colleagues[54] reported no significant superiority of FDG-PET/CT over MR imaging in staging endometrial cancer, although the sensitivity for lymph node involvement was 46.2% for MR imaging and 69.2% for PET/CT. Combination of PET/MR imaging could improve patient selection for primary lymphadenectomy, by allowing for assessment of myometrial invasion with MR imaging and lymph node involvement with PET.

Colorectal cancer

A retrospective study in a small cohort of 23 patients found no additional value of software-based PET/MR imaging fusion when compared with conventional investigations with MR imaging, CT, and chest radiography in the staging of patients with rectal carcinoma.[55]

Brændengen and colleagues[56] prospectively explored whether imaging with FDG-PET/CT provides additional information beyond that provided by MR imaging in delineation of gross tumor volume for radiation treatment planning of patients with locally advanced rectal cancer. The investigators concluded that PET/CT adds important information to standard delineation procedures, although the clinical significance is not known. New lesions were seen in 15% of patients, potentially changing treatment planning.

Prostate cancer

The clinical behavior of primary prostate cancer ranges from clinically indolent to aggressive, with an increased likelihood of local tissue invasion and early distant metastatic disease. It is essential to identify more aggressive disease to reduce morbidity and treatment costs in patients with indolent disease. Biopsy-based diagnosis is hampered by sampling error. FDG-PET has limited sensitivity for prostate cancer, because of low glucose uptake in early prostate cancer and artifacts created by high bladder radiotracer concentration. ^{11}C-Choline PET/CT and MR imaging with DW imaging are promising tools for the detection and characterization of lesions.[57] Park and colleagues[57] assessed the performance of post hoc PET/MR imaging fusion based on ^{11}C-choline PET/CT and ADC maps in 17 patients for the identification of primary prostate cancer, concluding that it is feasible and may improve identification of significant (Gleason score $\geq 3 + 4$) primary prostate cancer. However, another recent study found limited additional value of ^{11}C-choline PET/CT to T2-weighted MR images in the localization of intraprostatic tumor nodules.[58] Further studies are needed to reveal the additional value of ^{11}C-choline PET in combination with MR imaging.

Lymphoma

Current guidelines encourage the use of FDG-PET in staging and response assessment of FDG-avid lymphomas (Hodgkin lymphoma and diffuse large B-cell lymphoma).[59,60] Whole-body MR imaging is of high research interest and has promising results, with reported 94% concordance with the findings on FDG-PET/CT in the staging of lymphoma patients.[61] First experiences reported by Buchbender and colleagues[62] showed a good concordance for PET/MR imaging with findings on PET/CT. For potentially curable and young patients, the lack of radiation exposure of MR imaging makes PET/MR imaging an attractive alternative for the purposes of staging, response assessment, and restaging.

Sarcoma

Tateishi and colleagues[63] performed a retrospective analysis on 117 patients with bone and soft-tissue sarcomas, and concluded that the combination of FDG-PET/CT and conventional imaging (MR imaging of the primary site, chest radiography, whole-body CT, or bone scintigraphy) is the best preoperative staging method because of its significantly higher diagnostic accuracy, predominantly attributable to increased accuracy with N- and M-staging. Hybrid PET/MR imaging may offer optimizing TNM staging capability in a single session. T-staging, in particular, will primarily benefit from MR imaging, whereas N-staging will primarily benefit from FDG-PET, and M-staging will likely benefit from the combination of both.

N-STAGING

Several studies reported an increase in the diagnostic performance of post hoc fusion PET/MR imaging over that of FDG-PET/CT in the detection of local lymph node involvement in several tumor entities (head and neck,[37] pulmonary,[64] cervix[65]). However, when compared with histopathology as a reference standard, a significant number of pathologically proven lymph node metastases were not detected with PET/MR imaging, as reported by 2 studies.[37,65] Possible improvement of diagnostic accuracy in N-staging could be achieved by combining PET with functional MR imaging techniques that may increase lymph node characterization, such as DW imaging and/or ultrasmall superparamagnetic iron oxide (USPIO)-enhanced MR imaging. The ability of USPIO-enhanced MR imaging to identify metastatic deposits in lymph nodes depends on the uptake of USPIO by macrophages in normal lymph nodes and the nonuptake of USPIO by metastatic tumor deposits.[66] A meta-analysis revealed that USPIO-enhanced MR imaging offers better diagnostic performance than conventional MR imaging for the detection of lymph node metastases in different body regions.[66]

M-STAGING

Hepatic Metastasis

Liver metastases are common in various malignancies, and define a higher stage that is generally associated with a shorter survival. Accurate, sensitive detection is important in providing adequate treatment. Donati and colleagues[67] retrospectively compared the accuracy of lesion detection and diagnostic confidence between FDG-PET/CT, contrast-enhanced MR imaging, and post hoc fused PET/MR imaging in 37 patients. In this study, MR imaging and PET/MR imaging demonstrated higher sensitivity than PET/CT. PET/MR imaging yielded a nonsignificant higher sensitivity and increased diagnostic confidence in comparison with MR imaging alone. A retrospective analysis in 24 patients with histologically proven liver metastases from colorectal carcinoma compared CT, MR imaging, FDG-PET, and post hoc fused PET/CT and PET/MR imaging.[68] This study demonstrated a higher sensitivity for PET/MR imaging (98%) than with PET/CT (84%) and MR imaging (80%). Schreiter and colleagues[69] showed superiority of retrospectively fused PET/MR imaging over multiphase contrast-enhanced ^{68}Ga-DOTA-Phe^{1}-Tyr^{3}-octreotide PET/CT and MR imaging alone for the detection of hepatic neuroendocrine tumor metastases. In summary, it seems that MR imaging compensates more than CT for the drawbacks of PET in liver evaluation (**Fig. 4**).

Cerebral Metastasis

In general, patients with cerebral metastasis are known to have a relatively short survival. It is therefore essential to detect small lesions in providing adequate treatment. In a prospective trial to detect brain metastases in operable patients with non-small cell lung cancer, MR imaging detected a significantly greater number and smaller size of metastases compared with CT.[70] However, a prospective study in 32 patients diagnosed with solid tumors found that contrast-enhanced T1-weighted MR images of the brain embedded in a whole-body MR imaging protocol is less sensitive for detection of small (<5 mm) metastases than is dedicated brain MR imaging (27 vs 40 lesions).[71] Another prospective study compared the diagnostic accuracy of FDG-PET/CT and whole-body MR imaging for M-staging in 41 patients. Nine cerebral metastases were diagnosed with whole-body MR imaging (using contrast-enhanced T1-weighted and T2-weighted MR imaging of the brain) that were not demonstrated with PET/CT.[72] PET/MR imaging is expected to have an incremental value above PET/CT in assessing brain metastases during TNM staging, as FDG-PET does not compensate for the shortcomings of CT, given the high uptake of gray matter by FDG (**Fig. 5**).

Bone Marrow Metastasis

Accurate detection of bone marrow metastasis in staging and restaging is vital in assessing

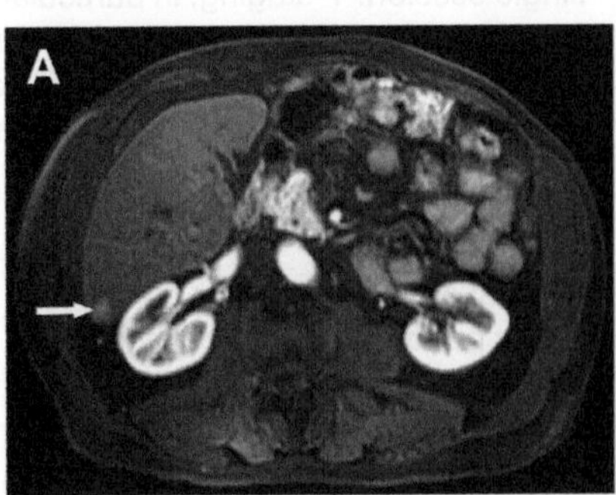

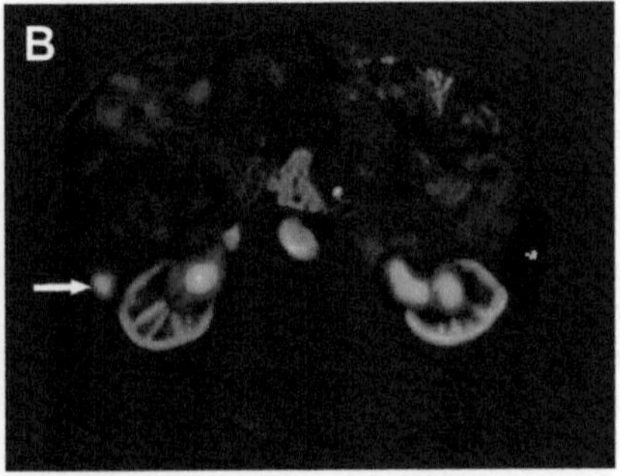

Fig. 4. A 71-year-old man with neck melanoma undergoing restaging evaluation following wide local excision. (*A*) Axial arterial-phase postcontrast fat-suppressed T1-weighted image through the abdomen shows a 1.3 × 1.1-cm homogeneously enhancing lesion (*arrow*) in the posterior inferior right hepatic lobe. (*B*) Axial fused PET/MR image at the same level reveals avid FDG uptake within lesion (*arrow*). Surgical resection was performed; the lesion was due to melanoma metastasis.

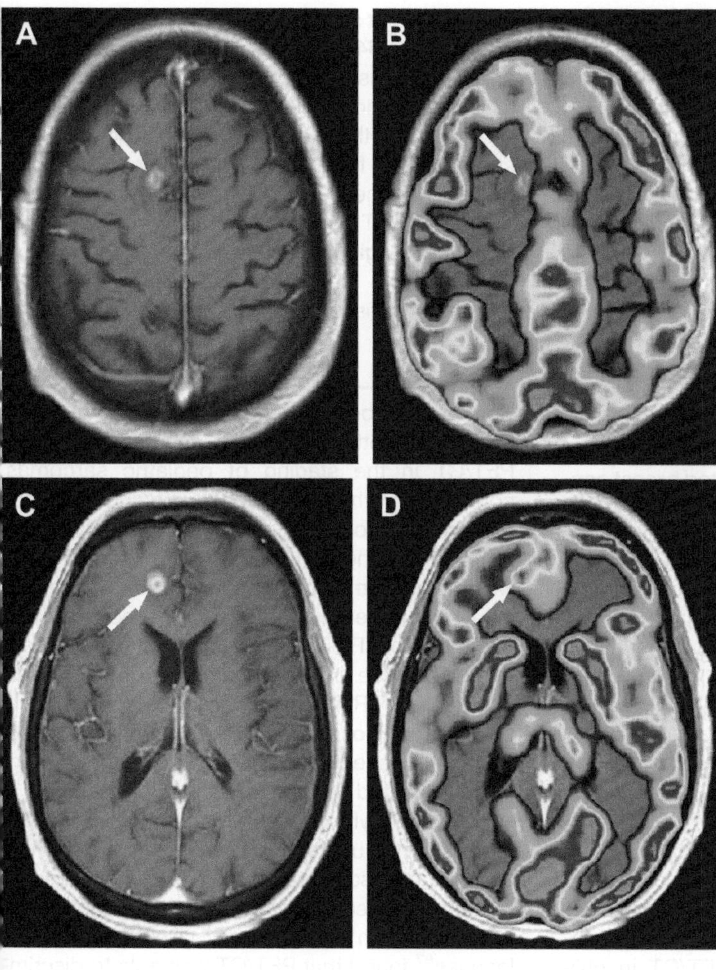

Fig. 5. A 59-year-old man with metastatic melanoma undergoing restaging evaluation. (*A*) Axial delayed-phase postcontrast T1-weighted image through the superior cerebrum shows a 1-cm enhancing lesion (*arrow*) in the right frontal lobe at the gray-white matter junction. (*B*) Axial fused PET/MR image at the same level demonstrates lack of FDG uptake within this lesion (*arrow*). (*C*) Axial delayed-phase postcontrast T1-weighted image through the midcerebrum shows a 1-cm enhancing lesion (*arrow*) in the right frontal lobe at the gray-white matter junction. (*D*) Axial fused PET/MR image at the same level reveals avid FDG uptake within this lesion (*arrow*). These findings are in keeping with melanoma metastases to brain, and were subsequently treated with gamma-knife therapy.

therapeutic options and prognosticating patients' outcomes. Several recent meta-analyses have compared the diagnostic performances of the different modalities for the detection of bone marrow metastasis in patients with a diverse set of primary tumor types. The broadest one has been provided by Yang and colleagues,[73] comparing FDG-PET, MR imaging, CT, and bone scintigraphy in more than 15,000 patients. This analysis demonstrated that FDG-PET, FDG-PET/CT, and MR imaging were significantly more accurate than bone scintigraphy and CT. Primary tumor type also affects the diagnostic accuracy of PET and bone scintigraphy.[73] For example, bone scintigraphy is known to be of limited value in detecting osteolytic lesions, whereas FDG-PET can identify bone marrow metastasis at an earlier stage by detecting increased glycolytic activity in tumor cells, although false-positive results resulting from FDG uptake in metabolically active processes such as infection or noninfectious inflammation do occur. Qu and colleagues[74] performed a meta-analysis in patients with lung cancer, and demonstrated a significantly better performance of PET/CT in comparison with MR imaging. Liu and colleagues[75] showed with their meta-analysis that MR imaging yields a better diagnostic accuracy than PET in patients with breast cancer. For imaging assessment of osseous lesions, hybrid PET/MR imaging may exceed the performance of PET/CT or MR imaging alone.

Pulmonary Metastasis

Despite considerable improvements in MR imaging sequences for assessment of the lung, CT is still superior to MR imaging for this purpose, especially in the detection of small lung nodules. Prospective studies demonstrated superiority of FDG-PET/CT over MR imaging for the assessment of pulmonary metastasis.[72,76] The better performance of PET/CT is based on CT rather than

PET. Liu and colleagues[77] performed a pilot study in 9 patients with renal cell carcinoma. In this series, all lesions larger than 7 mm were detected with MR imaging, including DW imaging. In conclusion, MR imaging shows some potential but is less sensitive than CT in detecting small pulmonary nodules. For this reason, additional CT of the chest remains necessary in certain indications.

SUSPECTED RECURRENCE

A first prospective study on the additional value of PET/MR imaging in the assessment of local tumor recurrence in 15 patients with head and neck malignancies demonstrated a sensitivity of 92% for PET/MR imaging, compared with 67% for MR imaging alone.[37] In the case of suspected breast cancer recurrence, a comparative study in 32 patients demonstrated that MR imaging and FDG-PET carry similar diagnostic accuracies.[78] The investigators found sensitivity of 79% and 100% and specificity of 94% and 72% for MR imaging and PET, respectively, suggesting a synergistic potential for PET/MR imaging. In conclusion, hybrid PET/MR imaging may be of potential benefit in the setting of tumor recurrence by combining the morphologic and functional MR imaging information with the molecular PET information.

PEDIATRIC ONCOLOGY

At present, FDG-PET/CT is a major diagnostic tool in adult oncology. Several studies have been published about the value of FDG-PET/CT in children.[79–81] However, an important disadvantage of CT is the additional exposure of patients to ionizing radiation. In the young population radiation exposure is of particular concern, because of an increased susceptibility to radiation-induced development of secondary malignancies relative to adults. In particular, in the oncologic setting with the frequent need for multiple follow-up examinations, children and young adults will benefit from imaging with PET/MR imaging, as MR imaging does not contribute to the overall dose of the combined examination, leading to a reduction in dose exposure. The effective dose in a 15-year-old for diagnostic whole-body CT depends on the protocol used, but is generally around 11.0 mSv, in contrast to PET with an effective dose of around 4.2 mSv.[82]

Oncologic Diseases

Pfluger and colleagues[83] retrospectively compared the diagnostic value of FDG-PET and MR imaging to coregistered fused PET/MR imaging for staging and restaging in pediatric patients with proven or suspected malignant disease (solid tumors [n = 64], systemic malignancies [n = 53], and benign diseases [n = 15]). For the detection of single tumor lesions, FDG-PET/MR imaging proved to be the most accurate methodology for staging. At follow-up assessment, however, FDG-PET alone was superior in diagnostic performance to PET/MR imaging, as MR imaging and PET/MR imaging resulted in a high number of false-positive results attributable to persistent morphologic tissue changes after therapy.

Sarcoma

Several prospective and retrospective studies showed a better diagnostic accuracy for FDG-PET/CT in the staging of pediatric sarcomas, compared with conventional imaging methods (MR imaging of primary site, CT, chest radiography, and bone scintigraphy).[84–86] This accuracy was mainly due to the superiority of PET in detecting lymph node involvement and osseous lesions. In conclusion, PET/MR imaging may be an attractive alternative in the staging of pediatric sarcomas, as MR imaging does not contribute to the radiation dose. In addition, because of the superb soft-tissue contrast with MR imaging, T-staging is expected to improve with MR imaging.

Compared with conventional imaging modalities (consisting of ultrasonography, CT, MR imaging, and/or bone scintigraphy), PET/CT appeared to be better in predicting response to chemotherapy in children with bone tumors.[81] Denecke and colleagues[87] found that PET/CT was able to discriminate between responders and nonresponders in children with osteosarcoma, and was superior to MR imaging. On the other hand, Uhl and colleagues[88] demonstrated that MR imaging with DW imaging could be of value in the assessment of response to therapy. The integration of PET and MR imaging with DW imaging could potentially offer the best diagnostic test in these indications.

Regarding M-staging, Cistaro and colleagues[89] evaluated 18 pediatric patients with bone sarcomas, and found that FDG-PET/CT is an accurate method for the characterization of lung nodules. Their data suggest that a maximum SUV value of greater than 1 is consistent with malignancy when a nodule is larger than 6 mm.

Neuroblastoma

Neuroblastoma is an embryonic tumor arising from neural crest cells that give rise to the adrenal medulla and sympathetic nervous system. At diagnosis, about 50% of patients have distant metastases with a long-term survival of less than

40%.[90] Tumor cells express the norepinephrine transporter, which makes MIBG, an analogue of norepinephrine, an ideal tumor-specific agent for imaging. Despite the high diagnostic accuracy of ^{123}I-MIBG scintigraphy, there are several disadvantages of this modality including limited spatial resolution, limited sensitivity for small lesions, planar technique, and the need for several acquisition sessions.[90] PET imaging using FDG or ^{11}C-hydroxyephedrine radiotracers in neuroblastoma has not been proved to be superior to ^{123}I-MIBG scintigraphy by recent studies.[91] However, recent pilot studies with ^{18}F-fluorodopa (FDOPA) PET/CT demonstrated promising results, with higher overall accuracy than ^{123}I-MIBG scintigraphy in patients with stage 3 and 4 neuroblastoma.[92] ^{18}F-FDOPA PET/MR imaging could evolve into the superior method for assessing neuroblastoma patients by combining an optimal molecular imaging method with the excellent morphologic information provided by MR imaging, while simultaneously limiting the radiation exposure of this combined technique in the pediatric setting.

Wilms Tumor

Wilms tumor is the second most common solid pediatric tumor. Overall, the 5-year survival rate is 91.7%.[93] In Europe, patients receive preoperative chemotherapy to facilitate resection of tumor and to treat distant metastases as early as possible. One potential important disadvantage is the inability to identify histologic subgroups at the time of diagnosis.[93] A noninvasive method for grading Wilms tumors at the time of diagnosis and during preoperative response assessment is desirable for adequate treatment planning. Begent and colleagues[94] performed FDG-PET/CT in 7 patients after induction chemotherapy and immediately before surgery, and concluded that active Wilms tumor is FDG avid and that higher SUVs are seen in histologically high-risk tumors. Restaging of suspected relapses is another area of possible application for functional or metabolic imaging, as suggested by a prospective study by Misch and colleagues.[95] PET/MR imaging could therefore be an interesting tool in early response assessment and for the restaging of suspected relapses of Wilms tumor.

Other Pediatric Applications

Langerhans cell histiocytosis

Langerhans cell histiocytosis (LCH) has a broad spectrum of disease manifestations ranging from a single osseous lesion to multisystem disease. It is characterized by uncontrolled monoclonal proliferation of activated dendritic cells and macrophages that may infiltrate nearly any tissue or organ. These infiltrates are accompanied by chronic inflammation and the formation of granulomas.[96]

FDG-PET and MR imaging have been reported as being able to identify multifocal disease. Mueller and colleagues[97] retrospectively reviewed PET and MR imaging performed in 15 patients with histologically proven LCH. Their analysis suggests improved sensitivity for the combination of PET/MR imaging during primary staging by decreasing the false-negative rate, whereas after treatment with chemotherapy they found a higher rate of false-positive findings for MR imaging and PET/MR imaging, indicating that PET alone is sufficient.

Neurofibromatosis

Neurofibromatosis type 1 (NF-1) is a common neurocutaneous syndrome. Two tumor types occur at high frequency in NF-1: optic-pathway gliomas and plexiform neurofibromas. MR imaging is currently the primary imaging method, but has limitations for the prediction of lesion progression in optic-pathway glioma and for assessment of malignant degeneration in plexiform neurofibromas.[98,99] Moharir and colleagues[100] performed a retrospective analysis on 18 children with NF-1 and optic-pathway glioma and/or plexiform neurofibroma. Their findings suggest that asymptomatic FDG-avid optic-pathway gliomas are more likely than those that are not FDG avid to become symptomatic. As in adults, PET/CT is useful for the detection of malignant transformation in plexiform neurofibromas in children with NF-1. The combination of PET with MR imaging is promising in this group of patients not only because of the expected additive value of hybrid PET/MR imaging but also because of the lower radiation exposure relative to PET/CT in this young population, in whom regular follow-up imaging studies are required.

SUMMARY

Current available literature reports that PET/MR imaging performance is at least as good as that of PET/CT. Potential indications for PET/MR imaging may lie in the realm of tumor entities for which MR imaging has traditionally been favored, resulting in a "1-stop shop" TNM staging method (**Table 3**). Compared with current available imaging methods, PET/MR imaging seems to be superior in detecting lymph node involvement, but the limited sensitivity of PET/MR imaging reflects the general problem of detecting lymph node micrometastases. M-staging will benefit from the combination of both modalities.

Table 3
Summary of the most important potential clinical applications of PET/MR imaging in oncologic imaging

Tumor Entity	Frequent Site of Metastases* Brain	Lung	Liver	Bone	PET/MR Imaging is Favorable in…	Special Objective
Intracranial tumors	NA	–	–	–	T	Ascertain extent and grade of infiltrating glioma Biopsy targeting Delineate post-therapy changes from recurrence
Head and neck	–	+	–	–	T/N	Assess locoregional spread
Breast cancer	+	+	+	+	T/N/M	Incremental value of PET over MR imaging for primary tumor assessment is questionable
Gynecologic malignancies	–	+	+	+	T/N/M	T-staging will benefit from MR imaging, N- and M-staging will benefit from the combination
Prostate cancer	–	–	–	+	T/N	Combination of DW imaging and PET may identify significant disease
Lymphoma	NA	NA	NA	NA		Staging and early response assessment
Sarcoma	–	+	+	–	T/N/M	T-staging will benefit from MR imaging, N- and M-staging will benefit from the combination
Neuroblastoma	–	–	+	+	M	FDOPA PET/MR imaging, especially for stage 3 and 4 disease
Wilms tumor	–	+	+	–	T	Additional metabolic and functional information in early response assessment, restaging, and suspected recurrence

Abbreviations: +, frequent; –, rare; NA, not applicable.
* Frequency of metastatic spread according to *AJCC Cancer Staging Manual*, seventh edition.

PET/MR imaging could be especially interesting for the evaluation of certain malignancies in patients for whom radiation exposure is a significant issue, such as children and pregnant women. Several reports suggest an additional value of PET/CT for pediatric oncologic indications. However, CT and FDG-PET/CT expose the patient to a considerable amount of ionizing radiation. This issue is especially important in childhood, as children are inherently more radiosensitive than adults and have more remaining years of life during which radiation-induced cancer could develop. PET/MR imaging therefore seems to be an attractive alternative to PET/CT in this radiosensitive population who may face repeated imaging sessions.

Functional MR imaging combined with PET using specific biomarkers bears potential to further increase the performance of PET/MR imaging. The possibility to combine anatomic with functional and molecular data is expected to further increase diagnostic accuracy during initial staging, and increase our ability to stratify patients into different therapeutic groups, assess early response to therapy, and identify recurrent disease earlier than with current methods.

PET/MR imaging provides a potential for a powerful "1-stop shop" combination of structural, functional, and molecular imaging technologies that may be superior to PET/CT or MR imaging for a wide range of clinical applications. Development of specific PET/MR imaging protocols will be the focus of ongoing studies. Further research will be needed to demonstrate whether the potential for improved diagnostic accuracy has significant influence on therapeutic management, and if this results in an overall reduction in cost.

ACKNOWLEDGMENTS

The authors would like thank Dr Maarten L. Donswijk for his contribution to the preparation of **Fig. 3**.

REFERENCES

1. Torigian DA, Zaidi H, Kwee TC, et al. PET/MR imaging: technical aspects and potential clinical applications. Radiology 2013;267(1):26–44.
2. Werner MK, Schmidt H, Schwenzer NF. MR/PET: a new challenge in hybrid imaging. AJR Am J Roentgenol 2012;199(2):272–7.
3. von Schulthess GK, Kuhn FP, Kaufmann P, et al. Clinical positron emission tomography/magnetic resonance imaging applications. Semin Nucl Med 2013;43(1):3–10.
4. Zaidi H, Del Guerra A. An outlook on future design of hybrid PET/MRI systems. Med Phys 2011; 38(10):5667–89.
5. Hofmann M, Bezrukov I, Mantlik F, et al. MRI-based attenuation correction for whole-body PET/MRI: quantitative evaluation of segmentation- and atlas-based methods. J Nucl Med 2011;52(9): 1392–9.
6. Platzek I, Beuthien-Baumann B, Schneider M, et al. PET/MRI in head and neck cancer: initial experience. Eur J Nucl Med Mol Imaging 2013; 40(1):6–11.
7. Drzezga A, Souvatzoglou M, Eiber M, et al. First clinical experience with integrated whole-body PET/MR: comparison to PET/CT in patients with oncologic diagnoses. J Nucl Med 2012;53(6): 845–55.
8. Mansi L, Ciarmiello A, Cuccurullo V. PET/MRI and the revolution of the third eye. Eur J Nucl Med Mol Imaging 2012;39(10):1519–24.
9. Boss A, Bisdas S, Kolb A, et al. Hybrid PET/MRI of intracranial masses: initial experiences and comparison to PET/CT. J Nucl Med 2010;51(8): 1198–205.
10. Arbizu J, Tejada S, Marti-Climent JM, et al. Quantitative volumetric analysis of gliomas with sequential MRI and ^{11}C-methionine PET assessment: patterns of integration in therapy planning. Eur J Nucl Med Mol Imaging 2012;39(5):771–81.
11. Neuner I, Kaffanke JB, Langen KJ, et al. Multimodal imaging utilising integrated MR-PET for human brain tumour assessment. Eur Radiol 2012; 22(12):2568–80.
12. Schwenzer NF, Stegger L, Bisdas S, et al. Simultaneous PET/MR imaging in a human brain PET/MR system in 50 patients—current state of image quality. Eur J Radiol 2012;81(11):3472–8.
13. Garibotto V, Heinzer S, Vulliemoz S, et al. Clinical applications of hybrid PET/MRI in neuroimaging. Clin Nucl Med 2013;38(1):e13–8.
14. Thorwarth D, Müller AC, Pfannenberg C, et al. Combined PET/MR imaging using (68)Ga-DOTATOC for radiotherapy treatment planning in meningioma patients. Recent Results Cancer Res 2013; 194:425–39.
15. Salamon N, Kung J, Shaw SJ, et al. FDG-PET/MRI coregistration improves detection of cortical dysplasia in patients with epilepsy. Neurology 2008;71(20):1594–601.
16. Herholz K, Carter SF, Jones M. Positron emission tomography imaging in dementia. Br J Radiol 2007;80(2):S160–7.
17. Hong-Qi Y, Zhi-Kun S, Sheng-Di C. Current advances in the treatment of Alzheimer's disease: focused on considerations targeting Aβ and tau. Transl Neurodegener 2012;1(1):21.
18. Kawachi T, Ishii K, Sakamoto S, et al. Comparison of the diagnostic performance of FDG-PET and VBM-MRI in very mild Alzheimer's disease. Eur J Nucl Med Mol Imaging 2006;33(7):801–9.
19. Cho ZH, Son YD, Kim HK, et al. Observation of glucose metabolism in the thalamic nuclei by fusion PET/MRI. J Nucl Med 2011;52(3):401–4.
20. Cho ZH, Son YD, Kim HK, et al. Substructural hippocampal glucose metabolism observed on PET/MRI. J Nucl Med 2010;51(10):1545–8.
21. Parker MW, Iskandar A, Limone B, et al. Diagnostic accuracy of cardiac positron emission tomography versus single photon emission computed tomography for coronary artery disease: a bivariate meta-analysis. Circ Cardiovasc Imaging 2012;5(6):700–7.
22. Klocke FJ, Baird MG, Lorell BH, et al, American College of Cardiology, American Heart Association; American Society for Nuclear Cardiology. ACC/AHA/ASNC guidelines for the clinical use of cardiac radionuclide imaging—executive summary: a report of the American College of Cardiology/American Heart Association Task Force on Practice Guidelines (ACC/AHA/ASNC Committee to Revise the 1995 Guidelines for the Clinical Use of Cardiac Radionuclide Imaging). J Am Coll Cardiol 2003; 42(7):1318–33.
23. Sharples L, Hughes V, Crean A, et al. Cost-effectiveness of functional cardiac testing in the diagnosis and management of coronary artery disease: a randomised controlled trial. The CECaT trial. Health Technol Assess 2007;11:49.
24. Kim WY, Stuber M, Börnert P, et al. Three-dimensional black-blood cardiac magnetic resonance coronary vessel wall imaging detects positive arterial remodeling in patients with nonsignificant coronary artery disease. Circulation 2002;106(3): 296–9.
25. Naghavi M, Libby P, Falk E, et al. From vulnerable plaque to vulnerable patient: a call for new definitions and risk assessment strategies: part I. Circulation 2003;108(14):1664–72.
26. Nekolla SG, Martinez-Moeller A, Saraste A. PET and MRI in cardiac imaging: from validation studies to integrated applications. Eur J Nucl Med Mol Imaging 2009;36(Suppl 1):S121–30.

27. Gerber BL, Rochitte CE, Bluemke DA, et al. Relation between Gd-DTPA contrast enhancement and regional inotropic response in the periphery and center of myocardial infarction. Circulation 2001;104(9):998–1004.
28. Schmidt M, Voth E, Schneider CA, et al. F-18-FDG uptake is a reliable predictor of functional recovery of akinetic but viable infarct regions as defined by magnetic resonance imaging before and after revascularization. Magn Reson Imaging 2004; 22(2):229–36.
29. Bengel FM, Ueberfuhr P, Schiepel N, et al. Myocardial efficiency and sympathetic reinnervation after orthotopic heart transplantation: a noninvasive study with positron emission tomography. Circulation 2001;103(14):1881–6.
30. Miese F, Scherer A, Ostendorf B, et al. Hybrid ^{18}F-FDG PET-MRI of the hand in rheumatoid arthritis: initial results. Clin Rheumatol 2011;30(9):1247–50.
31. Nawaz A, Torigian DA, Siegelman ES, et al. Diagnostic performance of FDG-PET, MRI, and plain film radiography (PFR) for the diagnosis of osteomyelitis in the diabetic foot. Mol Imaging Biol 2010;12(3):335–42.
32. Warmann SW, Dittmann H, Seitz G, et al. Follow-up of acute osteomyelitis in children: the possible role of PET/CT in selected cases. J Pediatr Surg 2011; 46(8):1550–6.
33. Koh DM, Collins DJ. Diffusion-weighted MRI in the body: applications and challenges in oncology. AJR Am J Roentgenol 2007;188(6):1622–35.
34. Kwee TC, Takahara T, Ochiai R, et al. Diffusion-weighted whole-body imaging with background body signal suppression (DWIBS): features and potential applications in oncology. Eur Radiol 2008;18(9):1937–52.
35. Gupta T, Master Z, Kannan S, et al. Diagnostic performance of post-treatment FDG PET or FDG PET/ CT imaging in head and neck cancer: a systematic review and meta-analysis. Eur J Nucl Med Mol Imaging 2011;38(11):2083–95.
36. Boss A, Stegger L, Bisdas S, et al. Feasibility of simultaneous PET/MR imaging in the head and upper neck area. Eur Radiol 2011;21(7):1439–46.
37. Nakamoto Y, Tamai K, Saga T, et al. Clinical value of image fusion from MR and PET in patients with head and neck cancer. Mol Imaging Biol 2009;11(1):46–53.
38. Huang SH, Chien CY, Lin WC, et al. A comparative study of fused FDG PET/MRI, PET/CT, MRI, and CT imaging for assessing surrounding tissue invasion of advanced buccal squamous cell carcinoma. Clin Nucl Med 2011;36(7):518–25.
39. Nagarajah J, Jentzen W, Hartung V, et al. Diagnosis and dosimetry in differentiated thyroid carcinoma using ^{124}I PET: comparison of PET/MRI vs PET/CT of the neck. Eur J Nucl Med Mol Imaging 2011; 38(10):1862–8.
40. Schwenzer NF, Schraml C, Müller M, et al. Pulmonary lesion assessment: comparison of whole-body hybrid MR/PET and PET/CT imaging—pilot study. Radiology 2012;264(2):551–8.
41. Bilsky MH, Vitaz TW, Boland PJ, et al. Surgical treatment of superior sulcus tumors with spinal and brachial plexus involvement. J Neurosurg 2002;97(Suppl 3):301–9.
42. Moy L, Noz ME, Maguire GQ Jr, et al. Role of fusion of prone FDG-PET and magnetic resonance imaging of the breasts in the evaluation of breast cancer. Breast J 2010;16(4):369–76.
43. Heusner TA, Hahn S, Jonkmanns C, et al. Diagnostic accuracy of fused positron emission tomography/magnetic resonance mammography: initial results. Br J Radiol 2011;84(998):126–35.
44. Uematsu T, Kasami M, Yuen S. Comparison of FDG PET and MRI for evaluating the tumor extent of breast cancer and the impact of FDG PET on the systemic staging and prognosis of patients who are candidates for breast-conserving therapy. Breast Cancer 2009;16(2):97–104.
45. Buchbender C, Heusner TA, Lauenstein TC, et al. Oncologic PET/MRI, part 1: tumors of the brain, head and neck, chest, abdomen, and pelvis. J Nucl Med 2012;53(6):928–38.
46. Hartung-Knemeyer V, Rosenbaum-Krumme S, Buchbender C, et al. Malignant Pheochromocytoma Imaging with [^{124}I]mIBG PET/MR. J Clin Endocrinol Metab 2012;97(11):3833–4.
47. Birchard KR, Semelka RC, Hyslop WB, et al. Suspected pancreatic cancer: evaluation by dynamic gadolinium-enhanced 3D gradient-echo MRI. AJR Am J Roentgenol 2005;185(3):700–3.
48. Tatsumi M, Isohashi K, Onishi H, et al. ^{18}F-FDG PET/MRI fusion in characterizing pancreatic tumors: comparison to PET/CT. Int J Clin Oncol 2011;16(4):408–15.
49. Epelbaum R, Frenkel A, Haddad R, et al. Tumor aggressiveness and patient outcome in cancer of the pancreas assessed by dynamic ^{18}F-FDG PET/ CT. J Nucl Med 2013;54(1):12–8.
50. Nakajo K, Tatsumi M, Inoue A, et al. Diagnostic performance of fluorodeoxyglucose positron emission tomography/magnetic resonance imaging fusion images of gynecological malignant tumors: comparison with positron emission tomography/ computed tomography. Jpn J Radiol 2010;28(2): 95–100.
51. Siegel CL, Andreotti RF, Cardenes HR, et al. American College of Radiology. ACR Appropriateness Criteria® pretreatment planning of invasive cancer of the cervix. J Am Coll Radiol 2012;9(6): 395–402.
52. Kitajima K, Murakami K, Sakamoto S, et al. Present and future of FDG-PET/CT in ovarian cancer. Ann Nucl Med 2011;25(3):155–64.

53. Kinkel K, Forstner R, Danza FM, et al. European Society of Urogenital Imaging. Staging of endometrial cancer with MRI: guidelines of the European Society of Urogenital Imaging. Eur Radiol 2009;19(7):1565–74.
54. Park JY, Kim EN, Kim DY, et al. Comparison of the validity of magnetic resonance imaging and positron emission tomography/computed tomography in the preoperative evaluation of patients with uterine corpus cancer. Gynecol Oncol 2008;108(3):486–92.
55. Kam MH, Wong DC, Siu S, et al. Comparison of magnetic resonance imaging-fluorodeoxyglucose positron emission tomography fusion with pathological staging in rectal cancer. Br J Surg 2010;97(2):266–8.
56. Brændengen M, Hansson K, Radu C, et al. Delineation of gross tumor volume (GTV) for radiation treatment planning of locally advanced rectal cancer using information from MRI or FDG-PET/CT: a prospective study. Int J Radiat Oncol Biol Phys 2011;81(4):e439–45.
57. Park H, Wood D, Hussain H, et al. Introducing parametric fusion PET/MRI of primary prostate cancer. J Nucl Med 2012;53(4):546–51.
58. Van den Bergh L, Koole M, Isebaert S, et al. Is there an additional value of ^{11}C-choline PET-CT to T2-weighted MRI images in the localization of intraprostatic tumor nodules? Int J Radiat Oncol Biol Phys 2012;83(5):1486–92.
59. Cheson BD, Pfistner B, Juweid ME, et al. International Harmonization Project on Lymphoma. Revised response criteria for malignant lymphoma. J Clin Oncol 2007;25(5):579–86.
60. Juweid ME, Stroobants S, Hoekstra OS, et al. Imaging Subcommittee of International Harmonization Project in Lymphoma. Use of positron emission tomography for response assessment of lymphoma: consensus of the Imaging Subcommittee of International Harmonization Project in Lymphoma. J Clin Oncol 2007;25(5):571–8.
61. Lin C, Itti E, Luciani A, et al. Whole-body diffusion-weighted imaging with apparent diffusion coefficient mapping for treatment response assessment in patients with diffuse large B-cell lymphoma: pilot study. Invest Radiol 2011;46(5):341–9.
62. Buchbender C, Heusner TA, Lauenstein TC, et al. Oncologic PET/MRI, part 2: bone tumors, soft-tissue tumors, melanoma, and lymphoma. J Nucl Med 2012;53(8):1244–52.
63. Tateishi U, Yamaguchi U, Seki K, et al. Bone and soft-tissue sarcoma: preoperative staging with fluorine 18 fluorodeoxyglucose PET/CT and conventional imaging. Radiology 2007;245(3):839–47.
64. Kim YN, Yi CA, Lee KS, et al. A proposal for combined MRI and PET/CT interpretation criteria for preoperative nodal staging in non-small-cell lung cancer. Eur Radiol 2012;22(7):1537–46.
65. Kim SK, Choi HJ, Park SY, et al. Additional value of MR/PET fusion compared with PET/CT in the detection of lymph node metastases in cervical cancer patients. Eur J Cancer 2009;45(12):2103–9.
66. Wu L, Cao Y, Liao C, et al. Diagnostic performance of USPIO-enhanced MRI for lymph-node metastases in different body regions: a meta-analysis. Eur J Radiol 2011;80(2):582–9.
67. Donati OF, Hany TF, Reiner CS, et al. Value of retrospective fusion of PET and MR images in detection of hepatic metastases: comparison with ^{18}F-FDG PET/CT and Gd-EOB-DTPA-enhanced MRI. J Nucl Med 2010;51(5):692–9.
68. Yong TW, Yuan ZZ, Jun Z, et al. Sensitivity of PET/MR images in liver metastases from colorectal carcinoma. Hell J Nucl Med 2011;14(3):264–8.
69. Schreiter NF, Nogami M, Steffen I, et al. Evaluation of the potential of PET-MRI fusion for detection of liver metastases in patients with neuroendocrine tumours. Eur Radiol 2012;22(2):458–67.
70. Yokoi K, Kamiya N, Matsuguma H, et al. Detection of brain metastasis in potentially operable non-small cell lung cancer: a comparison of CT and MRI. Chest 1999;115(3):714–9.
71. Thomson V, Pialat JB, Gay F, et al. Whole-body MRI for metastases screening: a preliminary study using 3D VIBE sequences with automatic subtraction between noncontrast and contrast enhanced images. Am J Clin Oncol 2008;31(3):285–92.
72. Schmidt GP, Baur-Melnyk A, Herzog P, et al. High-resolution whole-body magnetic resonance image tumor staging with the use of parallel imaging versus dual-modality positron emission tomography-computed tomography: experience on a 32-channel system. Invest Radiol 2005;40(12):743–53.
73. Yang HL, Liu T, Wang XM, et al. Diagnosis of bone metastases: a meta-analysis comparing ^{18}FDG PET, CT, MRI and bone scintigraphy. Eur Radiol 2011;21(12):2604–17.
74. Qu X, Huang X, Yan W, et al. A meta-analysis of ^{18}FDG-PET-CT, ^{18}FDG-PET, MRI and bone scintigraphy for diagnosis of bone metastases in patients with lung cancer. Eur J Radiol 2012;81(5):1007–15.
75. Liu T, Cheng T, Xu W, et al. A meta-analysis of ^{18}FDG-PET, MRI and bone scintigraphy for diagnosis of bone metastases in patients with breast cancer. Skeletal Radiol 2011;40(5):523–31.
76. Antoch G, Vogt FM, Freudenberg LS, et al. Whole-body dual-modality PET/CT and whole-body MRI for tumor staging in oncology. JAMA 2003;290(24):3199–206.
77. Liu J, Yang X, Li F, et al. Preliminary study of whole-body diffusion-weighted imaging in detecting pulmonary metastatic lesions from clear cell renal cell carcinoma: comparison with CT. Acta Radiol 2011;52(9):954–63.

78. Goerres GW, Michel SC, Fehr MK, et al. Follow-up of women with breast cancer: comparison between MRI and FDG PET. Eur Radiol 2003;13(7):1635–44.
79. Kleis M, Daldrup-Link H, Matthay K, et al. Diagnostic value of PET/CT for the staging and restaging of pediatric tumors. Eur J Nucl Med Mol Imaging 2009;36(1):23–36.
80. McCarville MB. PET-CT imaging in pediatric oncology. Cancer Imaging 2009;9:35–43.
81. London K, Stege C, Cross S, et al. ^{18}F-FDG PET/CT compared to conventional imaging modalities in pediatric primary bone tumors. Pediatr Radiol 2012;42(4):418–30.
82. Nievelstein RA, Quarles van Ufford HM, Kwee TC, et al. Radiation exposure and mortality risk from CT and PET imaging of patients with malignant lymphoma. Eur Radiol 2012;22(9):1946–54.
83. Pfluger T, Melzer HI, Mueller WP, et al. Diagnostic value of combined (18)F-FDG PET/MRI for staging and restaging in paediatric oncology. Eur J Nucl Med Mol Imaging 2012;39(11):1745–55.
84. Völker T, Denecke T, Steffen I, et al. Positron emission tomography for staging of pediatric sarcoma patients: results of a prospective multicenter trial. J Clin Oncol 2007;25(34):5435–41.
85. Eugene T, Corradini N, Carlier T, et al. ^{18}F-FDG-PET/CT in initial staging and assessment of early response to chemotherapy of pediatric rhabdomyosarcomas. Nucl Med Commun 2012;33(10):1089–95.
86. Tateishi U, Hosono A, Makimoto A, et al. Comparative study of FDG PET/CT and conventional imaging in the staging of rhabdomyosarcoma. Ann Nucl Med 2009;23(2):155–61.
87. Denecke T, Hundsdörfer P, Misch D, et al. Assessment of histological response of paediatric bone sarcomas using FDG PET in comparison to morphological volume measurement and standardized MRI parameters. Pediatr Radiol 2006;36(12):1306–11.
88. Uhl M, Saueressig U, Koehler G, et al. Evaluation of tumour necrosis during chemotherapy with diffusion-weighted MR imaging: preliminary results in osteosarcomas. Eur J Nucl Med Mol Imaging 2010;37(10):1842–53.
89. Cistaro A, Lopci E, Gastaldo L, et al. The role of ^{18}F-FDG PET/CT in the metabolic characterization of lung nodules in pediatric patients with bone sarcoma. Pediatr Blood Cancer 2012;59(7):1206–10.
90. Taggart D, Dubois S, Matthay KK. Radiolabeled metaiodobenzylguanidine for imaging and therapy of neuroblastoma. Q J Nucl Med Mol Imaging 2008;52(4):403–18.
91. Mueller WP, Coppenrath E, Pfluger T. Nuclear medicine and multimodality imaging of pediatric neuroblastoma. Pediatr Radiol 2013;43(4):418–27.
92. Piccardo A, Lopci E, Conte M, et al. Comparison of ^{18}F-dopa PET/CT and 123I-MIBG scintigraphy in stage 3 and 4 neuroblastoma: a pilot study. Eur J Nucl Med Mol Imaging 2012;39(1):57–71.
93. Owens CM, Brisse HJ, Olsen ØE, et al. Bilateral disease and new trends in Wilms tumour. Pediatr Radiol 2008;38(1):30–9.
94. Begent J, Sebire NJ, Levitt G, et al. Pilot study of F(18)-fluorodeoxyglucose positron emission tomography/computerised tomography in Wilms' tumour: correlation with conventional imaging, pathology and immunohistochemistry. Eur J Cancer 2011;47(3):389–96.
95. Misch D, Steffen IG, Schönberger S, et al. Use of positron emission tomography for staging, preoperative response assessment and posttherapeutic evaluation in children with Wilms tumour. Eur J Nucl Med Mol Imaging 2008;35(9):1642–50.
96. Schmidt S, Eich G, Geoffray A, et al. Extraosseous Langerhans cell histiocytosis in children. Radiographics 2008;28(3):707–26.
97. Mueller WP, Melzer HI, Schmid I, et al. The diagnostic value of (18)F-FDG PET and MRI in paediatric histiocytosis. Eur J Nucl Med Mol Imaging 2013;40(3):356–63.
98. Ferner RE, Gutmann DH. International consensus statement on malignant peripheral nerve sheath tumors in neurofibromatosis. Cancer Res 2002;62(5):1573–7.
99. Listernick R, Ferner RE, Liu GT, et al. Optic pathway gliomas in neurofibromatosis—1: controversies and recommendations. Ann Neurol 2007;61(3):189–98.
100. Moharir M, London K, Howman-Giles R, et al. Utility of positron emission tomography for tumour surveillance in children with neurofibromatosis type 1. Eur J Nucl Med Mol Imaging 2010;37(7):1309–17.

Index

Note: Page numbers of article titles are in **boldface** type.

PET Clin 8 (2013) 385–389
http://dx.doi.org/10.1016/S1556-8598(13)00045-X
1556-8598/13/$ – see front matter

Printed and bound by CPI Group (UK) Ltd, Croydon, CR0 4YY

03/10/2024

01040347-0011